YOGA THERAPY FOUNDATIONS, TOOLS, AND PRACTICE

of related interest

Yoga Therapy for Insomnia and Sleep Recovery
An Integrated Approach to Supporting Healthy Sleep and Sustaining Energy All Day
Lisa Sanfilippo
ISBN 978 1 84819 391 8
eISBN 978 0 85701 348 4

Yoga Therapy as a Creative Response to Pain
Matthew J. Taylor
Foreword by John Kepner
ISBN 978 1 84819 356 7
eISBN 978 0 85701 315 6

Yoga and Science in Pain Care
Treating the Person in Pain
Edited by Neil Pearson, Shelly Prosko, and Marlysa Sullivan
Foreword by Timothy McCall
ISBN 978 1 84819 397 0
eISBN 978 0 85701 354 5

Yoga Therapy as a Whole-Person Approach to Health
Lee Majewski and Ananda Balayogi Bhavanani
Foreword by Stephen Parker
ISBN 978 1 78775 092 0
eISBN 978 1 78775 093 7

Restorative Yoga for Ethnic and Race-Based Stress and Trauma
Gail Parker
Forewords by Octavia F. Raheem and Amy Wheeler
Illustrated by Justine Ross
ISBN 978 1 78775 185 9
eISBN 978 1 78775 186 6

YOGA THERAPY

FOUNDATIONS, TOOLS, AND PRACTICE

A Comprehensive Textbook

Edited by Diane Finlayson and
Laurie C. Hyland Robertson

Foreword by Matra Raj

SINGING DRAGON
LONDON AND PHILADELPHIA

First published in Great Britain in 2021 by Singing Dragon, an imprint of Jessica Kingsley Publishers
An Hachette Company

1

Disclaimer: The information contained in this book is not intended to replace the services of trained medical professionals or to be a substitute for medical advice. The complementary therapy described in this book may not be suitable for everyone to follow. You are advised to consult a doctor before embarking on any complementary therapy program and on any matters relating to your health, and in particular on any matters that may require diagnosis or medical attention.

A CIP catalogue record for this title is available from the British Library and the Library of Congress

ISBN 978 1 78775 414 0
eISBN 978 1 78775 415 7

Printed and bound in the United States by West Publishing Corp

Jessica Kingsley Publishers' policy is to use papers that are natural, renewable, and recyclable products and made from wood grown in sustainable forests. The logging and manufacturing processes are expected to conform to the environmental regulations of the country of origin.

Jessica Kingsley Publishers
Carmelite House
50 Victoria Embankment
London EC4Y 0DZ

www.singingdragon.com

Contents

Foreword

Yoga Therapy Foundations, Tools, and Practice: A Comprehensive Textbook not only lays down a strong theoretical foundation for yoga therapy, it also provides tools in abundance that therapists can incorporate into their practices.

Having worked in the field for over 45 years now, I can wholeheartedly recommend the topics selected by Diane Finlayson (MA, MFA) and Laurie Hyland Robertson (MS), both of whom are eminently qualified in the field of yoga therapy and its expert transmission. They have made insightful choices of material that will enhance the yoga therapist's knowledge in multiple fields.

These chapters represent a stimulating and informative body of knowledge contributed by experts with diverse approaches and skill sets. This book will provoke thought and enrich the reader's understanding and practice of yoga therapy in all its applications. The excellent resources listed at the end of each chapter will help to reach the depth of each subject.

The book encompasses many fundamentals and principles of the ancient holistic scriptures such as the Vedas, the Upanishads, the *Bhagavad Gita*, the Puranas, and ayurveda. Each of these has a universal and an individual elemental component, and an effect on the physical, emotional, and spiritual being. All emphasize the importance of the breath. Sage Patanjali's eight limbs of yoga, sutras, the Samkhya *gunas*, and the *koshas* weave through all the subject matter in the book. Sections on the Shaiva Tantra tradition of all-pervading consciousness and the energy principle of actualization by vibratory pulsation shed light on its use as a therapeutic modality that enables us to be well-balanced and at one with the universe.

Several chapters address the holistic philosophies of yoga in depth, and also the ways these philosophies can inform current practices. Yoga is increasingly recognized as a science as well as an art. It is heartening to see these bridges between quantum traditional and often-reductionist Western approaches to client care and treatment. Holism is increasingly in tune with today's understanding of the mind and body. For example, the interconnectivity of individual organ systems is now well-accepted, as is the importance of the mind in healing, in decreasing suffering and increasing wellness, and in creating inherent defenses against disease and disorder.

With greater understanding of Patanjali's sutras, a yoga therapist's role may include counseling clients based on authentic ancient wisdom to gradually modify kleshas and other mental errors to address maladaptive lifestyles that can contribute to suppression or overactivity of the immune system, thus exploring the root causes of how and why an individual's illness and suffering are occurring.

Salutogenesis is the name of a current medical approach that focuses on the processes of becoming healthy, rather than on factors that cause disease. It is an apt term for the panchamaya kosha model. Patanjali points out how cognitive errors lead to fluctuation of energy or breath (prana) and prescribes a generous course of treatment based on compassion, forgiveness, selfless service, self-study, asana, breathwork (pranayama), and meditation—all leading to what we might today call high emotional resilience and a high emotional intelligence quotient (EQ).

With this solid philosophical and theoretical foundation, yoga therapists can confidently apply critical thinking skills and attain research literacy in their pursuit of professional growth and development. Later chapters of the book address these needs with topics in current research relating to medicine, psychology, social factors, trauma care, inclusion, and community wellness. The client populations addressed span the years from birth and pediatrics to geriatrics and the end of life. These chapters will broaden the yoga therapist's spectrum of skills and depth of understanding.

Having gone through foundations and research topics, the book concludes with a wealth of use cases that enable the yoga therapist to explore their newly acquired theoretical knowledge in the context of potential real-life situations.

This book covers a variety of approaches, traditional and non-traditional, innovative and experimental, collaborative and complementary. The clear message throughout is one of building relationships with other para-professionals. And for the yoga therapist, the advice to connect first with SELF to improve efficacy of client care is most welcome.

As a rehabilitation and yoga therapist, I strongly recommend this book to rehabilitation therapists, yoga teachers, yoga therapists, and allied professionals alike. The text will long remain a highly respected resource in the field of yoga therapy. *Yoga Therapy Foundations, Tools, and Practice: A Comprehensive Textbook* is a most insightful and in-depth scholarly work. Each and every chapter merits rereading again and again. I have yet to leave off reading this book without a wonderful "Aha" moment!

Matra Raj

Acknowledgments

We owe a debt of gratitude to each of the expert contributors who so graciously shared their knowledge, patiently enduring multiple rounds of sometimes nitpicky revisions as we blended their varied perspectives into a cohesive whole. The contributors who authored the section introductions offered additional invaluable peer review.

To the faculty and administrators of Maryland University of Integrative Health (MUIH), thank you for believing in the Master of Science in Yoga Therapy program and committing to building it year after year. The words of many of these fine colleagues and mentors appear on these pages, including Marlysa Sullivan, Dorcia J. Tucker, Camille Freeman, and Steffany Moonaz. Additional MUIH faculty members are represented here, too: Thanks to Sarajean Rudman and Marybeth Missenda for offering additional perspective, which is one of the strengths of this book.

Thank you to the International Association of Yoga Therapists (IAYT) and its countless volunteers who tirelessly dedicate themselves to carving out a place for the profession of yoga therapy in contemporary healthcare—and have done so for more than 30 years. Many of these amazing individuals are featured in this work, including the current president of the board of directors, Matra Raj, who kindly wrote the Foreword, and the immediate past president, Amy Wheeler, who equally kindly and freely shared her deep knowledge. These beautiful beings are always willing to generously share their deep knowledge, but also upliftment through giving of their spirits.

To the Singing Dragon team, with special thanks to Claire Wilson and Maddy Budd: We are delighted to be aligned with a publisher whose aim is to change the world for the better. As their website notes, the company is "committed to publishing accessible books that make a difference." It took Claire 2 years to convince Diane to take on a project of this depth. Thank you for your persistence, Claire.

Diane

I would also like to express my own gratitude to the higher administration of MUIH for their forbearance as work on this textbook unfolded. I am additionally grateful to IAYT executive director John Kepner for keeping me informed of various meetings and movements in the yoga therapy community that are vital to my global understanding of the history and trajectory of the profession.

And it needs to be stated clearly here as well that, without Laurie Hyland Robertson's keen eye and attention to detail, this book would not exist.

Thank you to all my teachers and peers in the yoga therapy community. I am moved by your willingness to make space for young, fresh students to move forward into the roles of teaching, and I am honored to be able to now pass some of this legacy on to the next generations.

Thanks to all the students of yoga therapy who continue to believe in their teachers and this modality, with all its possibilities for healing the world. Thank you for trusting people like me to shine a light on the path, and for not being afraid to point out that there are additional legs to the journey for those who wish to take them.

Laurie

I would like to further express gratitude to all of my classmates in cohort 1 of the MUIH Master of Science in Yoga Therapy program—and to Diane Finlayson, who was largely responsible for conceiving the entire curriculum and invited me along on this sometimes wild and always illuminating ride.

Special thanks to my dear friends Tina Paul and Ann Swanson, members of that first cohort and accomplished yoga therapy professionals, who are always ready for a shot of aloe and a patient discussion of yogic science—and this ever-shifting concept of what it means to live a balanced life. (I promise I'm going out to sit under a tree soon, Tina!)

Thanks to the entire IAYT staff, most especially the other members of the management team, who are paragons of steady compassion and professionalism: Debra Krajewski, Devi Mueller, Marilyn Peppers-Citizen, Nancy Sinton, Annette Watson, and Beth Whitney-Teeple. Like any family we don't always agree, but also like the best of families, their support is invaluable and freeing. Marilyn's words appear in this book, and all of their influence is present as well.

Finally, profound thanks to my birth and assembled family, who unfailingly told me I could do whatever I set my mind to and never once batted an eye at the increasingly complicated projects I announced. To Mom, Dad, Bam, and everyone else, whether our love is in presence or in absence, endless humble gratitude. Particular thanks go to Kathy, Sharon, Rob, Becky, Robert, Tom D., and Peter, who so ably perform the essential task of bringing levity and joy to life. And Tom... There are no words to express how honored I am to walk this journey alongside you. Thank you for your unwavering support, your fearlessness, for encapsulating all that is sweet in the world.

Chapter Copyright Acknowledgments

The Editors, Contributors, and Reviewers

Editors

Diane Finlayson, MA, MFA, C-IAYT

Diane's history in education and writing includes time in radio copywriting, journalism, creative writing, and running a variety of schools and programs. After 20 years of teaching courses in writing, yoga, meditation, and ayurveda for Johns Hopkins University, in her own school, and at other yoga schools and universities, she was extended the opportunity to collaborate on the development of the MS Yoga Therapy program at Maryland University of Integrative Health where she now serves as department chair.

Laurie Hyland Robertson, MS, C-IAYT, E-RYT 500

After more than a decade in healthcare and business publishing, Laurie found her way to the transformative practices of yoga and then yoga therapy. She is now editor in chief of *Yoga Therapy Today* and managing editor of the *International Journal of Yoga Therapy*, and contributes editorial services to a variety of yoga and wellness publications. Laurie divides her time between the extremes of a Costa Rican rain forest and the Baltimore-Washington area, where she owns Whole Yoga & Pilates.

Contributors

Melinda Atkins, MSc, MEd, C-IAYT, E-RYT 500

Melinda Atkins is the founding director of AUM hOMe Shala, an IAYT-accredited, Miami-based non-profit yoga school. Atkins holds a Master of Education in administration and supervision and is on track to receive a Master of Science degree from the University of Maryland School of Pharmacy. She is proud to have served more than 6,000 individuals through group classes and individual clinics since AUM's founding in 2005, and she continues to oversee all aspects of the school's operations. As a grassroots organization, AUM is funded by grants, donations, and student tuitions and bolstered by strong partnerships with local and national organizations and foundations.

Sundar Balasubramanian, PhD, C-IAYT

Dr. Sundar Balasubramanian is a cell biology researcher currently studying cellular and molecular mechanisms involved in resistance to cancer therapy at the Medical University of South Carolina. Balasubramanian is also a yoga biology researcher and certified yoga therapist. As the founder and director of PranaScience Institute, Balasubramanian's yoga research has provided scientific evidence of the practices' efficacy to promote well-being. His books include *PranaScience: Decoding Yoga Breathing*, *Mind Your Breathing: The Yogi's Handbook with 37 Pranayama Exercises*, and *Murattu Kuthiraikku 37 Kadivalangal* (in Tamil). Balasubramanian's work has also appeared on the TEDx stage and National Public Radio and in *Discover* magazine, *The New York Times*, and Huffington Post.

Marsha D. Banks-Harold, C-IAYT, E-RYT 500

As the owner of PIES Fitness Yoga Studio, Marsha D. Banks-Harold utilizes all of the knowledge, skills, and experiences that were at first thwarted in her role as a supervisory electrical engineer practicing in intellectual property. Creator of the flagship class "My Body Don't Bend That Way" and an ambassador for Black Girl Yoga, Banks-Harold develops customized lifestyle and work plans. These strategies aim to help clients respond to interrupted work progress and move to the next level of success while manifesting internal peace and optimizing work/life balance. She has been featured as a presenter for organizations such as Black Therapists Rock, IAYT, and the Smithsonian and on broadcasts including "Aging Matters" and ABC7 News.

Judi Bar, C-IAYT, E-RYT 500

As lead yoga therapist and yoga program manager at Cleveland Clinic, Judi Bar has been developing yoga programs for patients and caregivers at the institution since 2007. Bar recently created a 200-hour-level Cleveland Clinic School of Yoga and is collaborating with the Cleveland Clinic Lerner College of Medicine to train medical students. As a certified yoga therapist, she works with all types of patients, including those with cancer, metabolic syndrome, epilepsy, digestive disease, multiple sclerosis (MS), chronic pain, and rheumatoid arthritis (RA). Bar has created two "Come As You Are" yoga DVDs, acts as a national yoga media resource for Cleveland Clinic, and speaks at medical symposia throughout the United States.

Kelli Bethel, DPT, PT, C-IAYT, E-RYT 500

Dr. Kelli Bethel is a practicing physical therapist, certified yoga therapist, and yoga instructor. Bethel is clinical director and the director of yoga therapy and yoga at the University of Maryland Center for Integrative Medicine. She also owns Tafiya Yoga and Wellness. Working in the field of yoga therapy since 2007, with an emphasis on stroke, brain injury, and cancer care, Bethel is committed to empowering patients, clients, and students along the course of their health and wellness journeys.

Leigh Blashki, C-IAYT

Leigh Blashki's life has been dedicated to the establishment of high, credible standards of education and professional practice for the fields of yoga, yoga therapy, and meditation. He is a member of the IAYT board of directors, has served on the organization's Standards, Accreditation, and Certification committees, and is a past president of Yoga Australia. Blashki came to yoga in the late 1960s and began teaching in the 1970s and practicing yoga therapy in 1991. His most influential teachers include A. G. Mohan, Richard Miller, and Swami Gitananda. He is passionate about people developing an authentic, personal, and experiential understanding of what yoga and meditation are and what they are not. In late 2017, Blashki transitioned into *vanaprastha*, the third stage of life according to the Vedic tradition, and spends his time in reflection, personal practice, and mentoring, while stepping back from many previous professional roles.

Courtney D. Butler-Robinson, C-IAYT, E-RYT 500

Courtney D. Butler-Robinson is a stress-management specialist for the Dr. Dean Ornish Reversal Clinic in intensive cardiac rehab and a certified yoga therapist working in cancer rehabilitation at Saline Wellness Heart Center, under the supervision of Dr. Allan B. Hatch. Butler-Robinson is the author of *The Mud &*

The Lotus: A Guide and Workbook for Students of Yoga and *The Mud & The Lotus Guide to Successful Workshops, Retreats, and Conferences*. She trains yoga teachers through her business, Balance Yoga and Wellness. She has worked extensively with the Veterans Administration and the University of Arkansas in training their staff to use yoga and meditation practices for the communities they serve. Butler-Robinson also presents sessions on yoga therapy for cancer and cardiac care at national conferences on behalf of organizations such as MD Anderson and the University of Arkansas for Medical Sciences.

Christopher Key Chapple, PhD

Dr. Christopher Key Chapple is Doshi Professor of Indic and Comparative Theology and Director of the Master of Arts in Yoga Studies at Loyola Marymount University in Los Angeles. Chapple has published more than 20 books, including many translations and analyses of Sanskrit texts about yoga, including the *Yoga Sutras*, the *Bhagavad Gita*, the *Yogavasistha*, and the *Yogadrishtisamuccaya*. In 2002, he established the first of several yoga-related certificate programs at LMU, including Yoga Philosophy and Yoga Therapy Rx. Chapple serves on numerous advisory boards and has lectured on yoga worldwide.

Madoka Chase Onizuka, MA, JYTS Certified Yoga Therapist

Madoka Chase Onizuka began meditation in 1996, after a career in environmental and human rights advocacy. In 2003, she began yoga and studied under Keishin Kimura, president of the Japan Yoga Therapy Society (JYTS), where she was certified as a yoga therapist in 2010. Her work has focused primarily on international networking and building JYTS's relationships with yoga therapy organizations around the world. She has translated two yoga therapy books published by Japan Yoga Niketan into English.

Theresa Conroy, C-IAYT, E-RYT 500

In 2007, after spending 26 years as a newspaper reporter, Theresa Conroy left journalism to pursue a career in yoga therapy. Conroy has owned and operated a traditional yoga studio, a yoga therapy clinic, and a yoga therapy studio and specializes in working with neurological disorders. She trains other teachers and yoga therapists in teaching yoga for Parkinson's disease, and is a faculty member teaching Yoga for Neurological Disorders at Inner Peace Yoga Therapy.

Marsha Therese Danzig, MEd, C-IAYT, RYT-500

Marsha Therese Danzig founded Y4A: Yoga For Amputees. A below-knee amputee herself, Danzig has been at the forefront of adaptive yoga for more than 30 years. A certified yoga therapist, Danzig believes that yoga is a pathway to re-remembering wholeness. She is the author of *Yoga for Amputees: The Essential Guide to Finding Wholeness After Limb Loss for Yoga Students and Their Teachers*, *Yoga for Busy Little Hands: Children's Book of Mudras*, and *From the Roots: The True Story of How I Beat Death and Learned to Live.*

Uma Dinsmore-Tuli, PhD, C-IAYT

Dr. Uma Dinsmore-Tuli is the founder of Total Yoga Nidra, Yoni Nidra (for women's health), and Wild Nidra: Radical Creative and Intuitive Yoga Nidra. In 2005, Dinsmore-Tuli co-created the annual Santosa Living Yoga and Bhakti Camp. She works internationally and online, training specialist teachers in Total Yoga Nidra, therapeutic yoga for fertility, menstrual health, pregnancy, birth, postnatal recovery, and healthy menopause. Dinsmore-Tuli is currently completing *Nidra Shakti: A Decolonising Encyclopaedia of Yoga Nidra.*

Jivana Heyman, C-IAYT, E-RYT 500

Jivana Heyman is the founder and director of Accessible Yoga, an international non-profit organization dedicated to increasing access to yogic teachings. He is also the creator of the Accessible Yoga Training School and author of *Accessible Yoga: Poses and Practices for Every Body.* For more than 25 years, Heyman has specialized in teaching yoga to people with disabilities; out of this work, the Accessible Yoga organization was created to support education, training, and advocacy with the mission of shifting the public perception of yoga.

Keishin Kimura

Keishin Kimura is director of Japan Yoga Niketan and president of the Japan Yoga Therapy Society. Kimura also serves as a member of the board of the Ayurveda Society in Japan, and is a member of the Working Group on Standards for Yoga Instruction organized by the World Health Organization. In August 2019, his work was recognized when Japan Yoga Niketan was awarded the Indian Prime Minister's Award for Outstanding Contribution Towards the Development and Promotion of Yoga, the first time the award was conferred at the international level.

Yana Kofman, DPT, C-IAYT

Dr. Yana Kofman is a physical therapist and certified yoga therapist. In 2009, Kofman founded The Yoga Way Therapy Center, a private practice in Morristown, New Jersey. Her clinical work incorporates yoga asana, positioning, and neuromotor breathing retraining techniques to optimize motor performance. She developed a neurointegrative therapy approach that incorporates biomechanics, body alignment, training nervous system regulation toward parasympathetic dominance, and myofascial release therapy. Kofman is a published author, researcher, and practitioner of Yoga for the Special Child.

Rachel Krentzman, PT, C-IAYT

Rachel Krentzman is both a physical therapist and certified yoga therapist. Krentzman is also codirector of Wisdom-Body Yoga Therapy School, an IAYT-accredited yoga therapy training program in Israel, where she now resides. She is the author of two books: *Yoga for a Happy Back: A Teacher's Guide to Spinal Health through Yoga Therapy* and *Scoliosis, Yoga Therapy and the Art of Letting Go.*

Jennie Lee, C-IAYT

Jennie Lee is the author of three books: *Spark Change: 108 Provocative Questions for Spiritual Evolution*, *True Yoga: Practicing with the Yoga Sutras for Happiness & Spiritual Fulfillment*, and *Breathing Love: Meditation in Action*. As a certified yoga therapist, Lee has taught classical yoga and meditation for more than 20 years and coached private clients in the practices that integrate life spiritually, mentally, emotionally, and physically. A recognized expert in the fields of yoga therapy and spiritual living, her writing is regularly featured in national magazines and other yoga-related publications.

Leigh Leibel, MSc, C-IAYT

Leigh Leibel is a journalist and integrative oncology specialist working at the intersection of cancer prevention, integrative cancer support, and lifestyle medicine. She has a mind-body practice at Columbia University Irving Medical Center in New York City, where she works with cancer patients and survivors at all stages of care and teaches the oncology mind-body curriculum to medical students in the Integrative Medicine elective. She is a 2020 TEDMED scholar and an alumna of the NIH/NCI Cancer Prevention and Control Summer Fellowship Program, and serves on the board of trustees of the Society for Integrative Oncology, where she founded and co-chairs the SIO Yoga Committee. She holds a Master of Science in Yoga with distinction from S-Vyasa University in Bengaluru, India. Formerly an executive producer with CNN, Leibel sits on the editorial advisory board of *Cancer Health Magazine* and is coeditor of the book *Yoga Therapy across the Cancer Care Continuum.*

Gina Macauley, C-IAYT

Gina Macauley is a senior registered teacher with Yoga Australia, a certified yoga therapist, and a certified iRest teacher. Macauley is codirector of the Australian Institute of Yoga Therapy and runs the YogaHara yoga studio in Bendigo, Australia. She mentors yoga teachers and therapists and offers workshops on yoga philosophy and yoga therapy. Macauley has served on various committees within Yoga Australia over many years and regularly presents at Yoga Australia events.

Michael J. de Manincor, PhD

Dr. Michael J. de Manincor is a registered psychologist and an academic researcher in mind-body-lifestyle integrative medicine. De Manincor is founding director of The Yoga Institute, a center dedicated to excellence in yoga teacher training and yoga therapy training, and is also founding director of The Yoga Foundation, a non-profit organization that provides yoga for disadvantaged and underserved people and communities. He served as president of the Executive Committee of Yoga Australia and is an invited expert advisor to the World Health Organization for the development of global standards for yoga in healthcare. De Manincor is passionate about supporting the highest professional standards for yoga teachers and therapists.

Molly McManus, C-IAYT

Molly McManus co-owns Yoga North International SomaYoga Institute. She is a past chair of the Accreditation Committee for the International Association of Yoga Therapists and holds certifications as a yoga therapist, somatic educator, and ayurvedic health counselor. As a speaker and trainer, McManus is sought out for her areas of interest in the resolution of chronic pain and creating systems for whole-person well-being. She has designed programs such as "Nourish Ayurveda—Feeding the Whole Person," "SomaYoga for Chronic Pain," "The Chemistry of Joy," and "Yoga for Stress, Anxiety and Depression."

Tracey Meyers, PsyD, C-IAYT

Dr. Tracey Meyers, a licensed clinical psychologist, leads national mindfulness and yoga programs, retreats, and yoga teacher training immersions. Meyers has spent most of her professional career working in inpatient and outpatient behavioral health settings. She has authored publications on holistic behavioral treatment for different mental health conditions and yoga for addiction. She is currently writing a book on yin yoga and mental health. Meyers is an assistant clinical professor at Yale University Department of Psychiatry and an adjunct faculty member at the University of Hartford Graduate School of Professional Psychology and Maryland University of Integrative Health.

Marybeth Missenda, RPh, CNS

Marybeth Missenda is a health system pharmacist in clinical pharmacy and transition of care with a specialization in parenteral nutrition. Her international experience as a pharmacy consultant for the Pan-American Health Organization in Port-au-Prince, Haiti, and the island of Montserrat in the Caribbean gave her an appreciation for integrative approaches to healthcare that recognize the value of traditional medicine. Missenda is an assistant professor and department chair for Integrative Health Studies at Maryland University of Integrative Health. She is published in the journal *Advances in Integrative Medicine* and runs a small practice collaborating with complementary health practitioners and clients on medication and dietary supplement therapy management (Bridges to Wellness, LLC).

Mamta Parikh, PharmD, BCPS, BCPP

Dr. Mamta Parikh is an assistant professor at Notre Dame of Maryland University, School of Pharmacy. Parikh implemented a pharmacy-led mental health consulting service for Gilchrist's Elder Medical Care—Home Care. She currently has a practice in the inpatient psychiatry service at Sinai Hospital of Baltimore.

Crystal L. Park, PhD

Dr. Crystal L. Park is Professor of Clinical Psychology at the University of Connecticut (UConn). Park has published nearly 300 articles and chapters on stress and coping, focusing especially on the roles of religious beliefs and religious coping, the phenomenon of stress-related growth, and the making of meaning in the context of traumatic events and life-threatening illnesses, particularly with cancer survivors, congestive heart failure patients, and military veterans. She is currently principal or co-principal investigator of NIH- and foundation-funded studies of religious beliefs and stressful experiences, resilience in cancer survivorship, and yoga for stress management. Park is coauthor or coeditor of six books, including *Empathic Counseling* and *Trauma, Meaning, and Spirituality*, and is editor of the American Psychological Association journal *Psychology of Religion and Spirituality*. At UConn, she maintains a research lab with graduate and undergraduate students and teaches health psychology at both the graduate and undergraduate levels.

Gail Parker, PhD, C-IAYT, E-RYT 500

Dr. Gail Parker, a psychologist and certified yoga therapist, is president of the board of directors of the Black Yoga Teacher's Alliance. Parker currently instructs and mentors behavioral healthcare providers, allied healthcare providers, yoga teachers, and yoga therapists in using restorative yoga as a therapeutic intervention that reduces stress and supports recovery from emotional trauma associated with race-based traumatic stress injury. She is the author of *Restorative Yoga for Ethnic and Race-Based Stress and Trauma*.

Nya Patrinos, C-IAYT

Nya Patrinos holds a diploma in yoga therapy from the Ghosh College of India in Kolkata (Muktamala Mita). A competitive athlete from the age of 6, she started practicing yoga to alleviate chronic knee pain after all else failed. Patrinos has been an editorial board member for the *Journal of Yoga Practice and Therapy* and serves as a practicum mentor at Kripalu School of Integrative Health. She educates yoga instructors through Art of Yoga teacher trainings and is passionate about yoga, meditation, and creativity as tools for healing and transformation.

Sarajean Rudman, MS, MA, E-RYT 500

Sarajean Rudman serves as adjunct faculty for ayurveda at Maryland University of Integrative Health. Rudman has more than 15 years of experience educating and developing curricula in yoga, ayurveda, multiple fitness and wellness modalities, and clinical nutrition.

Karen Soltes, LCSW, C-IAYT

Karen Soltes is a licensed clinical social worker and senior iRest instructor who served as Director of Therapeutic Programs at Circle Yoga in Washington, DC, specializing in working with children and young adults with developmental challenges. Soltes also served at the VA Medical Center in Washington, DC, as part of the integrative health and wellness program for veterans with posttraumatic stress disorder and other war-related conditions. She was a founding partner of Warriors at Ease, whose mission has been to bring the healing practices of yoga and meditation to military communities.

Robert H. Stucky, MDiv

Robert H. Stucky earned a Master of Divinity degree from Yale University and a Master of Anglican Studies degree from the Berkeley Episcopal Divinity School at Yale. He lived and studied under the direct tutelage of Swami Muktananda Paramahamsa of Ganeshpuri, India. Stucky cofounded the Faith in Diversity Institute to combat religious ignorance and intolerance and is on the faculty of Al Basheer Institute and the Civilizations Exchange and Cooperation Foundation. He has taught at the University of Maryland, Baltimore County (UMBC), Goucher College, and the Johns Hopkins Hospital. He has lectured and run workshops and retreats on six continents. Stucky authored *The Tantric Jesus: Christ as God, Guru and Self* and *Paradigms: Why We Believe, What We Believe, and How It Can Change*, and he coauthored *Reductionism, Globalization, and Faith*.

Marlysa Sullivan, DPT, C-IAYT

Dr. Marlysa Sullivan is a physical therapist and certified yoga therapist working with people suffering with chronic pain. Sullivan, an assistant professor in Yoga Therapy and Integrative Health Sciences at Maryland University of Integrative Health, also holds an adjunct position at Emory University, where she teaches the integration of yoga and mindfulness into physical therapy practice in the Doctor of Physical Therapy program. She is the author of *Understanding Yoga Therapy: Applied Philosophy and Science for Health and Well-Being* and coeditor of *Yoga and Science in Pain Care: Treating the Person in Pain* as well as several peer-reviewed articles. Sullivan has been involved in the professionalization of the field of yoga therapy through the Educational Standards Committee of the International Association of Yoga Therapists, which helped to define the competencies for the field, and in characterizing the yoga therapy workforce through research.

Robyn Tiger, MD, C-IAYT, RYT-500

Dr. Robyn Tiger, physician and certified yoga therapist, integrates Western and Eastern philosophies into her care for complete physical, mental, and emotional well-being. Tiger specializes in self-care programming for those touched by anxiety, stress-related disorders, and cancer and founded Yoga Heals 4 Life for the public and StressFreeMD for physicians. She is on the faculty of Trauma Informed Yoga Therapy, serves on the Advisory Council of *Yoga Therapy Today* and yogatherapy.health, is the medical resource director for Journey to Be FREE, and is an O2X Human Performance Specialist for first responders. During years in medical practice, she witnessed firsthand the need for more complete patient care and physician self-care education. Through classes, workshops, and private sessions, Tiger guides individuals to holistically achieve optimal health and become the best versions of themselves.

Dorcia J. Tucker, PsyD, MS, C-IAYT

Dr. Dorcia J. Tucker is a licensed clinical psychologist and certified yoga therapist. Tucker has served on the faculty of the Yoga Therapy and Integrative Health Sciences departments at Maryland University of Integrative Health. Tucker previously served as an active-duty military psychologist in the US Air Force, where she integrated complementary modalities such as biofeedback, yoga, meditation, and breathwork into her clinical practice.

Amy Wheeler, PhD, C-IAYT

Dr. Amy Wheeler is a professor of kinesiology at California State University, San Bernardino. Wheeler was a subject matter expert to the National Ayurvedic Medical Association for setting standards for ayurvedic yoga therapy. She is the founder and director of the Optimal State of Living programs, which provide both yoga and yoga therapy training programs. Wheeler served as president of the board of directors for IAYT from 2018 to 2020.

Vignette Contributors

Courtney D. Butler-Robinson, C-IAYT, E-RYT 500, RCYT, RPYT
Crystal L. Park, PhD
Dorcia J. Tucker, PsyD, MS, C-IAYT
Durga Leela, C-IAYT, AP (NAMA), AYT (NAMA)
Erin Byron, MA, RP, C-IAYT, E-RYT 500
Göran Boll
Jana Long, C-IAYT, E-RYT 500
Jivana Heyman, C-IAYT, E-RYT 500
Judi Bar, C-IAYT, E-RYT 500
Keishin Kimura
Kelli Bethel, DPT, PT, C-IAYT
Laura Schmalzl, PhD, RYT-500
Leigh Blashki, C-IAYT
Lucia Plata, C-IAYT
Lynne Valdes, MS, C-IAYT
Madoka Chase Onizuka
Matthew J. Taylor, PT, PhD, C-IAYT
Pamela Stokes Eggleston, MBA, MS, C-IAYT, E-RYT 500
Reverend Lakshmi Barsel, PhD
Shelley K. Goldman, MS, RN, LICDC-CS, CCM, MAC, C-IAYT
Shelly Prosko, PT, C-IAYT
Takakazu Oka, MD, PhD
Tawanna J. A. Kane, RYT-500
Tina Paul, MS, C-IAYT, E-RYT 500
Uma Dinsmore-Tuli, PhD, C-IAYT

Reviewer/Foreword Author

Matra Raj, OTR/L, C-IAYT, E-RYT 500

Matra Raj is the president of the board of directors of the International Association of Yoga Therapists. Ms. Raj is a somatic yoga and mudra teacher as well as a perinatal educator. She is the author of *Yoga for Pregnancy, Birth and Vibrant Life.*

Section Reviewers and Introduction Authors

Camille Freeman, DCN, LDN

Dr. Camille Freeman is a professor in the Department of Nutrition and Herbal Medicine at Maryland University of Integrative Health (MUIH), where she teaches physiology and pathophysiology. She holds a doctoral degree in clinical nutrition from MUIH, as well as degrees from Rice University, the Tai Sophia Institute, and Georgetown University. Freeman is a licensed nutritionist who specializes in reproductive health and fertility, as well as a trained yoga teacher.

Stephanie Lopez, LISW-S, C-IAYT

Stephanie Lopez is the senior director of Teachings, Trainers, and Community, and senior iRest trainer and retreat leader for the iRest Institute. A psychotherapist, meditation teacher, and certified yoga therapist, Lopez also serves on the Certification Committee for the International Association of Yoga Therapists, helping to promote yoga therapy standards and credentialing. With an embodied understanding of meditation informed by over 25 years of immersion in the non-dual teachings of yoga, she leads retreats and trainings internationally.

Steffany Moonaz, PhD, C-IAYT

Dr. Steffany Moonaz is a certified yoga therapist and researcher who focuses on the effects of yoga for chronic pain and joint conditions. She is the director of research at Maryland University of Integrative Health. Dr. Moonaz also founded and directs Yoga for Arthritis, which provides training and content to improve the safety and accessibility of yoga practices for people with arthritis worldwide. She is also the author of *Yoga Therapy for Arthritis: A Whole Person Approach to Movement and Lifestyle.*

Marilyn Peppers-Citizen, PhD, NBC-HWC, C-IAYT, E-RYT 500

Dr. Marilyn Peppers-Citizen has more than 35 years of military and business leadership experience in various senior-level capacities. With a PhD in public policy, specializing in interdisciplinary policy, and master's degrees in business and national resource strategy, Dr. Peppers-Citizen is experienced in strategic planning, international and interagency collaboration, logistics planning and integration, and program management. As a certified yoga therapist and health and wellness coach, she supports clients in applying yoga and lifestyle choices to age well.

Preface

The teacher and psychologist Richard Alpert, better known as Ram Dass, liked to tell stories. One of those stories had to do with life being like a Monopoly game. If a person is not engaged and playing the game, it is not much fun. By the same token, if one gets attached and starts jumping around, thumping their chest, and yelling "I'm the top hat!" that is also not much fun. Somewhere in between lies the truth.

Expression of the instincts of greed and lust (both related to power and masculinity in many cultures) can ultimately bring humans to their knees. This is an era in which many individuals, primarily men, who have been playing that game of Monopoly are exclaiming confidently that they are the top hat. And because of the power they are perceived to hold, seekers follow them, usually to a bad end. This is an age when discernment and solid spiritual footing are more important than ever.

Back to Ram Dass: He felt that one needed to be "somebody" before they could be "nobody." It is important to consider how yoga therapists come to their *dharma* of service. Is this the means by which the person will finally become "someone"? If so, some additional reflection may be warranted. As Dass and coauthor Paul Gorman put it:

> So we are called upon to take what is valuable from our training, but not let it constrict the helping relationship itself. We need to enlist the service of the intellect, but not let it block the intuitive compassion of the heart...
>
> Once we have acquired all this knowledge, it's hard to keep it in perspective. It may dazzle us and make us forget the bedrock of wisdom to which all are privy. It gives us one kind of power but cuts us off from our birthright, the wisdom that comes directly from our common humanity and divinity.
>
> Finally, when we identify with our special knowledge, we may develop a vested interest in being "right."... In professions we defend schools of thought. Helping often slips through the cracks.[1]

This gentle yet pointed reminder to continually reexamine our motives, seeking ever-greater clarity and humility, is reminiscent of a poem written in 1872 by John Godfrey Saxe, "The Blind Man and the Elephant."[2] In this short theological treatise, a variety of men who cannot see insist on defining an elephant, a metaphor for God, by their individual experiences touching a single part of the animal. Their attachment to their own circumscribed perceptions (and lack of vision) meant that none of them accurately took in the enormity of the experience. They were blinded by their ego and personal limitations.

As "householder" yogis and as professionals, yoga therapists have a great need for *sangha*, community. Individuals, be they gurus or *sadhakas* (seekers), cannot see their own backs. Eyes must stay open, with everyone willing to take a step back from the elephant to perceive what is actually there.

As Dass and Gorman continued:[3]

> Many times we may be alert to the risk of the role. Out of the corner of our eye we catch ourselves acting out our private agendas or see our attachment to certain self-images… Our conditioning, our motives, our training, our attachment to our ideas, the vested interest of organizations…all these, then, can seduce us into believing we've got the help, we are the "helpers." The self-image is very compelling.

Motivated initially by the desire to serve, individuals can be seduced by the desire for name and fame to develop protocols, sequences, and methods. Likewise, in yoga and yoga therapy are those who would have things done only by their prescription. Others think yoga and yoga therapy are synonymous and inseparable ("Isn't all yoga therapeutic?").[4]

This textbook presents the best information available from a variety of respected schools so that students can review "all the parts of the elephant" and discover, using their own critical thinking skills, alongside engaged dialogue with their yoga therapy faculty and fellow students, how the various pieces of therapeutic yoga fit together. The future clients of yoga therapists who adopt this style of education stand to benefit tremendously from the depth and breadth provided by knowledge of a variety of traditions within the wide ocean of yoga.

Notes on Cultural Appropriation and Abuse

This approach may sound like sacrilege to students who have been exhorted to stay with one school or lineage to avoid watering down the medicine. We have seen—starkly and with dismaying frequency in recent years—how this insistence on allegiance sometimes plays out in the abuse of the guru-disciple relationship around the world. Often, too, when students shift from being "true believers" to practitioners who recognize the gift of their *sadhana* (practice) and want to share that authentically with others they have faced repercussions from so-called lineage holders. Such retribution can include excommunication or defamation as erstwhile students present "adulterated" versions of the practices they learned, divulge secret teachings, or disclose instances of fraud and abuse in the communities of which they had been a part. Aside from being cruel and sometimes outright criminal, the misapplications of yoga by so-called gurus are antithetical to the liberation the practices have always promised—and to the societal liberation that seems in many ways now more possible than ever when aided by such supports.[5]

As editors of this text, we acknowledge that yoga is an Indian tradition and that we do not wish to make it something other than it is, a tradition developed and designed for the culture from which it sprang. We do wish to present ways to approach this tradition that make it applicable to a variety of cultures, in the same way that global religions have adapted to the needs of various cultures—or indeed the ways in which various medical practices have come to be adapted to different settings.[6]

In this text, we have chosen to forgo Sanskrit diacritics.[7] The point of this textbook is not to teach Sanskrit, but rather the philosophies, principles, and practices that are represented by Sanskrit words. We find that understanding this material is already a sufficiently arduous endeavor without an additional layer of scholarly pursuit more appropriate to a linguist than a clinician. To that end, we have chosen to use the most standard transliterations possible for the Devanagari text.

The delivery of good yoga therapy, for which we hope to build a foundation with this text, is about sound integrative clinical skills. This has more to do with development of critical thinking, as modeled in the *Samkhya Karika*, than with learning Sanskrit or adhering to a particular lineage or protocol. The original terms are generally given at first mention within a chapter, and practices and concepts are subsequently referred to by their English equivalents, unless the term is most widely known in its Sanskrit form or no accurate and reasonably brief equivalent exists. Diacritics that appear in source materials have been retained where possible.

We also aim to present a textbook that may be broadly adopted across a range of educational settings, including both academic and community-based programs. We have therefore attempted to balance honoring the philosophical tradition and the origins of the practices with adaptations needed to align them to contemporary settings. We contend that in such cases persisting with the Sanskrit would not only thwart this aim but also constitute cultural appropriation in the sense of pretending that such rich traditions do not themselves evolve and adapt as they remain relevant through history.

Similarly, although cogent arguments have been made on either side of this debate, we have elected to use the more secular lowercase *yoga* and *yoga therapy* as a further means of encouraging wide adoption and adaptation of these practices in healthcare settings. Specific forms of the practice, for example Hatha Yoga, are capitalized, as are major philosophical schools including those from which yoga and ayurveda arose.

Because yoga therapy is a holistic modality, this book sometimes guides students to consider the spiritual experience of the client. In considering the *panchamaya kosha* (five sheaths) system, many yoga therapists skip over *anandamaya* with a nod toward bliss, making it seem more like a mind-blowing drug that provides a happiness trip than an experience that brings the individual into union with the ocean of which they are a drop. In the *Bhagavad Gita* (11.8–51), Krishna must wipe Arjuna's anandamaya experience of being with All That Is from his mind because of its all-encompassing intensity.[8] Such experiences surpass mere "bliss" or "joy"—they are the awe that alters and reshapes dharma.

These explorations are not inherently "religious," although they may involve means that are essentially yogic in origin. This book, for example, refers to Shiva consciousness in Kashmir Shaivism (Chapter 5) as well as ways to use the tools of this system through the client's religion of origin so that they may find a way to connect to the experience of Awe.

We feel that this postlineage approach moves the traditions forward in a way that emphasizes equal empowerment, avoids appropriation, and encourages deep and critical thinking about yoga therapy while allowing students to put to appropriate use the tools needed to serve a suffering world. See Chapter 22 for a full discussion of the term *postlineage yoga*—which does not mean antilineage—and the rationale for its use. This exploration constitutes one of many unique features of this book, which deliberately includes a range of perspectives and a full discussion of the feminine power of *Shakti* and of women's health issues (Chapter 15).

The gender-neutral pronouns "they/their/them" have been consciously employed in this text.

How to Use this Book

The book is laid out in four sections, each aligned with the educational competencies set down by the International Association of Yoga Therapists for accredited yoga therapy training programs. We have chosen not to present the fifth competency, practicum, as the experience and needs of the variety of schools training yoga therapists are too varied and remain too fluid for such an inclusion to make sense at this time.

The first section presents an academic perspective on the history and philosophies that provide the foundation for the contemporary work of yoga therapy. We hope that the reader will perceive how the threads of the foundational philosophies begin to create the fabric by which individuals over the millennia have sought to engage this variety of paths with the singular goal of better understanding themselves and others through the connection of body, breath, mind, and spirit. Although this is an academic text, it is intended to provide practical starting points that the beginning yoga therapist must have to understand the tradition that they are carrying forward.

The book is intended to be used in the context of a comprehensive yoga therapy training program, although individuals will find useful points for departure to guide their further studies, and perhaps also perspectives to which they had not previously been exposed. Contributors to this collection are many and varied. Presenting different perspectives on the material is a deliberate choice to encourage faculty and fellow students to work together to understand the many paths that lead to the one Source.

We have assumed that readers who are students in yoga therapy training programs will already have a solid working knowledge of yoga's basic physical and respiratory practices (*asana* and *pranayama*), along with an ability to offer appropriate variations to suit a range of non-clinical populations. This book is therefore not a how-to manual, nor does it present clinical protocols or exhaustive recommendations.

Readers will note entreaties from a number of contributors to attend to their own personal work, building in the laboratory of their dedicated practices a foundation for conscientiously guiding others. This not only facilitates resilience and personal growth, but aids in clinical acumen as the practitioner engages with and unfolds the possibilities of the practices, particularly those outside of their normal sadhana. Readers who need additional background on the mechanics of yogic practices are encouraged to work with their program directors to identify appropriate means of filling knowledge and skill gaps. The hybrid reference/endnote style employed is intended to enable quick identification of such needs as well as starting points for addressing them. To aid schools and students in their development, most chapters, including this Preface, also offer resources for further study.

Note that at the time of writing, the long-term impact of COVID-19 on yoga and the practice of yoga therapy remains to be seen. Please adjust any practices suggested in this book to comply with ongoing guidelines and regulations.

Additional Resources

Dass, R., & Gorman, P. (1985). *How can I help? Stories and reflections on service*. Alfred A. Knopf.

Desikachar, T. K. V. (1999). *The heart of yoga: Developing a personal practice*. Inner Traditions.

Easwaran, E. (2007). *The Upanishads*. Nilgiri Press.

Fields, G. P. (2001). *Religious therapeutics: Body and health in yoga, ayurveda, and tantra*. State University of New York Press.

Mallinson, J., & Singleton, M. (2017). *Roots of yoga*. Penguin Classics.

Sargeant, W. (2009). *The bhagavad gītā*. State University of New York Press.

Sullivan, M., & Robertson, L. C. H. (2020). *Understanding yoga therapy: Applied philosophy and science for health and well-being*. Routledge.

Cultural appropriation: What yoga therapists promote and why

Antony, M. G. (2016). Tailoring nirvana: Appropriating yoga, resignification and instructional challenges. *International Journal of Media and Cultural Politics, 12*(3), 283–303.

Bapuji, H., & Chrispal, S. (2020). Understanding economic inequality through the lens of caste. *Journal of Business Ethics, 162*(3), 533–551.

Gemar, A. (2020). Cultural capital and emerging culture: The case of meditation, yoga, and vegetarianism in the UK. *Leisure/Loisir, 44*(1), 1–26.

McCartney, P. (2019). Stretching into the shadows: Unlikely alliances, strategic syncretism, and de-post-colonizing yogaland's "yogatopia(s)." *Asian Ethnology, 78*(2), 373–401.

Medhananda, S. (2020). Was Swami Vivekananda a Hindu supremacist? Revisiting a long-standing debate. *Religions, 11*(7), 368–396.

Surmitis, K. A., Fox, J., & Gutierrez, D. (2018). Meditation and appropriation: Best practices for counselors who utilize meditation. *Counseling & Values, 63*(1), 4–16.

Endnotes

1 Dass, R., & Gorman, P. (1985). *How can I help? Stories and reflections on service* (pp. 130–131). Alfred A. Knopf.

2 Saxe, J. G. (1876). *The poems of John Godfrey Saxe: Complete in one volume* (pp. 259–261). Ticknor and Fields.

3 Dass & Gorman, *How can I help?* (p. 133).

4 The "prescriptive approach to yoga therapy" described by physical therapist and yoga therapist Matthew Taylor has much in common with the yoga practice experiences provided in many contemporary studio settings. Taylor instead recommended a "process approach to yoga therapy" that distinguishes group yoga from group (or individual) yoga therapy: "The goals of a group Yoga therapy program are not only to teach the techniques of Yoga, but also to invite students to experience a healing process within a community. In this community, students' voices are heard, experiences are honored, beliefs and actions are transformed, and the lessons learned are sustainable beyond the walls of the group meetings": Taylor, M. J. (2006). Harvesting the full potential of group yoga therapy classes. *International Journal of Yoga Therapy, 16*, 33–37. See also this further exploration of the distinct purposes and orientations of general yoga practice and the provision of yoga therapy: Bhavanani, A., Sullivan, M., Taylor, M. J., & Wheeler, A. (2019). Shared foundations for practice: The language of yoga therapy. *Yoga Therapy Today*, Summer, 44–47.

5 Despite having arisen in an institution that enabled a long-term, widespread culture of abuse, materials from the Bihar School of Yoga remain widely cited, including in this book. Many of these teachings remain relevant and useful, albeit sometimes overly rigid or hyperbolic, and readers may prefer to borrow or locate second-hand copies of these works for their own explorations. As always, the cultivation of discernment is of paramount importance.

6 Yoga therapists need to fully understand the complex cultural heritage that has produced this modality. They should also recognize the impact of colonization on India and be able to locate within these historical repositories all the meaning that comes along with their interventions. In 2017, professor Shreena Gandhi and antiracism advocate Lillie Wolff framed this history and called for Western yogis to consider their relationship to the practices (Gandhi, S., & Wolff, L. (2017, Dec. 19). Yoga and the roots of cultural appropriation. Praxis Center. www.kzoo.edu/praxis/yoga): "The reasons why yoga became popular, and why various Indian yogis started travelling to England and the United States to 'sell' yoga, [are] tied up with colonialism. Yoga was often used as a tool to show the British that Indians were not backwards or primitive, but that their religion was scientific, healthy, and rational. This was a position they were coerced into, and unfortunately [one that] reified colonial forms of knowledge—that knowledge must be proven or scientific to be worth anything.

"Beyond its utility, yoga became popular, in part, because it reinforced European and Euro-American ideas of India. Early Indian yoga missionaries played on the orientalist construction of the 'west' as progressive and superior and the 'east' as spiritual but inferior. Yoga became—and remains—a practice which allows western practitioners to experience the idea of another culture while focusing on the self."

Practitioners are obliged to examine the tension between cultural appreciation and cultural appropriation, between inclusivity and dishonoring by erasure. The yoga therapist may find themselves in a hospital providing yoga therapy to someone in an acute-care bed who has no desire to understand the history that informs the work they are doing together, or in a behavioral health organization where the client's need for stability overrides their capacity to take in what they are receiving.

Even if the client served is not cognizant of the rich tradition that informs the care in which they are engaged, it is important that the yoga therapist is, and is capable of sharing that information with the client as they become ready to hear it. If the client asks the yoga therapist about the tools of yoga therapy, the yoga therapist must be able to draw on accurate knowledge of the origins of the tools being used—and the way in which they are being employed. This understanding can be especially helpful in situations where institutional or setting-based restrictions limit the ability to deliver a full plan of care based on the traditions of the profession.

The Additional Resources list above the Endnotes offers further starting points in a discussion of cultural appropriation in yoga; yoga therapists are encouraged to explore the additional educational resources that abound.

7 Sanskrit, an Indic language that dates to the second millennium BCE, is a primary language of Hindu liturgy. Because it is written in the Devangari alphabet, Sanskrit has no direct or universally agreed-upon transliteration to the Latin alphabet of English. Resources abound for students who wish to pursue further Sanskrit studies.

Is it better to read a text in the original language? Probably. If we limit yoga therapy to include only those who can read Sanskrit, however, we will lose people who have excellent observation skills and limit the field to intellectuals and linguists.

8 Sargeant, W. (2009). *The bhagavad gītā* (pp. 460–503). State University of New York Press.

1

Introduction: An Inclusive Style that Encourages Critical Thinking

DIANE FINLAYSON

This textbook comprehensively addresses the who, what, when, where, and why of the profession of yoga therapy and the training of competent practitioners, moving section by section through the educational competencies laid out by the International Association of Yoga Therapists.

Because learning and practicing yoga therapy with integrity from a postlineage perspective (see Chapter 22) requires students to engage in critical thinking, the book starts with the why and what of the profession. Approached from this perspective, the Socratic method, in which students and faculty question the material and one another's perceptions of that material, is useful. Yoga therapy is a profession that requires more than the mere digestion of facts; it requires the ability to observe and discern prior to action.

This Book's Approach to Yoga Therapy

The primary texts of the major yogic lineages serve as the foundation for these discussions. It is important to know and engage with these texts to truly understand "what" the yoga therapist is charged with doing (serve the individual by supporting liberation) and "why" (to ease suffering). Section I provides much of the content beginning yoga therapists will need to understand to enable them to move forward into conscious care of the suffering client and the conscientious support of self-empowerment. This section includes material that offers the Indian philosophies used in yoga as a therapeutic modality, presented by scholars, academics, and those who have steeped themselves deeply in their respective traditions. Each of these authors has been actively contributing to their field for an extended period.

The yoga traditions sourced here are rooted in one or more of the following texts or philosophies: the Vedas, the *Bhagavad Gita*, the Upanishads, the *Yoga Sutras*, the Puranas, Kashmir Shaivism, Samkhya, Yoga, and Ayurveda. Look for similarities as well as differences to get the most out of this reading.

Transcendence and embodiment: Dual and non-dual philosophies

A primary consideration is the ability to comprehend the difference between dualistic and non-dual systems. Those who may be curious about the ways in which European, or Continental, philosophy approaches dualism can look through the lens of René Descartes: "I think, therefore I am."[1] This statement clearly delineates mind from body, prioritizing the former and dismissing embodied life. The Cartesian aim is to transcend the body and identify with mindstuff. From a simplistic angle, in this logic, the activity of the mind is what determines the presence of life. This is similar to various yoga schools (or Western theologies) that focus on liberation as transcendence of this world, or this body, rather than on the embodied assimilation of this world's material. One could say that there are schools of transcendence (dual) and schools of embodiment (non-dual).

Alternatively, at the beginning of the 20th century CE a group of primarily French philosophers became curious about what it means to be embodied. Much insight is to be gained through exploration of the branch of philosophy called phenomenology, which gives a non-dual view through the Continental lens. Of particular use for this exploration are the writings of Michel Foucault.[2]

Another Western author who may help with the understanding of these ideas is Ken Wilber. Wilber has been thinking and writing about this material over the course of two generations in an effort to make it more accessible. Wilbur's Integral Theory (which can be complex) focuses on the individual moving through lines and levels of development. Similarly, there are yogic practices (e.g., meditation) that allow the individual to rise along established pathways (more dualistic or transcendent, leading to what Wilber calls the "dual mystical state") and practices (e.g., Hatha Yoga) that allow the integration of material of each level as part of present-moment embodied experience (more non-dual, or embodied).[3]

The importance of understanding the roles of dual and non-dual material relates not only to knowledge of yoga therapy's foundational traditions, but also to the yoga therapist's ability to correctly assess a client's need and capacity to effectively work within their own interoceptive map—to be able to recognize and liberate themselves from the net of *samskara* (deeply ingrained patterns) in which they may find themselves entangled.

Also contained in this text are discussions of the various yoga *margas*, or yogic paths, especially Raja (classical) Yoga, Hatha Yoga, Tantra, and Laya Yoga. Most students will be familiar with the eight-limbed path of Raja Yoga as presented in Patanjali's *Yoga Sutras*. Additionally, many will have some familiarity with the origins of Hatha Yoga and its importance to the delivery of yoga therapy.

There is ongoing discussion throughout the yoga community as to whether Patanjali's Sutras are dual or non-dual. The more common approach is to teach that the *Yoga Sutras* are dualistic; however, that may be influenced by the more dualistic nature of male-dominated Western Abrahamic traditions (the non-mystical approaches of the religions of "People of the Book," as evidenced in Judaism, Christianity, and Islam) and the interpretation and teaching of the material from the perspective of these different faith traditions.

It should be noted here, too, that debate exists as to the appropriate placement of the *Yoga Sutras* within a hierarchical framework of the origins of contemporary yoga practice. Given a complete historical understanding of the context in which modern practice arose, the relative importance of this work in the canon may not reach the level ascribed to it by some traditions. Nevertheless, the ideas presented in the *Yoga Sutras*, and the many commentaries they have inspired, provide robust jumping-off points for yogic explorations of the human system.

Tantra, which developed out of Hatha Yoga, provides an abundance of useful dual and non-dual material for the yoga therapy student. The development of the ability to recognize pairs of opposites and feel those opposites simultaneously, to experience a unified wholeness that exists as one's essential nature, allows for both movement along developmental lines and pauses for integration of the material, as presented in practices like yoga nidra. Bringing together opposing qualities in this way allows the individual to recognize the disparate elements of existence while usefully balancing them.

Laya Yoga, a practice that makes use of both these lines, or pathways, and levels of development, moves the elemental energies represented in the subtle body. These practices allow the yogi to dissolve their embodiment when the moment of death and "ultimate transcendence" is upon them, moving toward union with the whole. Note that different traditions, for example yoga and ayurveda, have different views of the subtle "yogic body," and contemporary practice may present composites of these conceptions.

Section II of this book provides more of the "what" information through the lens of biomedical foundations. Such an understanding is needed to work in collaboration with licensed healthcare providers and to ensure that *ahimsa* (non-harming) is the primary determinant in the yoga therapy provided. This section is also a starting point for moving the yoga therapist and the practice of yoga therapy into the realm of evidence-informed practice.

In the modality of yoga therapy, specific effects of the intervention (as elucidated by research) and non-specific effects (of therapeutic relationship, small-group communities, etc.) are both valid and important. Research that helps to clarify the value of particular yoga practices and the limitations of others is key to the global adoption of this modality as a means of care that is larger than the sum of its *panchamaya* (five sheaths) parts.

Some may feel that this sort of approach is inauthentic to the practice of yoga therapy, that it is similar to what has come to be known (sometimes derisively) as evidence-based practice. Evidence-based practice, in the original and patient-centered intent of the term,[4] is clearly delineated in texts from the yoga traditions as well.

Consider the *Samkhya Karika*, which neatly lays out the yogic equivalent of the scientific method, advising the reader to begin their investigation with direct perception (2.5–8).[5] Next comes the process of inference: Once the reader, perhaps a yoga therapist, has made an evaluation (done an assessment), discernment must be engaged to infer what may be true about what has been observed. Finally, one may engage with valid testimony to deepen understanding. As Richard Miller wrote in his translation of the *Samkhya Karika*, "*Valid Testimony* occurs when what we read, hear, or observe is deemed to be true and irrefutable based on the writings or statements that come from persons or sources that we regard as reliable and trustworthy."[6] This approach aligns with the work of peer-reviewed research and considerations for inclusion of practices that have been investigated in randomized clinical trials or even written up as case reports. Yoga therapists who are well-versed in evidence-informed practices can work in clients' best interests to create uniquely integrated and holistic plans of care to best serve individual needs.

BOX 1.1 INJURY IN YOGA

As noted in the Preface, this text assumes that those enrolled in yoga therapy training programs will already have a sound understanding of basic *asana* and *pranayama*, along with an ability to offer safe and appropriate variations for a range of non-clinical populations.

As with any modality that aims to affect the body-mind-spirit, injuries may be associated with the practice of yoga or yoga therapy. Contraindications and red flags are noted at several points in the book, although these listings are not intended to be exhaustive or taken as such.

Each generation of yoga therapists has the ethical duty to be diligent about following the latest, and best, research available on the effects of various tools of yoga therapy, used alone and combined, to understand what may be beneficial, ineffective, or even detrimental for individual clients. Staying abreast of research serves and protects clients, furthers the profession, and promotes the tenet of *ahimsa*, non-harming.

The following studies on adverse events in yoga are among those highly recommended for yoga therapy professionals:

Cramer, H., Quinker, D., Schumann, D., Wardle, J., Dobos, G., & Lauche, R. (2019). Adverse effects of yoga: A national cross-sectional survey. *BMC Complementary and Alternative Medicine*, 19(1), 190.

Cramer, H., Ward, L., Saper, R., Fishbein, D., Dobos, G., & Lauche, R. (2015). The safety of yoga: A systematic review and meta-analysis of randomized controlled trials. *American Journal of Epidemiology*, 182(4), 281–293.

Lee, M., Huntoon, E. A., & Sinaki, M. (2019). Soft tissue and bony injuries attributed to the practice of yoga: A biomechanical analysis and implications for management. *Mayo Clinic Proceedings*, 94(3), 424–431.

Section III of this book presents information that informs the where, when, and how of the practice to augment the beginning yoga therapist's toolkit. The section includes ideas on ethics, appropriate use of energetics, ideas for delivery of care of the subtler panchamaya sheaths, and a variety of tools from different traditions. Working with yoga therapy clients on behavior change requires both a distinct therapeutic skill set (Section IIIA) and tools that can be manipulated to meet the client at the level of their needs (Section IIIB). Here and elsewhere in the text, all client and patient names and details have been changed to protect individuals' privacy.

A note on meditation

Often, beginning yoga therapists are either overly confident or afraid of working with the subtler levels of being. These subtler levels involve the recognition of clients' instinctual habits or samskara. Rest assured that the yoga traditions provide a variety of scope-appropriate tools to aid clients in overcoming reactivity in *manomaya kosha* (the mind, or mental/emotional body) while developing discernment or witness consciousness in *vijnanamaya kosha* (intelligence, or the wisdom body).

Two of the primary tools yoga therapy has to offer clients in search of behavior change and peace of mind are mindfulness and meditation. This book discusses both. As with the other tools presented in this book, the methods and perspectives particular to each chapter author are showcased as jumping-off points for further study.

When considering the appropriate intervention to support self-agency, it is useful for yoga therapists to assess whether the client will be better served by a cognitive inquiry, or top-down approach, or interoceptive means and inquiry into their ability to accurately assess for themselves the meaning of the internal sensation cues that motivate their behavior, or a bottom-up approach. Returning to the need to understand and be able to work within dual and non-dual systems, does the client need to move in a more transcendent way, or to integrate what is currently present so that they may move again? In either case, yoga therapists who learn both the foundation of the tradition and its tools will be equipped to assist clients in deconstructing prediction errors, or samskara, that may have built up over a lifetime of habitual behaviors.

BOX 1.2 ADVERSE MENTAL HEALTH EFFECTS IN MEDITATION

As with asana and physical injury, the potential for adverse mental health effects of meditation must not be overlooked. Although they may be time-honored, techniques in various lineages are not suitable for every individual in every context. Based in the Theravada Buddhist tradition, mindfulness meditation, for example, has been researched as a treatment for conditions from chronic pain to substance-use disorders; mindfulness remains one of the most studied modalities, but its practice can be detrimental for certain populations. The Additional Resources in Chapter 23 list research drawn from a number of traditions as well as cautionary studies.

Side-effects and adverse reactions to meditative modalities do occur, and yoga therapists need to be prepared for these events. It is vital that yoga therapists continue their own practices—and their education—to ensure that they are able to respond appropriately to client needs. The non-profit Cheetah House, founded by researcher Willoughby Britton, is one resource for teachers and "meditators-in-distress" (www.cheetahhouse.org). Yoga therapists should also maintain current lists of trusted mental health providers to whom they can refer clients for additional support.

Beginning in the 1990s, the most popular and most widely studied means of working with the mind in the West has been "mindfulness" as designed and promoted by Massachusetts General Hospital and Jon Kabat-Zinn. This form of meditation is an offshoot of the Buddhist tradition and in the forms most commonly engaged would be considered a non-dual, bottom-up, or interoceptive approach to well-being.

A great deal has been written by a great many people on the integration of mindfulness into yoga and other complementary and conventional healthcare modalities. In Section III, subject-matter experts from various traditions present additional approaches, both top-down (cognitive, mind-matter, more dualistic) and bottom-up, and all appropriate to the development of discernment and within yoga therapy's scope of practice. Section IIIA considers key therapeutic skills through a broader lens, and Section IIIB covers tools that employ those competencies. (Although clinical applications are concentrated in these sections, they are presented throughout the book.) The tools in Section IIIB are presented from the chapter authors' particular points of view, partly because by the time they reach a yoga therapy training students will already presumably be familiar with these tools; these chapters therefore represent an opportunity to dive deeper into selected ideas and critically apply knowledge from the other sections.

Real-world applications

Finally, Section IV offers chapters on cultivating ethically minded and entrepreneurial perspectives. As yoga teacher trainers and future leaders in yoga education, yoga therapists will need such a mindset to successfully navigate the varied settings in which their skills will be employed.

This section also provides stories of seasoned professionals who have been working in the field for some time. These are meant to help students to understand the possibilities within various avenues of practice and to identify practicing individuals who have already begun to pave the way in their chosen niches.

Additionally, accounts of "a day in the life" for many of these professionals who are out in the world providing care showcase for students the skills and attitudes their future lives may require.

These yoga therapists, whose practices span five continents, offer inspiration and encouragement to those beginning on the professional path.

Endnotes

1 See, e.g., Nolan, L. (Ed.). (2016). *The Cambridge Descartes lexicon*. Cambridge University Press.

2 See, e.g., Rabinow, P. (Ed.). (1984). *The Foucault reader*. Pantheon.

3 Wilber, K. (2000). *Integral psychology*. Shambhala.

4 Sackett, D. L., Rosenberg, W. M., Gray, J. A., Haynes, R. B., & Richardson, W. S. (1996). Evidence based medicine: What it is and what it isn't. *British Medical Journal, 312*(7023), 71–72.

5 Miller, R. C. (2012). *The Sankhya Karika: A new translation with embedded commentary* (pp. 14–17). Integrative Restoration Institute.

6 Miller, *Sankhya Karika* (p. 14).

Section I

YOGA FOUNDATIONS: TRADITIONS AND TOOLS OF YOGA, AYURVEDA, AND TANTRA

By its very nature, the aim of yoga is to relieve suffering and support realization of one's essential nature. Yoga therapy empowers the individual to realize their inherent wholeness and promotes freedom from suffering through the application of yogic principles and practices. Understanding the history and foundations of yoga-informed philosophy is essential for critical thinking and skillful therapeutic practice.

This section offers a breadth of wisdom spanning many yogic traditions that inform contemporary yoga therapy, beginning with an overview of source texts. Although one could devote a lifetime of study to any one of these, their key elements illuminate how healing unfolds through body, breath, mind, and spirit. A four-step model derived from Patanjali's *Yoga Sutras* covers assessment, goal setting, and practical tools of yoga therapy to create balance. In this tradition as taught through the Krishnamacharya Yoga Mandiram, the development of a heartfelt therapeutic relationship, a theme returned to from a clinical perspective in Section III, is imperative to facilitate healing and transformation. Grounded in Samkhya philosophy, the essential principles of yoga's medical sister science of *ayurveda* offer another lens for yoga therapy assessment and the application of particular yogic practices.

Finally, this text uniquely presents key underpinnings of the Trika tradition of Shaiva Tantra (Kashmir Shaivism). The 36 *tattvas* offer a model for understanding reality and how matter and consciousness relate to embody awakening. Yoga therapy is enhanced by developing skills to work with *spanda*, the “motive impulse” behind every movement, emotion, and thought, as it expresses itself in all of existence.

Stephanie Lopez

2

Textual Sources for Yoga Therapy

CHRISTOPHER KEY CHAPPLE

Yoga therapy relies on a theory and practice of the body and mind grounded in three main principles: (1) the elemental components of earth, water, fire, air, and space; (2) the emotional, affective constitution, comprising habits and impressions that manifest in thought and action; and (3) the breath, which energizes, mixes, and moves the elemental and subtle components. This chapter presents the primary literature from India that outlines this dynamic and offers an overview of Hatha Yoga texts that prescribe specific breathing and movement exercises.

The earliest literature that outlines the above worldview can be found in the 1,008 hymns of the *Rig Veda* (ca. 1500–900 BCE), the principal *Upanishads* (ca. 800–200 BCE), and the epic *Mahabharata* (ca. 600 BCE) (Figure 2.1 offers a brief timeline of principal yogic texts). Key ideas from these texts, augmented with insights from Buddhism and Jainism and the *Bhagavad Gita*, become codified in two primary sources, the *Yoga Sutras* (ca. 300 CE) and the *Samkhya Karika* (ca. 400 CE). In the years following, additional details regarding energetic flows can be found in the *Markandeya* and other Puranas, starting in the 8th century. Next came texts such as the *Yogasastra* (11th century) and the *Dattareyayogasastra* (13th century), which contain themes and practices recognizable as Hatha Yoga. By the 18th century, many texts, including the *Hatha Yoga Pradipika*, the *Gheranda Saṃhita*, and the *Hathatatvakaumudi*, were widely available.

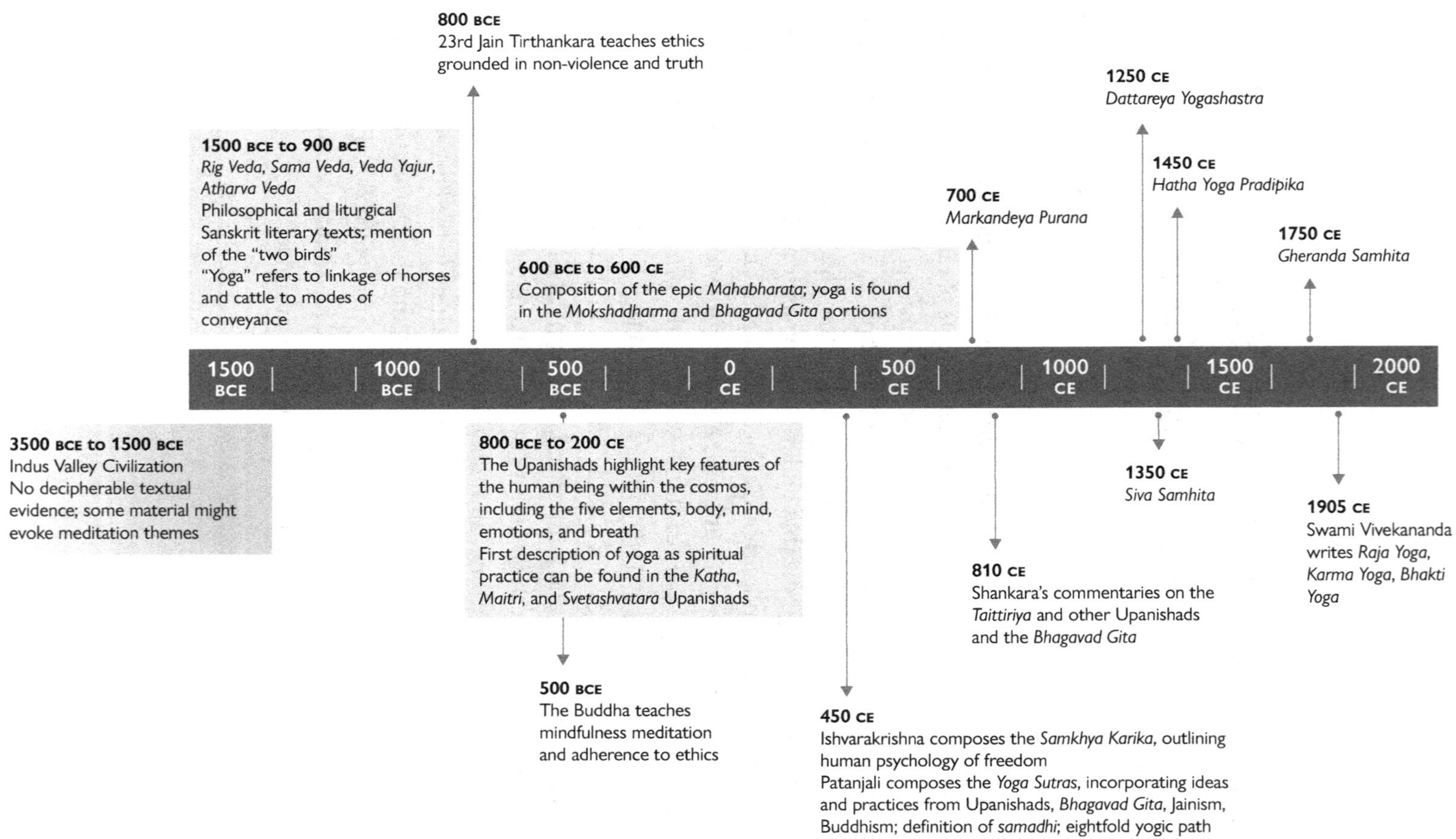

FIGURE 2.1 TIMELINE OF KEY YOGIC TEXTS

All dates are approximate.

Many of the ideas in this chapter form the substratum for the system of health known as ayurveda—literally "knowledge of life." Ayurveda, which is explained fully in the *Charaka Samhita* (ca. 200 CE), involves the use of medicine and surgery as well as attentiveness to a healthy lifestyle.

Early Literature

The Vedas

The Vedas comprise the earliest literature composed in the Sanskrit language. They date to more than 3,500 years ago and describe gods and goddesses in the *Rig Veda* and *Sama Veda*, rituals in the *Yajur Veda*, and tools for healing in the *Atharva Veda*.

The *Rig Veda* praises the earth, water, fire, and wind. It also identifies the core importance of breath and desire. Through the breath we live; through desire and the power of speech (*vac*) we seek and obtain what is needed for a life well-lived. The goal of life is to enter into a rhythm (*rta*) that brings fulfillment, a process that requires dedication and sacrifice. These poetic stanzas from the *Rig Veda* convey a sense of the awe and questioning that can be found at the ground of Vedic wisdom:

Lost in thought I wander.
Then came to me Vāc, Ṛta's first born.
Of her, I got a portion. (I.164)

When humans created language with wisdom...
They followed the path of Vāc through sacrifice...
They drew her out, distributing her in every place,
Vāc, which Seven Singers her tones and harmonies sing. (X.71)

Only I, Vāc, utter the word that brings joy...
I give my power to the persons I favor,
Making them divine, the seer, a perfect sacrificer. (X.125)[1]

Although the language sounds archaic even in the original Sanskrit, the message is clear: The mastery of speech, and before that thought, brings power and great capacity. Thoughts and words with good intent can engender health and wholeness as well as societal harmony.

The *Mokshadharmaparvan*, one of the books of the *Mahabharata* epic, summarizes the relationship between body and cosmos first articulated in the *Rig Veda* and the *Brihadaranyaka Upanishad*:

The Lord, the sustainer of all beings, revealed the sky.
From space came water and, from water, fire and the winds.

From the mixture of the essence of fire and wind arose the earth.
Mountains are his bones, earth his flesh, the ocean his blood.
The sky is his abdomen, air his breath, fire his heat, rivers his nerves.
The sun and moon, which are called Agni and Soma, are the eyes of Brahman.
The upper part of the sky is his head. The earth is his feet and the directions are his hands. (182.14–19)[2]

This vision of the relationship between the body, divinity, and the overall order of things became both descriptive and prescriptive in terms of the human relationship with nature. The world cannot be separated from the human body, nor can the human body be separated from the world.

The Upanishads

The Upanishads arose after the Vedas were completed, starting around 2,800 years ago. Philosophical and speculative in nature, they present divergent views on the nature of the world and the structure of the universe. However, three themes recur: (1) the correlation between the human body and the larger cosmic order, (2) the primacy of the breath, and (3) the importance of food.

Various narratives in the Upanishads assert the superiority of the breath among all the bodily functions (*Brihadaranyaka* I.2.1–21 and 5.21–23; *Chandogya* V.1.1–15). The *Taittiriya Upanishad* praises food:

From food, indeed, beings are born.
All beings who dwell on the earth, by food, in truth, they live.
Into food (earth, the source food), they pass at the time of death.
Food is the chief of beings. It is called a panacea.
Those who worship the highest as food obtain all food.
... By food, all things that are born grow! (II.2)[3]

Food and breath allow all beings to flourish. A deep understanding of food and breath allows one to prosper.

The *Taittiriya Upanishad* (I.8) describes human experience by correlating environmental and mind-body phenomena (Figure 2.2).

By understanding these various relationships, the text proclaims that a human being can arrive at a place of abiding tranquility, a significant marker of good health:

[One becomes] the lord of the mind, lord of the voice, lord of the eye, lord of the ear, lord of understanding...this, and more: one's body (*śarīra*) becomes space (*ākāśa*), one's self (*ātman*) becomes authentic (*satya*), one finds pleasure in the breath itself, the mind becomes filled will bliss (*mana-ānanda*), and one abounds in tranquility (*śānti-samṛddha*). (*Taittiriya Upanishad* I.6)[4]

Earth (*bhur*)	Atmosphere (*bhuvas*)	Heaven (*suvar*)	Four cardinal directions	Intermediate directions
Fire (*agni*)	Wind (*vayu*)	Sun (*surya*)	Moon (*candra*)	Stars (*astra*)
Water	Plants	Trees	Space	Human body
Inhale	Exhale	Down breath	Up breath	Side breath
Sight	Hearing	Mind	Speech	Touch
Skin	Flesh	Muscle	Bone	Marrow

FIGURE 2.2 CORRELATIONS FROM THE *TAITTIRIYA UPANISHAD* DESCRIBE HUMAN EXPERIENCE

The *panchamaya kosha* model has come to be associated with the conceptualization of the relationships among body, mind, and spirit in yoga therapy (see Chapter 3). Although it is commonly assumed that the word *kosha* first appeared in the *Taittiriya Upanishad*, it gained recognition through its use by the Advaita Vedanta philosopher Sri Adi Shankaracharya (788–820 CE). Shankara wrote commentaries on the Upanishads, the *Bhagavad Gita*, and the *Brahma Sutras*. Over the course of five chapters in his commentary on the Valli segment of the *Taittiriya Upanishad*, Shankara lists the now well-known sequence of the five (*pancha*) koshas, or sheaths: food (physical; *annamaya*), breath (energy; *pranamaya*), mind (mental/emotional; *manomaya*), intelligence (wisdom; *vijnanamaya*), and bliss or awe (spiritual; *anandamaya*).[5] Additionally, Shankara writes about the koshas in verses 165–168 and 183–189 of *The Crest Jewel of Discrimination* (*Viveka-Chudamani*), advising that they must all be stripped away to reveal the divine state.[6]

The Mahabharata and Bhagavad Gita

The *Bhagavad Gita*, part of the epic *Mahabharata*, explains the philosophical approaches of knowledge-based (*jnana*), action-based (*karma*), and devotional (*bhakti*) forms of yoga. In addition, the *Bhagavad Gita* explains in several chapters the threefold constituent forms of reality (*gunas*): heaviness and lethargy (*tamas*), often a cause of disease; fiery passion (*rajas*), an energizing force that can move upward or downward; and illumination and buoyancy (*sattva*), the factor that brings one toward an enlightened state (see Chapter 3).

Building on the emphasis between body and food in the Upanishads, and serving as a template for moderation in all things, the *Bhagavad Gita* urges the cultivation of knowledge in regard to the effects of food:

> *Foods increasing life, vitality, strength, health, happiness and joy,*
> *Tasty, rich, lasting and agreeable: these are dear to the sattvic.*
> *Foods which are pungent, sour, salty, very hot, spicy, astringent, burning,*
> *Which cause pain, grief and sickness: these are desired by the rajasic.*
> *Food which is spoiled, tasteless, foul-smelling, stale, which is left-over or unclean:*
> *This is the food dear to the tamasic. (XVII.8–10)*[7]

As noted earlier, food constitutes the human body. To enhance wellness, it is important to be mindful of the origins and effects of food and to seek food that promotes "happiness and joy" not only in the short term but to ensure strength and longevity.

Philosophy by the 8th Century

By the time of Shankara, six major schools of Indian philosophy had emerged from the Vedas and Upanishads, each with a specific focus:

- ***Nyaya*** (logic)
- ***Vaishesika*** (description of physical realities)
- ***Mimamsa*** (ritual instructions)
- ***Samkhya*** (philosophical psychology)
- ***Yoga*** (practice instructions)
- ***Vedanta*** (theology)

The final three philosophies in particular highlight tools for self-improvement and are the most helpful to the yoga therapist. Vedanta, as seen above, emphasizes the need to separate the unreal from the real, illusion from the ultimate reality. Samkhya places great emphasis on the purification of the mind and the discernment of the difference between change and the changeless.

The resources of two other philosophical systems that originated in India can be useful for the yoga therapist as well: Buddhism and Jainism, which focus on meditation and ethics.

Buddhism and Jainism

Breath to facilitate healing

Buddhism, similar to the Upanishads, emphasizes the importance of the breath. The Buddha established the breath as the gateway to meditation. It is important for the yoga therapist to be familiar with mindfulness practice as found in the *vipassana* (insight) meditation of early Theravada Buddhism. The foundational text for meditation on the breath, the *Satipattana*, documents the Buddha's direct instructions for contemplation:

> *And how, monks, does one contemplate the body?*
> *Whether in the forest, or at the base of a tree, or in an empty hut, one sits down with legs crossed, body erect, and establishes mindfulness, mindfully breathing in and mindfully breathing out.*
> *Breathing in long, one notes, "I breathe in long."*
> *Breathing out long, one notes, "I breathe out long."*
> *Breathing in short, one notes, "I breathe in short."*
> *Breathing out short, one notes, "I breathe out short."*
>
> [The meditator goes on...]
>
> *I shall breathe in experiencing the whole body. I shall breathe out experiencing the whole body. I shall breathe in calming the body. I shall breathe out calming the body*
> *In this way, [the meditator] contemplates the body internally and externally, contemplates the nature of the arising and the passing away of the body...not clinging to anything in the world.*[8]

These words provide instruction on how to enhance the awareness of body and breath, an important part of the healing process. The "mindfulness movement" has introduced breath practice to millions worldwide, with ample scientific evidence of its efficacy.[9]

An ethical code to facilitate self-regulation

Ethics plays a central role in the development of a self-regulated lifestyle. To achieve a healthy, balanced life, arguably one must adopt an ethical code. The first detailed account of the five ethical precepts of Buddhism can be found in the *Acharanga Sutra*. This Jain text from the 3rd century BCE provides the earliest list of vows that enhance a life well-lived: non-violence, truthfulness, not stealing, appropriate sexual behavior, and non-possession. These vows can be reinterpreted for contemporary everyday life. They are practiced by yogis as the *yamas* (restraints) and *niyamas* (observances) (see Chapter 24) but can be found in variant forms in ethical codes from the biblical ten commandments to the cultivation of Confucian virtues.

In the observance of non-violence (*ahimsa*), one must guard against any thought that "produces cutting or splitting or division and dissension, quarrels, faults, and pains, injures living beings, or kills creatures"; one must also avoid speech that is "sinful and blamable," and take care to not "hurt or displace or injure or kill all sorts of living beings" (*Acharanga Sutra* II.15.i.1–5).[10] The second vow, holding to truth (*satya*), requires speaking only after deliberation; not speaking from anger, greed, or fear; and not speaking for the purpose of ridicule. The third vow, not stealing (*asteya*), entails the pronouncement that "I shall neither take myself what is not given nor cause others to take it, nor consent to their taking it" (II.15.iii). The fourth vow, *brahmacharya*, involves restraint from sexual thought and activity. Acknowledging the range of ways in which sexual desire can manifest, the *Acharanga Sutra* proclaims "I renounce sexual pleasures, with gods or humans or animals" (II.15.iv).

The fifth vow, non-possession (*aparigraha*), requires a person to renounce all attachments. Jain monks and nuns are allowed to own only a bare minimum of possessions, generally a change of robes, a begging bowl, and small satchel for carrying books. Male members of some Jain monastic communities wear no clothes and carry only a begging bowl and satchel. Adherence to the fifth vow in Buddhism requires not taking any intoxicants.

The practice of these five vows equips a person with an adherence to behavioral limits and promotes self-regulation. Discussion of these five vows comprises the most sustained series of verses within the *Yoga Sutras* (2.29–39). So many difficulties in life could be avoided if people could agree to be gentle, authentic, honest, and respectful of the bodies of others, and to stop hoarding!

Yoga Sutras

By the middle of the first millennium of the common era, a non-denominational yoga was codified by Patanjali in 196 short statements known as the *Yoga Sutras*. Patanjali is believed to have composed this text to have a broad appeal, and it includes and alludes to ideas from Vedanta, Buddhism, and Jainism. He incorporated the philosophy and psychology of Samkhya throughout the text.

Patanjali organized yoga into four aspects, dedicating a chapter to each:

- contemplation/meditation (*samadhi*)

- practice (*sadhana*)
- powers (*vibhuti*)
- freedom (*kaivalyam*)

In the first chapter, the practitioner of yoga comes to understand the mind and learn various techniques to focus and purify one's mental and emotional landscape. The second chapter describes how karma operates and lays out eight primary steps for undertaking yoga:

- ethics (identical to the Jain practices described above)
- observances
- posture
- breath control
- inwardness
- concentration
- meditation
- the state of being absorbed (samadhi)

The third chapter of the *Yoga Sutras* describes various benefits and powers of yoga. The text states that with regular yoga practice, one can become virtuous, empathetic, beautiful, and discerning. The fourth chapter reiterates the role of each person in shaping their own reality, encouraging the yogi to ascend to a state of abiding freedom. Although not a medical text, the *Yoga Sutras* outline a basic philosophy of healthy mindedness that has many therapeutic applications.

Patanjali designed his text to be understandable to all without being tied to one particular theological view. By invoking an eightfold path, this yoga appealed to Buddhists. By requiring adherence to a strict fivefold code of non-violence, truthfulness, not stealing, sexual propriety, and non-possession, it spoke directly to the Jains. By introducing the practice of choosing one's own favorite deity as a focal inspiration, it echoed the Hindu celebration of multiple gods and goddesses. By grounding these insights and practices within the landscape of human psychology, yoga came to develop a universal appeal.

The Samkhya-informed philosophical foundation of yoga rests on the articulation of an ongoing relationship between two ways of being human. The person houses a place of silent awareness (*purusha*) that remains untouched regardless of circumstance. The realm of activity (*prakriti*) presents to the consciousness of purusha a wide range of experiences, along with the opportunity to unravel the ups and downs that obscure awareness (see Chapter 11). Yoga claims that the key to freedom lies in sorting out these two aspects, one from the other, through the repeated entry into states of absorption. Defined as a moment where the distinction between subject and object collapses, the ensuing states of bliss serve to recondition prior inclinations and cultivate self-improvement.

Patanjali also sketched out an energetic physiology. The *Yoga Sutras* contain perhaps one of the earliest records of the centers in the body (*chakras*) that become well-known in the texts of Tantra. The *Yoga Sutras* discuss bodily energy sparingly and strategically, landing at the center of the heart. After achieving samadhi, the yogi re-enters the world, first through one-pointed return into the realm of transformation and change (*parinama*; 3.11) and then through control over the senses, the body, and the elements (3.13, 3.47–48). Patanjali describes energetic control of the body as follows:

On the navel cakra, knowledge of the ordering of the body...
On the hollow of the throat, cessation of hunger and thirst...
On the tortoise point-of-flow (nāḍī), stability...
On the light in the head, vision of perfected ones...
Or from intuition, everything. (3.29–33)[11]

This ascent from the lower realm of the body up to the throat and head signals an energetic process leading to a sublime connection with the realm of freedom (*siddhaloka*). However, Patanjali, in the spirit of explaining how elevated experiences can inform reengagement with the transactional realm, asserts the following statement as the culmination of human energetic exploration: Through focus "on the heart [comes] understanding of the mind" (3.34). Rather than escaping the world and staying in the realm of the transcendent, the yogi returns to the everyday, taking up a life of happiness, compassion, joy, and equanimity.

These four qualities are also lauded as the hallmark of enlightened living (*brahma vihara*) in Buddhism and Jainism. Patanjali describes the application of the four qualities as follows: "With clarification of the mind (*citta prasāda*) arises the cultivation of happiness toward the happy, compassion for those who suffer, sympathetic joy for the good, and equanimity toward those who lack goodness" (1.33).[12]

The ongoing discernment expressed through these practices reduces stress, paving the way for a balanced, healthy lifestyle.

Samkhya

As noted above, the philosophical foundation of yoga rests on the articulation of an ongoing relationship between the silent awareness (purusha) that remains untouched regardless of circumstance and the realm of activity (prakriti), which presents a wide range of experiences. The *Rig Veda* expresses this relationship through the metaphor of two birds on the same tree: "One bird eats the sweet berries of the tree, while the other merely looks on," also echoed in the *Shvetashvatara Upanishad*.[13] The Samkhya system explores the relationship in detail between the two realms of the silent witness and the world of change and activity. By the 5th century, the principles and premises of Samkhya were encapsulated in the 72 verses of the *Samkhya Karika*, written by the philosopher Ishvarakrishna. Its main ideas are also found in verses 2.12–26 of the *Yoga Sutras*. Both texts emphasize the central role of discerning the gunas on the path to understanding and freedom. A brief summary of Samkhya follows.

1. The Samkhya system posits two interfacing energies, purusha and prakriti.
2. Their co-presence allows the flourishing of all experience, individual and collective, sullied and sublime.
3. As prakriti, known by the many names of the many goddesses, performs her dance for the sake of the ever-present witness (purusha), the whole human drama unfolds.
4. The human drama takes us from the moment of the first flaring forth, the first cry emitted as the baby emerges from the womb, to the last whimper, the last breath. In between, the human person lives so many births, compiling and destroying, emitting and releasing experience after experience.
5. The question arises: How can one find rest? Peace? Repose? According to the *Samkhya Karika*, freedom can only be known through reflection on the 25 constituents of reality (*tattvas*) (see Chapter 5).
6. Starting from the foundation, one can walk the path of Samkhya through knowledge of
   - earth, and its connection with the sense of fragrance through the nose, and with the anus;
   - water, and its connection with flavor through the mouth, and with the genitals;

- fire, and its connection with color and form through the eyes, and with the hands and arms;
- air, and its connection with feel and touch through the skin, and with the feet and legs; and
- space, and its connection with sound through the ears, and with the voice.

7. Mind (*manas*) names and navigates perceived experience.
8. Ego (*ahamkara*) receives and lays claim.
9. The place of emotionality and past impressions, sometimes referred to as the intellect (*buddhi*), flavors and colors the outward flow of mind and senses. (Chapter 11 outlines the constituents of mind.) Its states (*bhavas*) determine the quality of human experience, moving from weakness toward strength (*aishvarya*), from attachment to repose (*vairagya*), from ignorance to knowledge (*jnana*), and from viciousness to virtue (*dharma*).
10. The dance of prakriti manifests through the three gunas (tamas, rajas, and sattva).
11. Moving ever upward and forward with knowledge, one attains freedom.

In terms of human health and the application of yoga therapy, Samkhya provides a roadmap that contextualizes the human body and mind within the greater embrace of the elemental and the cosmic.

Early Tantra and the *Markandeya Purana*

The beginning of this chapter explored the correlations and correspondences between the parts of the human body and the cosmos. This worldview eventually developed into the tradition known as Tantra by the 8th century of the common era and is taught and practiced in various ways by Hindus, Buddhists, and Jains. In contrast to Shankara's Advaita Vedanta, which emphasizes that the body and mind must be negated, Tantra proclaims that the body must be used as the vehicle for purification. The body contains energies that must be understood, elevated, and transformed; it is the means of transcendence rather than its enemy.

One of the earliest detailed accounts of the relationship between the external, macrophase elements and the microphase human body and its system of ascending energies can be found in the *Markandeya Purana* (ca. 450 CE). These ideas later blossomed into a school of thought and practice known as Tantra. The Puranas are vast books that generally tell the story of a god or goddess or a sage, interlaced with philosophical insights and instructions on the practices of yoga.[14] The *Markandeya Purana* describes an inward journey that culminates in a state of rapture. Beginning with earth and increasing in subtlety through water, fire, air, and space, this text teaches about a sevenfold progression through the five elements, the mind, and beyond, each associated with energy centers (chakras). The yogi of the *Markandeya Purana* begins with the *muladhara chakra* at the base of the spine and disappears at the seventh stage into supreme bliss:

> *Thinking about the highest Brahman, having inclined the mind toward that goal,*
> *the Yogi is always yoked by Yoga,*
> *abstemious in regard to food and in control of the senses.*
> *One should hold seven subtle concentrations in the head, starting with the earth.*
> *The Yogi should hold to the earth and enter its subtle quality.*
> *[The Yogi] thinks on its expansive nature and moves beyond its fragrance.*
> *Likewise in regard to the subtle flavor in water and the form [revealed by] fire.*
> *This concentration extends similarly to the touch of the wind.*
> *In the subtle activity of the sky, one moves beyond sound.*
> *Thus one enters all of the elements of the mind through the mind.*
> *Carrying this mental concentration, the subtle mind is born.*
> *The one who knows Yoga, having associated the intellect (buddhi)*
> *with those states of illumination free of karmic residue (sattva)*
> *renounces all that has been obtained with an unsurpassed, super subtle intellect.*
> *The knower of Yoga rises above these seven subtleties.*
> *O Alarka, worldly existence is not known for that person*
> *with this even minded wisdom.*
> *With these seven concentrations, one possesses a subtle self.*
> *This person would stride with accomplishment beyond the seen and the unseen,*
> *beyond that which has been renounced, and that which has not yet been renounced.*
> *O King, even the one who experiences pleasure in the elements, having*
> *obtained even-mindedness in the midst of attachment, destroys [attachment].*
> *Therefore, having known the various subtle attachments,*
> *the embodied one who renounces, would attain the next step.*
> *O Parthiva, one gathers all seven subtleties and quells all these elements*
> *[earth/smell, water/taste, fire/sight, wind/touch, space/hearing, manas, buddhi—*
> *correlating to the seven chakras] and frees the knower of true existence.*

The one who re-attaches to the senses perishes and returns again to the human realm.
O King, that person separates from Brahman.
Having mastered these seven concentrations,
the Yogi attains whatever is desired becomes absorbed, O Nareśvara,
into any of the subtle elements.
That person can become absorbed into the realms of the gods, demons,
celestial beings, serpents, and protective spirits,
without becoming attached in any way.
One obtains the eight powerful qualities, becoming minute, light, great,
accomplished, powerful, lordly, magical, and self possessed leading to Nirvana.
(40.16–331)[15]

The chakra system

This text provides an early account of what later develops in the subtle-body theories of Tantra. At the base of the body, one finds earth, associated with the muladhara chakra at the bottom of the spine in the area of the anus, and water, associated with the *svadhisthana chakra* in the realm of the genitals (named *linga* for males and *yoni* for females). In the central part of the body, one finds the heat and fire of digestion in the abdomen, referred to as *nabhi* (cognate with the word *navel*) or *manipura*, "the city of jewels," indicating the internal organs. Above the belly, one finds the operations of the respiratory system, the lungs and heart, which connect with the element of air. The names for the heart chakra include *hridaya* and *anahata*. The realm of space starts in what is later designated as the *vishuddha chakra*, located in the throat, and extends up into the head, the realm of discernment and eventually transcendence, associated with the *ajna* and *sahasrarha chakras*, respectively. In Hindu and Tibetan Buddhist narratives, the spiritual life unfolds as the adept moves the energy coiled at the bottom of the spine up through the realms of power and love into the realms of non-attachment and insight, culminating in freedom.

The knots (*granthi*) of karma and patterns of past conditioning (*samskara* and *vasana*) impede an individual, keeping the energy in the lower realms. (See Chapter 21 for more on granthi and Chapter 3 for contextualization of these concepts of patterning.) Through practices (*sadhana*) found in various forms of Hindu, Buddhist, and Jain Yoga, one purifies the gross body, which in turn purges the subtle body of its habitual impulses. With this release of tightly held patterns, one is able to ascend to the realm of the heart, gain discernment, and move toward freedom, an ascent from anus, gonads, and stomach to heart, throat, forehead, and finally a sense of bliss and freedom beyond even the confines of the human skull.

Texts of Hatha Yoga

By the time of the full emergence of the Hatha Yoga tradition in the 13th century CE, the language shifted from metaphysical talk of freedom to specific bodily benefits made possible by yogic practice. Although some ayurvedic medical and food-based practices are discussed in Hatha Yoga texts, contemporary yoga therapy does not include the use of medicines.

The *Yoga Sutras* list sickness (*vyadhi*) as the first of ten obstacles to be overcome through yoga. The later Hatha Yoga texts name specific disorders for which purifications (*shatkarmas*), *asana*, various forms of *pranayama*, *mudra*, *bandha*, *dharana*, foods (*ahara*), and herbs (*osadhi*) may be prescribed.[16] *The Encyclopedia of Traditional Asanas* lists numerous disorders and the specific texts that suggest remediation. The disorders include conditions ranging from lethargy and acid reflux to heart ailments, fever, skin diseases, mental disorders, epilepsy, snake bite, headache, and pain in childbirth.[17] Editor M. L. Gharote gives citations from more than 150 texts that address these maladies.

For the yoga therapist, familiarity with at least three texts of Hatha Yoga can be very helpful. The *Siva Samhita*, composed in the 14th century, teaches a form of Kundalini Yoga that entails asana, the movement of energy through the breath, and various meditations and visualizations.[18] The *Hatha Yoga Pradipika*, most likely composed by Svatmarama in the 15th century, lists various poses and instructions for the performance of breath control. It states that of the 84 traditional asana, four are the best for the avoidance of all diseases: the sitting postures of *siddhasana* (easy seated pose), *padmasana* (lotus pose), and *bhadrasana* (butterfly pose), and the kneeling *simhasana* (lion pose).[19] The *Gheranda Samhita*, most likely composed in Bengal in the 18th century, provides the most comprehensive treatment of the three,[20] giving details on various asana, specific pranayama instructions, and meditation instructions regarding the five elements.[21] All three texts speak of the importance of the *tribandha*—the application of *mula bandha*, *jalandhara bandha*, and *uddiyana bandha*, the closure and holding of the pelvic floor, throat lock, and navel lock, respectively (see Chapter 21).

Summary

The psychological and philosophical foundations of yoga recognize that actions of the past leave residues known as samskara that condition one's experience of the present and the future. Many of these residues take root in the body, which can become tight and contorted, and in the breath, which can become irregular and shallow. Yogic practices work at healing and releasing body and breath, which in turn improves mental outlook and emotional state.

Yoga, practiced by a person of any faith or no faith, works to enhance physical, respiratory, emotional, psychological, and spiritual well-being. Regular practice can help caregivers find a space of safety and stability. Those who cultivate yoga on a daily basis will be better equipped to recognize symptoms of stress, which has become a near-universal epidemic. The tools of yoga allow one to lengthen the breath and to relax the musculature that contracts and contorts one's posture and overall comportment. Yoga teaches an important human skill: the ability to recognize adversity; feel it in one's body, mind, and breath; and use the body, thoughts, and breath to move into a space of calm and acceptance. By acquainting themselves with the traditional literature of yoga, yoga therapists can come to understand the context, history, and philosophy of this effective restorative practice.

Additional Resources

Gharote, M. L. (Ed.). (2013). *Encyclopedia of traditional asanas* (pp. liii–lx). Lonavla Yoga Institute.

Gharote, M. M., Jha, V., & Devnath, P. (Eds.). (2015). *Therapeutic references in traditional yoga texts.* Lonavla Yoga Institute.

Mallinson, J., & Singleton, M. (2017). *Roots of yoga* (p. 389). Penguin Random House.

Endnotes

1 de Nicolás, A. T. (1976). *Meditations through the Ṛg Veda: Four-dimensional man* (pp. 193–235). Nícolas-Hays, Inc.

2 Adapted from Dwivedi, O. P., & Tiwari, B. N. (1987). *Environmental crisis and Hindu religion* (p. 126). Gitanjali Publishing House.

3 Adapted from Hume, R. E. (1921). *The thirteen principal Upanishads* (p. 284). Oxford University Press.

4 Adapted from Hume, *Thirteen principal Upanishads.*

5 See Shastri, A. M. (Trans.). (1903). *The Taittiriya Upanishad with the Commentaries of Sankaracharya, Suresvaracharya, and Sayana (Vidyarana)* (pp. 387–502). G. T. A. Printing Works.

6 Prabhavananda, S. (Trans.). (1970). *Shankara's crest jewel of discrimination: Viveka-chudamani* (2nd ed.). Vedanta Press & Bookshop.

7 de Nicolás, A. T. (Trans.). (2004). *The Bhagavad Gita: The ethics of decision-making* (p. 114). Nicolas-Hays, Inc.

8 Adapted from the translation of the *Satipaṭṭhāna Sutta* by Anālayo as found in Goldstein, J. (2013). *Mindfulness: A practical guide to awakening* (p. 406). Sounds True.

9 Two practical resources include the following: Goldstein, *Mindfulness*; Salzberg, S. (2011). *Real happiness: The power of meditation*. Workman.

10 Jacobi, H. (Trans.). (1884). *Sacred books of the East: Jaina Sutras, part I*, Vol. 22 (pp. 203–204). Oxford University Press.

11 Chapple, C. K. (2008). *Yoga and the luminous: Patanjali's spiritual path to freedom* (pp. 192–193). State University of New York Press.

12 Chapple, *Yoga and the luminous* (pp. 154–155).

13 *Rig Veda* I.164.20, *Mundaka Upanishad* III.1.1, and *Shvetashvatara Upanishad* IV.6. See Hume, *Thirteen principal Upanishads*.

14 Examples are the *Bhagavata Purana* (the life of Krishna), the *Devi Bhagavatam* (tales of the goddess), the *Siva Purana* (tales of Shiva), and the *Agni Purana* (tales of Agni).

15 This translation by Christopher Key Chapple was completed in collaboration with Jodi Shaw, Christopher Miller, Griffin Guez, Amparo Denney, and Wijnanda Jabobi: Chapple, C. K. (2020). *Living landscapes: Meditations on the five elements in Hindu, Buddhist, and Jain Yogas* (pp. 8–11). State University of New York Press.

16 Gharote, M. M., Jha, V., & Devnath, P. (Eds.). (2015). *Therapeutic references in traditional yoga texts*. Lonavla Yoga Institute.

17 Gharote, M. L. (Ed.). (2013). *Encyclopedia of traditional asanas* (pp. liii–lx). Lonavla Yoga Institute.

18 Mallinson, J. (2007). *The Shiva samhita: A critical edition and English translation*. YogaVidya.com.

19 Svatmarama. (2002). *The Hatha yoga pradipika* (B. D. Akers, Trans.). YogaVidya.com.

20 Mallinson, J. (2004). *The Gheranda samhita: The original Sanskrit and an English translation*. YogaVidya.com.

21 For a translation of this practice as found in the *Gheranda Samhita*, see Chapple, *Living landscapes* (pp. 64–66, 82–84, 106–107, 121–123, 169–170).

3

Foundations of Yoga as Therapy: Assessment and Healing Approach

AMY WHEELER

One of the longstanding yoga therapy traditions of India is that of the Krishnamacharya Yoga Mandiram (KYM), a non-profit organization established by T. K. V. Desikachar in 1976 as a gift to his father, T. Krishnamacharya.

In this lineage, yoga therapy is first and foremost about creating healthy and sustainable relationships.[1] Without a strong, compassionate connection between the client and the yoga therapist, a connection the KYM lineage might describe as "heart-based," the yoga therapy process will not produce the intended healing effects. It is taught that one of the strongest tools of healing in yoga therapy is the shared intention of the two people involved to listen, to understand, and to feel and become comfortable in each other's presence. According to Desikachar, "Yoga is relationship."[2] The connections to which he refers include the relationship to Self and to one's breath, as well as relationship to something that causes joy or suffering, including relationships with loved ones. Ultimately, yoga therapy is about the profound relationship established between the teacher and student to facilitate healing (Figure 3.1).

Patanjali's *Yoga Sutras* provide a foundational understanding of how to do this work, along with clues about how to view this unique relationship. For instance, Yoga Sutra 4.2 explains the process of transformation: "Change from one set of characteristics to another is essentially an adjustment of the basic qualities of matter."[3]

An effective yoga therapist is one who is deeply connected to themselves and understands the process of transformation because they have gone through their own inner rearrangement. Having walked the road oneself is an essential precursor to guiding someone else along the same path. Once a certain level of transformation has happened in the yoga therapist over many years, they can share the fruits of this labor in a natural way with clients.

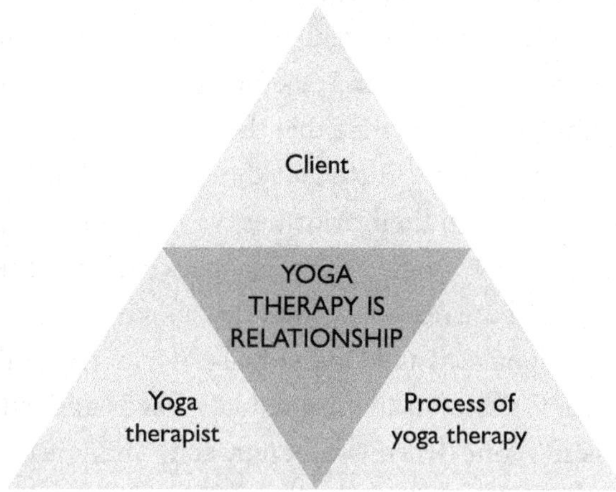

FIGURE 3.1 RELATIONSHIP AT THE HEART OF YOGA THERAPY

Yoga Sutra 4.3 continues this thought, illustrating that the yoga therapist must understand the client's inner terrain and help them to transform in a way that is consistent with the unique expressions of their own potential: "[S]uch intelligence can only remove obstacles that obstruct certain changes. Its role is no more than that of a farmer who cuts a dam to allow water to flow into the field where it is needed."[4] Just like a farmer taking care of their plants, the yoga therapist interacts with the client on a heart-to-heart level. The healing that occurs within each client is nothing more than a rearrangement of the potentials that already exist within them.

The job of the yoga therapist is in guiding the client in the removal of obstacles to their flow of consciousness, to experience this rearrangement and allow it to filter through all the layers of their system. These five layers, *panchamaya koshas* (sheaths), represent all aspects of physical, energetic, mental/emotional, personality/intelligence, and spiritual development and comprise the human system. (See Chapter 2 for a discussion of panchamaya's origins.)

Yoga Sutra 4.4 suggests that transformation happens only when something beyond the mind is empowered in the seeker.[5] The heart of the client must transform over time, not just the mind or lifestyle habits forced by sheer willpower. According to the KYM approach, this heart connection between yoga therapist and client is the driving force of transformation.

A Multidimensional, Individualized Approach to Self-Empowered Healing

Yoga therapy must be a self-empowered process. After the initial yoga therapy assessment, the client works with a personalized and evolving yoga practice that addresses the symptoms of dis-ease. The multidimensional assessment and daily practice address the entire human system, with a goal of alleviating suffering in a progressive and non-invasive manner. Yoga therapy is a self-empowering process for the client; therefore, it is imperative that they take responsibility to heal from the inside out. More importantly, the client should be willing to do serious self-analysis and ready to question their priorities, values, motives, personality, and communication style. Usually, yoga therapy practices evolve over time and require a commitment to making the necessary lifestyle changes.

Yoga therapy is personalized and "individual-centric" rather than "technique-centric"; the practice focuses on the individual's needs and symptoms, not on generic yogic tools in a one-size-fits-all approach. This means that how yoga therapy is presented is entirely contextually sensitive and unique to the needs of the individual. In a way, this approach is akin to the patient- or person-centered care that has been increasingly emphasized in conventional medicine during the beginning of the 21st century.[6]

Yoga therapy is oriented to healing rather than curing. Yoga therapists work in a complementary fashion with other medical professionals who might be working to cure the individual—to eliminate the symptoms of a disease or condition. The level of healing employed by a yoga therapist involves acceptance of the present moment. Healing, associated with the client's feelings and perceptions associated with the illness or present condition, can only aid the curative process. Curing often relies on external interventions like medicine or surgery; healing involves using one's own internal resources and potentials to cultivate "salutogenesis," the ability to manifest and sustain a sense of well-being from the inside out. Salutogenesis focuses on supports to health rather than on causes of disease.

The definition of healing in yoga is unique compared to other modalities and professional fields. One can juxtapose the feelings and sensations that come from dis-ease at multiple layers of the human system with the enduring inner experience of being healthy and well. Table 3.1 describes the experience of healing from the perspective of yoga therapy.

Table 3.1 Yoga therapy and the definitions of healing

Dis-Ease	Healing
Duhkham That which causes suffering Feeling of contraction and restriction Lack of satisfaction, unhappiness	*Suhkham* That which creates lightness and happiness Feeling of space in the body and mind
Vyadhi Extraordinary suffering, of the physical body, mind, and senses Strong connection with identity/conditions Disconnection from Self	*Svastha* Ability to sustain oneself Ability to abide with the Self Finding balance/health
Rogam (roga) Strong desire, desperate want to get out of a painful situation	*Arogyam* No pain or illness
Citta viksepa Mind is disturbed, agitated	*Citta sthairvam* Mind is stable, steady
Visamatran Agitation of mind and body	*Samatran* Tranquility, peace *Dvandva sahanam* To remain balanced, even in extreme situations
Ama Food, thoughts, and emotions are "uncooked"—not digested well, improperly processed Poor digestion is an indication of ill health	*Pakva* Food, thoughts, and emotions are well-digested, well-cooked/well-conceived, and nourishing

The Four-Step Model of Healing

The Krishnamacharya tradition relies heavily on the *Yoga Sutras* as the theoretical foundation for client assessment, negotiation of short- and long-term goals, and development of an appropriate practice to promote salutogenesis. The KYM tradition teaches a four-step model of healing derived directly from Patanjali.

The care provider approaches the care-seeker individually according to their needs. The process unfolds in the following way.

1. ***Heyam*** (Yoga Sutra 2.17): What symptoms of suffering is the client experiencing?

2. ***Hetu*** (Yoga Sutras 2.17, 2.23, 2.24): How did it happen? What is the cause of this suffering?

3. ***Hanam*** (Yoga Sutra 2.25): Short- and long-term goals with the input and desires of the client.

4. ***Upayam*** (Yoga Sutra 2.26): The tools or means of achieving the co-created goals are chosen.

Step 1: Heyam, assessment of symptoms of suffering

In yoga therapy from the KYM perspective, one does not evaluate or identify the client only by the label of the disease they are displaying. Instead, the yoga therapist attempts to perceive the client as a whole person, to uncover and define patterns of imbalance in the body and mind that do not support them. The yoga therapist also takes inventory of healthy and functional patterns that nourish the client. The yoga therapist carefully considers all of these patterns in the physical body, physiology, mind, personality, emotions, and even spiritual outlook (Figure 3.2). The goal is to determine which symptoms are causing suffering, then to help the client discern how they can change themselves from the inside out.

The symptoms or patterns of illness are listed concisely in the *Yoga Sutras*: "All these interruptions [to developing mental clarity] produce one or more of the following symptoms: mental discomfort, negative thinking, the inability to be at ease in different body postures, and difficulty in controlling one's breath" (1.31).[7] The presence of any of these four symptoms should be an alert signaling the need to pay attention.

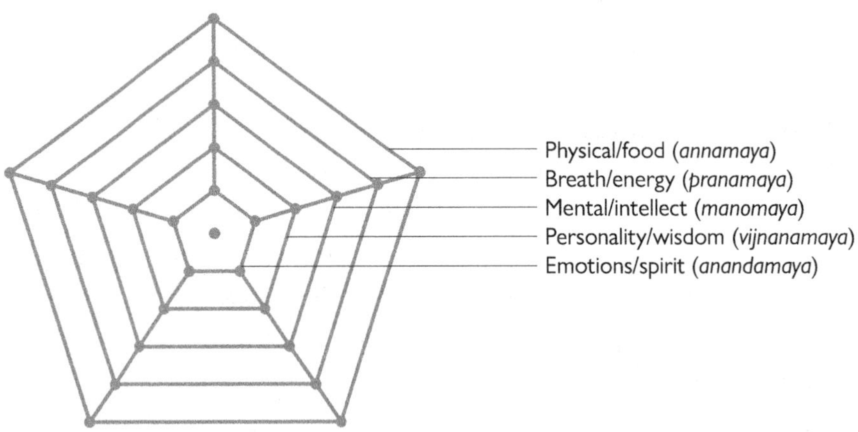

FIGURE 3.2 FIVE LEVELS OF THE HUMAN SYSTEM (PANCHAMAYA KOSHA)

Often, the care-seeker attempts to numb symptoms or cover them up to continue living in the way that has caused the illness in the first place. Unfortunately, for a host of reasons, many people do not pay close attention to signs of dis-ease; they may not realize how much they are suffering, or even that they are suffering. This lack of self-awareness is precisely what leads to greater suffering in the future.

Self-awareness is the first step toward achieving salutogenesis. Humans are resilient and often push through, using and abusing their bodies and minds until they cannot push any more. This is usually the point at which a diagnosis of serious illness occurs in Western medicine. The diagnosis is often a surprise to the patient, who wonders how it happened. However, according to the yogic tradition, one can learn to become aware of the early warnings outlined in Yoga Sutra 1.31 and pay close attention to these signals on a moment-by-moment basis.

Four symptoms of suffering and their opposites

There are four symptoms of suffering:

- ***duhkham:*** feeling of contraction and restriction in the body and the mind
- ***daurmanasya:*** negative attitude, critical, dark mind
- ***angamejayatva:*** changes in physiological patterns, restlessness, insomnia, digestive problems, etc.
- ***avasa prasvasa:*** shortness of breath, hyperventilation

Although Patanjali does not describe the opposites of these symptoms of suffering, one can extrapolate and see what it means to suffer less or detach from suffering. This does not mean that one's environment or relationships will magically change, or that life will be golden every day. Instead, detaching or de-linking from suffering means that external circumstances no longer hold the same influence. The individual perceives differently and becomes able to observe the painful events of life as the witness.[8]

According to the KYM tradition, possible opposites of the four symptoms of suffering are

- ***suhkham:*** happy, spacious, and comfortable in the body and the mind
- ***saumanasya:*** positive thinking and outlook
- ***anga sthairyam:*** good physiological functioning
- ***dirgha sukshma prana:*** quiet, smooth, and refined breathing patterns

There are many ways an individual might come to understand that they are suffering according to the yoga therapy paradigm and decide to more closely examine how they could rearrange their internal landscape.

The nine obstacles to salutogenesis: A paradigm for assessment

Another method often used in the KYM tradition is the model of the nine obstacles, again derived from the *Yoga Sutras*:

> There are nine types of interruptions to developing mental clarity: illness, mental stagnation, doubts, lack of foresight, fatigue, overindulgence, illusions about one's true state of mind, lack of perseverance, and regression. They are obstacles because they create mental disturbances and encourage distractions. (1.30)[9]

The nine-obstacles paradigm can help both yoga therapist and client understand what is happening for the client and why they are suffering. This model is employed via a phenomenological interview methodology that requires the client to have self-awareness and the capacity for self-analysis. The nine-obstacles model is a helpful paradigm to use when clients can examine their feelings and experiences and be honest about the symptoms and causes of their suffering. Addressing and overcoming these obstacles (*antarayas*) that prevent salutogenesis is the goal of participating in yoga therapy:

- ***vyadhi:*** physical illness, disconnection from body, imbalance in body
- ***styana:*** mental exhaustion, mental burnout
- ***samsaya:*** confusion or doubt in self or direction of life
- ***pramada:*** haste in many activities
- ***alasya:*** laziness, tiredness, inability to think properly
- ***avirati:*** excess of sensual temptation
- ***bhrantidarsana:*** delusion of grandeur or state of denial
- ***alabdhabhumikatva:*** despite practicing, not reaching the goal
- ***anavasthitattva:*** falling back, regression after meeting a goal

The gunas and salutogenesis: A paradigm for assessment and healing

A third example of how an individual might come to understand that they are suffering comes from the model of the *gunas* (constituents of reality). The KYM tradition encourages careful consideration of Patanjali's definition of the mental gunas of *rajas*, *tamas*, and *sattva*.

The theoretical underpinnings of yoga come from the five-element theory as outlined by Samkhya philosophy (see Chapter 2). The essence of Samkhya is that every object, person, thought, and emotion is made up of some combination of the five elements of earth, water, fire, air (wind), and space (ether) (Figure 3.3).

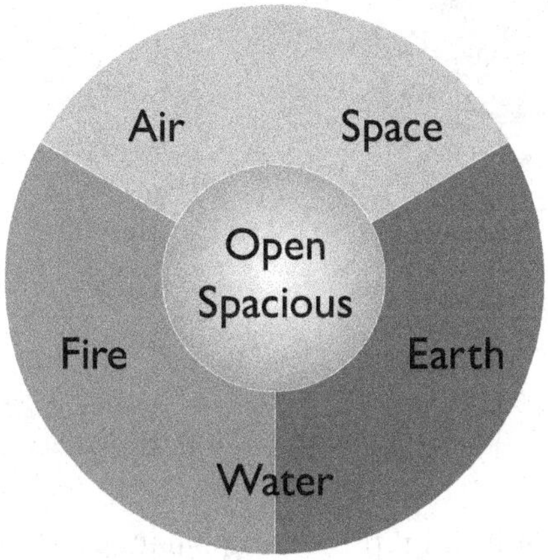

FIGURE 3.3 ELEMENTS OF THE GUNAS

Denser objects have a higher percentage of heavy materials like earth and water. The more subtle objects have higher proportions of fire, air, and space. These concepts are easy to comprehend when referring to actual physical objects. Although it can be difficult to imagine that even thoughts, speech, and emotions have an elemental nature, they can be understood as simply comprising more of the subtle elements than gross, tangible objects.

When considering the world, society, and human behavior through the lens of Samkhya, how the five elements combine to make up the natural world becomes apparent. In addition to ayurveda, many other traditional medicines, including shamanism and Native American healing arts, use an elemental worldview to inform their understanding of health/disease and illness/wellness models. Interestingly, quantum physics is theorized to correlate with many of the underpinnings of Samkhya philosophy.[10]

Patanjali compresses the five-element theory from Samkhya into the mental states of tamas, rajas, and sattva. The tamasic state of mind, comprising the elemental qualities of earth and water, is heavy, dull, lethargic, and slow-moving. The rajasic state of mind is excited, fast-moving, and often distracted; defined by the qualities of fire, air, and space, it is light and dry. Both tamasic and rajasic states of mind are considered to be out of balance (Figure 3.4), although excess sattva is also possible. A mind that has excess sattva may lend itself to enlightened states of being but sometimes has difficulty being present to the inevitable real-world problems that occur as a result of being human.

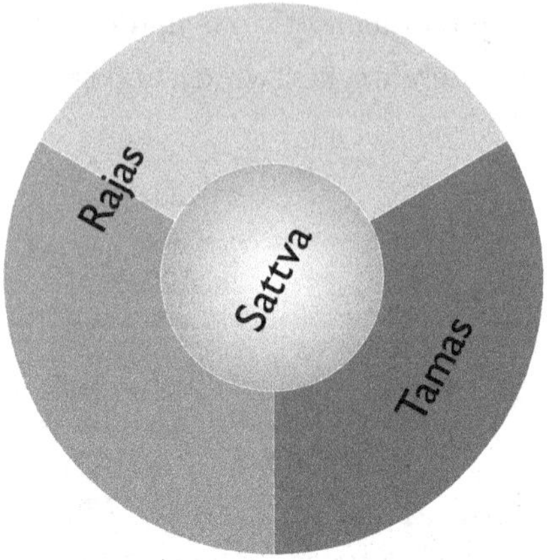

FIGURE 3.4 MENTAL GUNAS

Sattva is the quality of mind representing balance or harmony of the five elements. Other traditions consider true sattva to be the absence of all five elements. The goal of Patanjali's yoga is to assist in finding this sattvic state of mind, in which the gunas no longer affect the enlightened being, in meditation and daily life.[11]

A sister school of yoga and Samkhya, ayurveda, further breaks down the five elements into pairs of opposites (see Chapters 4 and 20). For example, air is light and earth is heavy; fire is hot and space is cool; air is mobile, earth is static. Every quality in the universe has an opposite. Ayurveda's ten pairs of opposites are simply a pared-down version of hundreds of thousands of pairs of opposites. That said, these 20 qualities and how they can be layered over the elements are easily understood (Figure 3.5). It is said that only when one recognizes these opposites and accommodates for excess or deficiency can balance be created in mind, thoughts, words, and body.

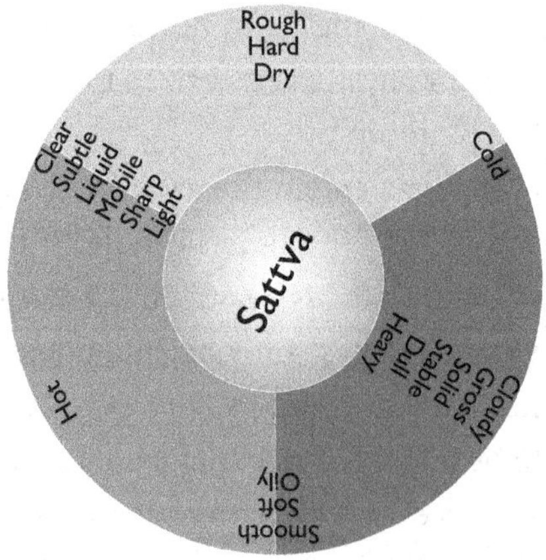

FIGURE 3.5 QUALITIES OF THE GUNAS: PAIRS OF OPPOSITES

Ayurveda, knowledge of life, is said to have been revealed directly by Brahma, the creator. According to the narrative of the *Charaka Samhita*, this Vedic knowledge was passed down to the terrestrial level and eventually refined by Charaka (see Chapter 2).

In short, the yoga therapist observes these 20 qualities (or ten pairs of opposites) to assess the symptoms of balance or imbalance in the physical, energetic, mental, wisdom, and spiritual levels. When an imbalance is observed, they determine which elements or qualities need to be increased or decreased to create a more harmonious mind and body—a salutogenic system.

The above are just three examples of how a yoga therapist might assess the symptoms of suffering on multiple layers of the human system. From these examples, one can clearly see how different this unique process is from that of diagnosis in conventional medicine. Yoga therapy's goal is to encourage the care-seeker toward deep self-connection. The foundation of healing is built on yoga therapists themselves being in balance, so that they can connect with clients in a way that bypasses the intellect and goes right to the heart of both people involved.

Step 2: Hetu, investigation of causes of suffering

Yoga therapy clients are asked to reflect on where their suffering originates. The yoga therapist then helps the client to determine what is within their power to change.

Adhyatmika duhkham

Adhyatmika means that the source or cause of suffering comes from within. Such diseases may be the result of lifestyle choices, made over time, that cause physical or mental forms of suffering. Examples are cancer caused by smoking or cirrhosis caused by alcoholism. Another might be a person with diabetes who cannot stop eating sugar even after diagnosis. Lifestyle choices might appear on the surface to represent a lack of willpower when variables such as epigenetic profile or residual effects of childhood trauma make it nearly impossible for the person to sustain health behavior changes.

It should be noted that in Patanjali's time suboptimal choices appeared to be self-inflicted wounds. Contemporary understanding of adverse childhood experiences (ACE)[12] indicates that childhood suffering has a significant impact on adult coping mechanisms, and thus on health outcomes. In other words, causes of suffering related to adhyatmika duhkham are not necessarily due to lack of willpower; they may also be related to *adhibhautika duhkham*.

Adhibhautika duhkham

Adhibhautika duhkham is suffering caused by the behavior of another being. This includes diseases caused by external factors like sexual abuse in childhood by a family member, a dog bite, physical assault by a robber, or parental neglect. There may be crossover between adhyatmika duhkham and adhibhautika duhkham, as mentioned above.

Adhidaivika duhkham

Adhidaivika duhkham is suffering caused by a divine force or nature. This might include diseases caused by a pandemic, a tornado, or an earthquake.

Yoga and yoga therapy are based on a self-realization system that asks each person to take responsibility for their lives. Both adhibhautika duhkham and adhidaivika duhkham exist and are definite causes of suffering. However, the yogic path considers the parameters of well-being that are within an individual's control. Yoga therapy clients are encouraged to master their lives to the best of their ability within these constraints. Much of the work of yoga therapy is done on the level of adhyatmika duhkham through observation and assessment of where the suffering emanating from within the body-mind system can be influenced.

The kleshas

One common example of such observation in yoga therapy is asking the client to do self-analysis pertaining to the five *kleshas*, or causes of suffering, outlined in Yoga Sutras 2.3–2.9: "The obstacles are misapprehensions, confused values, excessive attachments, unreasonable dislikes, and insecurity" (2.3).[13] The kleshas are

- ***avidya:*** wrong understanding or misperception, sometimes translated as "ignorance"
- ***asmita:*** false/incorrect identification, false image, sometimes translated as "ego"
- ***raga:*** desire, unfulfilled or leading to addiction, sometimes translated as "attachment"
- ***dvesha:*** aversion, suffering due to avoiding things good for the individual
- ***abhinivesha:*** fear at the deepest layers of one's being (i.e., of death)

These kleshas can be thought of as parts of a large oak tree. When an individual is suffering, the roots of the tree are made from abhinivesha, or fear. When one lives from a place of fear of death, loss, or not being able to sustain themselves, this foundation for perception affects how one moves through life. Imagine if the individual instead had roots constructed of unwavering faith, trust, strength, expansive thoughts and feelings, and joy. This is essentially salutogenesis, and the tree would grow in a very different fashion.

The trunk of the tree is avidya. When an individual lives from a place of fear (consciously or unconsciously), misperception and wrong understanding result. The senses take in information from the outside world differently when a person is contracted in fear. The mind, in turn, perceives the sensory information differently and attempts to explain the strange somatic sensations (of fear) occurring in the body. Misperception is all around and quickly leads to thoughts, words, and actions that sprout out in all areas of life to cause suffering.

The branches of the tree of fear blossom into more misperception, strong aversions to things that cause uncomfortable sensations and thoughts, strong attachments to what one thinks will bring happiness, and overidentification with a false image of Self.

Sources of suffering and opportunities for healing

Although volumes could be written on the kleshas as a cause of suffering, additional adhyatmika duhkham (causes of suffering arising from one's own actions) are needed to give a more well-rounded view of the types of assessment and therapeutic planning that a yoga therapist might undertake. Following is a brief list of the areas they might consider:

- ***ayukta ahara:*** inappropriate dietary practices according to ayurveda (type of food, amount, company for eating; food must be appropriate for an individual's constitution)
- ***ayukta vihara:*** inappropriate lifestyle (sleep patterns, work habits; lifestyle must be appropriate for an individual's constitution)
- ***asatmya indriya samyoga:*** a strong link with sensual objects or excessive attachment to sensual pleasures
- ***ayukta svatmika gaurava:*** low self-esteem or arrogance
- ***asat sanga:*** spending time with inappropriate company or community (e.g., people who are always pessimistic or using drugs)
- ***parinama:*** change will inevitably happen inside and outside the individual

- ***tapa:*** obsession with a person, material thing, or idea
- ***svabhava:*** the nature of the individual, their predispositions, genetic inheritance, and other influential factors
- ***vasana:*** experiences and the feelings that remain (positive and negative) after the initial event (e.g., traumatic experiences may cause lingering emotions/feelings for years to come)
- ***samskara:*** conscious or unconscious patterns of thought, communication, and behaviors

The above list offers an overview of the types of assessment and analysis in which both yoga therapist and client engage. These concepts also help clients to take responsibility for the causes of suffering in their lives, so that salutogenesis can be experienced to the fullest.

Step 3: Hanam, goal setting

According to the KYM tradition of yoga therapy, healing is a process of creating new patterns that will facilitate a change from *vyutthana samskara* to *nirodha samskara*: These patterns are clearly outlined in Patanjali's *Yoga Sutras*. "The mind is capable of having two states based on two distinct tendencies. These are distraction [vyutthana] and attention [nirodha]. At any one moment, however, only one state prevails, and this state influences the individual's behavior, attitudes, and expressions" (3.9).[14]

Sutras 3.9–3.14 essentially tell us that when the mind is in vyutthana samskara, the whole system is in a sympathetic-dominant state characterized by the fight/flight response. When the mind is in nirodha samskara, the system is dominated by the parasympathetic nervous system: the relaxation response (Figure 3.6 and Chapter 7). A modern scientific view of these teachings is outlined by Porges in his polyvagal theory, which Sullivan et al.[15] have melded with the yogic healing paradigm.

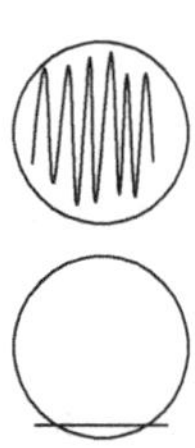

Vyutthana samskara: agitation, imbalance, lack of focus, unstable mind

Nirodha samskara: stability, comfort, focus, calm, alert mind

FIGURE 3.6 THE GOAL OF YOGA: CONVERSION OF VYUTTHANA TO NIRODHA

One can think of yoga therapy as a healing modality that directs and assists clients to change the samskara that are no longer serving them. Old habits and patterns need to be replaced with new habits through effort. The more the individual develops new and more functional patterns of perceptions, thoughts, and behaviors, the more the old patterns diminish. Over time, this process reduces suffering and increases salutogenesis.

The following questions, based on the *Yoga Sutras*, address the role of creating new and more positive samskara in the healing process.[16] The yoga therapist sets both short- and long-term goals with the client in a joint process driven by the client. The client's beliefs, values, and priorities are considered when making the daily plan of action, also called the *therapeutic lifestyle intervention*. A few additional considerations that might be included in the goal-setting process are as follows.

- What is the main goal of the daily therapeutic plan?
- What is the priority in the present moment?
- Which goals, if achieved, would have the quickest impact?
- What are the client's mental, emotional, and physical abilities?

One of the first priorities of the care provider is to identify a realistic plan for the client. This often involves first referring them to another therapist (e.g., acupuncturist, psychiatrist, nutritionist, ayurvedic practitioner), in preparation for beginning a yoga therapy practice. Because yoga therapy requires self-empowerment, it has a high bar for entry. Clients must be ready to create sustainable change in their lives. (See Chapter 13 on stages of change.)

Yoga therapists might weigh the following factors when co-negotiating goals with clients.

1. Begin with the client's most critical issue when possible.
2. Start with the issue that is easiest to show improvement in, thus inculcating inspiration for the client to continue their treatment plan.
3. The size of the steps taken is important. It may be necessary to break down a short-term goal into smaller short-term goals. Most permanent and sustainable change derives from a sequence of short-term goals.[17]
4. Yoga therapy is a process that evolves step by step. Most often, not all of the

information is revealed at the first meeting. This process needs to be fluid, as the client's life is constantly evolving and changing.

5. Sometimes the client's suffering is too great, overpowering the strength and balance needed to work on the psyche, spirit, and body. The KYM tradition recognizes this state as one in need of *samanam*, or pacification, and recommends setting goals to soothe and comfort before proceeding.
6. Other times, clients are ready to address the root causes of their suffering. They are willing to do the work of looking inward deeply and interested in finding new ways to perceive life, communicate needs, change lifestyle habits, and support personal salutogenesis. In this case, the goals would be set for a *sodhanam*-type practice, or purification to get to the heart of the suffering. This process is akin to taking the weed out of the ground with the roots still connected. Clients must have a certain amount of strength, vigor, and honesty to go in this direction.
7. A client's enthusiasm about trying yoga therapy should not be confused with readiness to do the actual work of healing. Their stage of change should be considered carefully when setting goals together. It is better to start small and be successful than to start with big changes and engender feelings of failure.
8. The yoga therapist's goal is not to make the client dependent; the goal is to make the client independent and responsible for their own salutogenesis.

Once the short- and long-term goals are set, they can be modified in a fluid process at any time. However, if the yoga therapist has done a thorough assessment of the symptoms and properly evaluated their causes, and if they have clarity in their own mind and heart, a smooth path forward will have been laid.

Step 4: Upayam, the tools of yoga therapy

The yoga therapist must know how to choose the appropriate yogic tools for the nourishment of each layer of the human system to give effective individualized daily practices for healing. Following are examples of ways to think about nourishment that might pertain to each layer of the panchamaya model.

- ***Annamaya***

  Nourishment from appropriate food and liquid

Proper exercise for the physical body

Taking good care of the physical body

- ***Pranamaya***

  Nourishment from proper breathing

  Adequate fresh air and sunshine

- ***Manomaya***

  Nourishment for the mind and emotions

  Sufficient opportunities for learning and development

- ***Vijnanamaya***

  Nourishment from experiential knowledge

  Expression of personality, life experience, behavior

  Healthy, fulfilling relationships

- ***Anandamaya***

  Nourished by bliss

  Connected with the divine or a sense of awe

Yoga therapy's toolbox

It follows that the toolbox of yoga and yoga therapy offers the perfect technology for helping clients to find balance, obtain nourishment, and finally come into a place of salutogenesis. Yoga therapy's tools include

- ***Yama and niyama:*** *Vihara* (lifestyle) samskara (pattern).
- ***Asana:*** *Sarira* (body) samskara. Asana's physical postures change body habits and set up new patterns, creating positive energetic changes in faculties of the mind and body.
- ***Pranayama:*** *Prana* (breath/energy) samskara. Pranayama's conscious breathing creates new patterns and pathways in the brain and body.
- ***Pratyahara:*** *Indriya* (senses) samskara. Withdrawal from sensual attractions.

- ***Dhyana:*** *Citta* (mind) samskara. Meditation repatterns the mind and is a form of self-medication.
- ***Bhavana:*** Emotional attitude, self-reflection, visualization.
- ***Nyasam:*** To place attention and focus on a gesture to help remember a concept (e.g., putting hands over the heart to reflect self-love or touching one's own feet to help in grounding or in gratitude for their support).
- ***Mudra:*** Symbolic gesture, often with a spiritual focus.
- ***Mantra:*** Symbolic sounds.
- ***Japam:*** Repetition of mantra.
- ***Svadhyaya:*** A process of self-discovery and self-understanding.
- ***Yajna:*** Ancient Vedic rituals performed around the full moon, new moon, and nature were done to heal particular situations or conditions (e.g., a forgiveness ritual for the release of guilt or an attempt to balance the menstrual cycle to mirror the phases of the moon for increased fertility).

Summary

This chapter encapsulates the process of healing according to the yoga therapy tradition of T. Krishnamacharya. The KYM approach incorporates the four-step model of healing as extrapolated from Patanjali's *Yoga Sutras*. These steps can be broken down extensively using models for assessing the symptoms and causes of suffering, setting goals with the client, and choosing the appropriate yogic tools for creating balance.

The most salient point to be made and remembered here is that yoga therapy is not focused on the pathology of a disease or on what is "wrong" with an individual. In yoga therapy the focus most importantly is on salutogenesis, the process of becoming healthy and whole on multiple layers of the human system.

Endnotes

1 Note that the KYM approach to yoga therapy differs from the classical approach to yoga in the KYM tradition. This chapter is written from the KYM yoga therapy perspective rather than from a *siksana* (perfection of each posture or breathing technique) approach to asana and pranayama.

2 Desikachar, T. K. V. (1999). *The heart of yoga: Developing a personal practice* (p. xxvi). Inner Traditions.

3 Desikachar, *Heart of yoga* (p. 204).

4 Desikachar, *Heart of yoga* (p. 204).

5 Desikachar, *Heart of yoga* (p. 204).

6 Rathert, C., Wyrwich, M. D., & Boren, S. A. (2013). Patient-centered care and outcomes: A systematic review of the literature. *Medical Care Research and Review, 70*(4), 351–379.

7 Desikachar, *Heart of yoga* (p. 158).

8 Patanjali discusses the witness or perceiver and that which is perceived in Yoga Sutras 2.17 and 2.18. See also the discussion of the Samkhya concepts of *purusha* and *prakriti* in Chapter 2.

9 Desikachar, *Heart of yoga* (p. 158).

10 See, e.g., Capra, F. (2010). *The tao of physics: An exploration of the parallels between modern physics and Eastern mysticism* (5th ed.). Shambhala.

11 Yoga Sutra 4.34, in Desikachar, *Heart of yoga* (p. 215).

12 See the long-term studies conducted by the US health maintenance organization Kaiser Permanente and the US Centers for Disease Control and Prevention: Felitti, V. J., Anda, R. F., Nordenberg, D., Williamson, D. F., et al. (1998). Relationship of childhood abuse and household dysfunction to many of the leading causes of death in adults: The Adverse Childhood Experiences (ACE) Study. *American Journal of Preventive Medicine, 14*(4), 245–258.

13 Desikachar, *Heart of yoga* (p. 166).

14 Desikachar, *Heart of yoga* (p. 187).

15 Sullivan, M. B., Erb, M., Schmalzl, L., Moonaz, S., Noggle Taylor, J., & Porges, S. W. (2018). Yoga therapy and polyvagal theory: The convergence of traditional wisdom and contemporary neuroscience for self-regulation and resilience. *Frontiers in Human Neuroscience, 12*, 67.

16 See Yoga Sutras 1.13, 1.50, 3.9, and 3.10 for more information on how samskara-replacement theory can rearrange an individual's internal map over time.

17 Desikachar, *Heart of yoga* (p. 123).

4

Ayurveda for the Yoga Therapist

SARAJEAN RUDMAN

Ayurveda, often referred to as the sister science of yoga, is indigenous to India. This medical approach was systematized between the 6th and 7th centuries BCE. Hindu philosophy is organized around six philosophies, one of which gave rise to ayurveda, that undertake to explain the very nature of existence. Four primary topics are covered in each of these systems:

- ***brahman:*** the nature of existence
- ***jiva:*** the individual soul
- ***jagat:*** creation of the world
- ***moksha:*** liberation and how to reach it

The six widely recognized systems of belief are called the *Shad Dharshana*:

- ***Nyaya*** is the system of philosophy based strongly in logic.
- ***Vaisheshika*** is a study of naturalism and the existence of God in tandem. Nyaya and Vaisheshika schools of thought merged and are studied as one.
- ***Samkhya*** is the system of study that observes dualism based in *prakriti* (physical matter) and *purusha* (the subtle but omnipresent and eternal spirit).
- ***Yoga***, based in the teachings of Patanjali's *Yoga Sutras*, is an eight-limbed practice toward wellness and betterment of mind, body, and spirit.
- ***Mimamsa*** is the school of thought based in reflection (mimamsa) and the observance of the rituals offered in four Vedic texts: the *Rig Veda*, *Sama Veda*, *Yajur Veda*, and *Atharva Veda*. Mimamsa is thought to be the oldest Darshan.

- ***Vedanta*** focuses on the study of the Upanishads, or classical texts that arose from the original Vedas.

These six systems are considered part of orthodox Hindu thought (*astika*) because of their reliance on the authority of the Vedas and their belief in a soul and the existence of Brahman. The heterodox schools of thought (*nastika*)—primarily Jainism and Buddhism—arose from Hinduism but do not rely on the authority of the Vedas nor presuppose the existence of a soul or Brahman.

Of the Shad Darshana, ayurveda is based in Samkhya. Samkhya and yoga are complementary and thus often studied in tandem (see also Chapter 2).[1]

If yoga serves as the path toward a sense of oneness or enlightenment, ayurveda is a catalyst that creates a physical body well enough to traverse the path of yoga. Ayurveda is a five-elemental approach to etiology, pathology, healing, and existence. The qualitative approach to human health is based on the understanding and balance of 20 *gunas*, or qualities, and five elements that inform the three *doshas*, referred to as the *tridosha*, or constitutional makeup (see Chapter 3).

As noted, ayurveda is based in Samkhya philosophy, which helps to explain embodied human experience (see Chapter 2). In Samkhya, purusha, which is unmanifested energy beyond the bounds of physical existence, comes to meet prakriti, which is the source of form and action and promotes manifestation. Purusha and prakriti interact in a manner that allows the creation of *Mahad*, the cosmic intelligence sometimes called *Mahad Buddhi*. From Mahad Buddhi, the *ahamkara*, or ego and sense of "I am," is born. The ahamkara is the sense of separation and otherness (see Chapter 11).[2]

Ahamkara births the three *maha gunas*, or big gunas, the major qualities of the *manas* (mind): *sattva*, *rajas*, and *tamas*. (The maha gunas are separate from the 20 attributes used to identify the elemental qualities that comprise the individual doshas; see Chapter 3 and Figure 3.4 for more information on this definition of the gunas and how the elemental properties build on each other to create specific effects in individuals and in nature.) Sattva is the ethereal space of balance, creation, and expansion. Tamas is inertia or the end of all processes. Rajas is the mobile and hot maha guna of creation. These maha gunas can be understood through a song-writing analogy: Sattva is the open and ethereal space that allows for creative expansion. In this space the essence of the song is born; it is subtle and perfect. Rajas is the energy to move forward and create the song, understand the notes and rhythm, and put it down on paper or transmit it through an instrument. Finally, tamas is the inertia needed to end the song, to bring it to a final measure so it does not become "the song that never ends."[3]

In Samkhya, sattvic ahamkara comes from the manas, or the "lower mind," and the ten *indriyas* (powers/capabilities). The indriyas include the five *karmendriyas* (active senses)—the organs in charge of creating speech, hands, feet, reproductive organs, and organs of elimination—and the *buddhindriyas*, the cognitive sense organs of ears, skin, eyes, tongue, and nose. From tamasic ahamkara the five *tanmatras* and five *bhutas* are born. The tanmatras are the five senses, also recognized as the five subtle elements: *shabda* (sound), *sparsha* (touch), *rupa* (sight), *rasa* (taste), and *gandha* (smell). The bhutas, or gross elements, are *akasha* (space or ether), *vayu* (air or wind), *agni* (fire), *jala* (water), and *prithvi* (earth).[4] Figure 4.1 illustrates the indriyas, tanmatras, and bhutas.

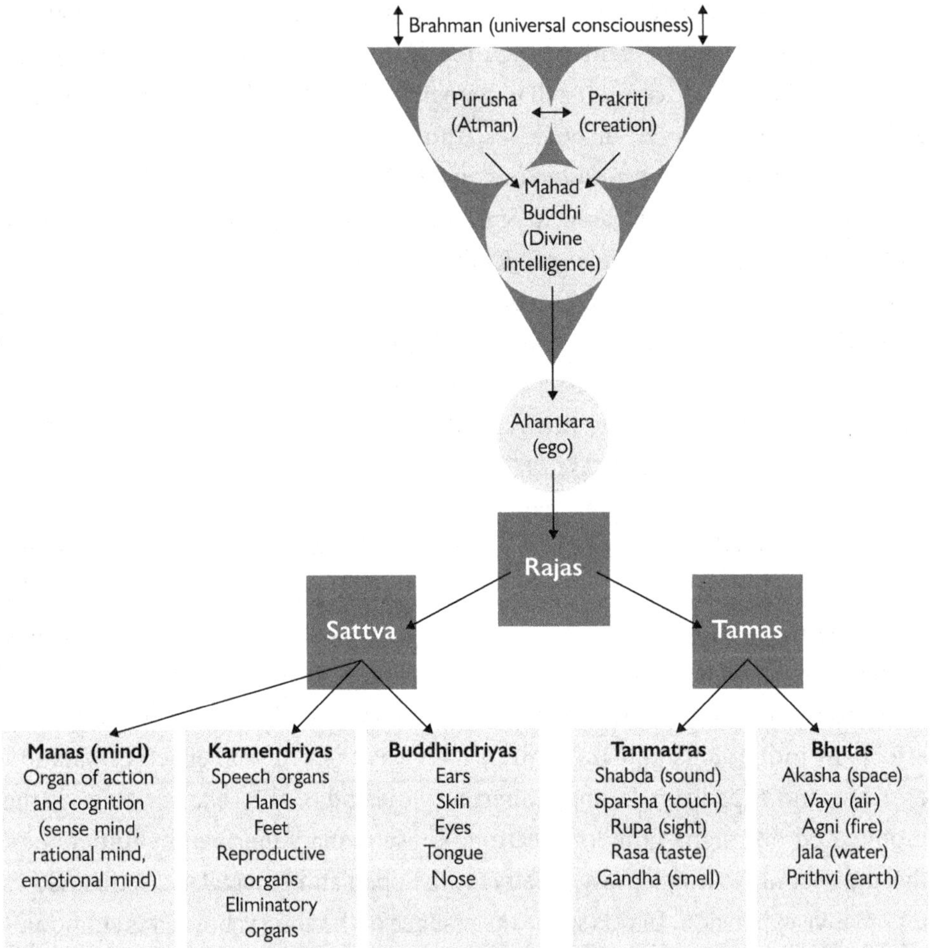

FIGURE 4.1 SOURCES OF EMBODIED HUMAN EXPERIENCE ACCORDING TO SAMKHYA

Rajasic ahamkara is the maha guna that impels both sattvic and tamasic ahamkara to create the manas, indriyas, tanmatras, and bhutas. It is important to note that in Samkhya philosophy, creation occurs from *sukshmna* to *sthula*, or subtle to gross. Tamas is the most *guru*, or heavy, guna; it compels prakriti to forever be changing, whereas purusha is unchanging and unwavering. This is important to both the study and practice of yoga and ayurveda, as both intend to evoke a more sattvic, and thus peaceful and balanced, state of the ahamkara and of the physical, mental, and spiritual bodies.

Tridosha

Everything observed in ayurveda, and thus in yoga, can be attributed to the five elements, which inform the makeup of the three doshas. Dosha translates to "that which moves," reflecting the constantly shifting state of ayurveda's three doshas (*vata*, *pitta*, and *kapha*). The three main doshas determine the constitutional makeup of people in their natural and balanced state as well as their imbalanced state. The state of relative balance at birth is *prakruti*, and the imbalanced state that results from lifestyle, diet, and exposure to life is *vikruti*. Through diet and lifestyle interventions and yogic practice, one can start to come back "home" to their prakruti by honoring the elements and qualities that naturally bring about homeostasis. The two major principles used in these therapies, or *chikitsas*, are *like increases like* and *opposites balance*.[5]

Vata dosha comprises a combination of air and ether elements, pitta is made up of fire and water elements, and kapha is made up of earth and water elements. These three doshas each have their own set of gunas, or innate qualities. A verse from the *Ashtanga Hridyam*, a foundational ayurvedic text compiled in 500–600 CE, describes the 20 gunas: "Heavy, slow, cold, unctuous, smooth, dense, soft and stable. These qualities, as well as subtle and clear, and their opposites, make up the twenty qualities" (1.18).[6]

The 20 qualities recognized in ayurveda are described in Chapter 3. As mentioned above, each person has a constitutional prakruti, or natural balance of the tridosha with which they are born, and a vikruti, or state of imbalance in which they currently live. When addressing someone's imbalance, it is important to consider their natural state and tendencies and to use both prakruti and vikruti to develop a therapeutic yoga approach that will balance them in their own unique constitution.

Ayurveda recognizes ten prakrutis: vata, pitta, kapha, vata-pitta, vata-kapha, pitta-kapha, pitta-vata, kapha-pitta, kapha-vata, and vata-pitta-kapha. The prakrutis are examined from the perspective of developing a yoga therapy plan in Chapter 20.

The three doshas each comprise five subdoshas, of which the five vayus of vata are the most important for a therapeutic yoga approach. The five vayus are *prana*, *apana*, *samana*, *udana*, and *vyana*. The five subdoshas of pitta are *pachaka*, *ranjaka*, *sadhaka*, *alochaka*, and *bhrajaka*. The five subdoshas of kapha are *avalambaka*, *kledaka*, *bodhaka*, *tarpaka*, and *slesaka*. Each subdosha is also associated with an element and serves as a function in the body. Vata is the only dosha that moves, so the five vayus or subdoshas of vata are worth exploring because they can be addressed using *asana* and *pranayama*.[7]

Ayurveda in Yogic Practice

The ayurvedic clock, dinacharya

In a 24-hour cycle, ayurveda recognizes six 4-hour cycles. Each of these 4-hour cycles is ruled by one of the three doshas. During that time of day, the gunas of that particular dosha predominate.

- 2 a.m.–6 a.m. and 2 p.m.–6 p.m. are ruled by vata dosha.
- 6 a.m.–10 a.m. and 6 p.m.–10 p.m. are ruled by kapha dosha.
- 10 a.m.–2 p.m. and 10 p.m.–2 a.m. are ruled by pitta dosha.

In the context of ayurveda for yoga therapy, different practices are best received at different times of the day. As mentioned above, ayurveda recognizes people as the microcosm of the macrocosm, so to align into balance it is important to align with nature. A basic *dinacharya* (daily practice routine) for balanced and optimal health would be designed around these different 4-hour cycles.

According to these principles, the best time for meditation or spiritual yogic practice is in the early morning hours of vata dosha. The qualities of the elements ether and air establish an expansive place of receptivity.

Pranayama is best done at the *kala sandhi*, or joints of time, meaning at dawn and again at dusk. This recommendation is predominantly for those with vata and pitta prakruti. Those who are predominantly kapha prakruti can practice pranayama and asana at various times of the day.

Asana is best practiced during the morning hours of kapha dosha, as the movement abates the guru guna, or heavy quality, and instills a *chala guna*, or mobile quality.

The middle of the day is pitta dosha time, so physical asana and pranayama would be contraindicated. Nature meditations; peaceful, meditative walks; and even resting are considered proper mid-day practices.

Ideally, the yoga practitioner rises with the sun and sets with the sun for optimal energy. Ayurveda considers waking during the time of vata and going to sleep during the evening hours of kapha to be an ideal practice.[8]

The seasons, ritucharya

Just as each 4-hour cycle of the day is associated with a specific dosha, so is each season. At the joints of each season, especially those between summer and fall and between winter and spring, the earth undergoes notable changes. As humans are the microcosm of the macrocosm, the practice of shifting one's own routines at these times creates further alignment with nature. In the summer, for example, the sun rises earlier and so, too, should people. Winter's increased hours of darkness make it appropriate to sleep more and stay in more. Listening to and following nature's lead offers everything needed to "treat with opposites" through the energies of each season. Just as springtime brings fresh bitter greens and sprouts to cleanse the heaviness of winter, cool fruit is plentiful to cool down from the hot summer sun, and so on. These principles should also inform any yoga therapy practice.

Late fall and early winter are associated with vata dosha, late winter and spring are associated with kapha dosha, and summer is associated with pitta dosha. The qualities ascribed to each dosha are higher during their associated seasons, so it is important to adjust therapeutic protocols to meet the client in a balanced place, taking into consideration not only their prakruti (constitution) and vikruti (imbalance), but also the time of year. For example, offering hot yoga in the high heat of summer would be contraindicated for all doshas. This individualized approach to yoga therapy, taking into consideration all elements and external factors, will help to create the specific practices best for the client. Generally, practices in the late fall and early winter should include elements to pacify vata dosha, practices in the late winter and spring should include elements to pacify kapha dosha, and practices in the summer should include elements to pacify pitta dosha.[9]

Subdoshas of Vata: The Pranavayus

The subdoshas of vata—the vayus, or winds, of movement within the body—are each responsible for different actions.[10]

Prana vayu is related to the element of ether and is seated in the heart and head. The areas of movement related to prana vayu are the head, throat, chest, and all of the sense organs (skin, eyes, ears, nose, and tongue). The direction of movement is downward and inward. Prana vayu governs inhalation, the life function of all cells, respiration, movement of intelligence, and vital force. This subdosha is even responsible for a sense of elation and joy, general happiness, and the heart-mind-body connection.

Apana vayu is related to the element of earth and is seated in the colon. As the colon is also the main seat of vata dosha in general, it is important to pay close attention to apana for the overall balancing of vata dosha. If a client's apana is imbalanced, all other subdoshas are likely imbalanced as well. The areas of movement related to apana vayu are the reproductive organs, hips, thighs, abdomen, and colon, as this subdosha is related to elimination as well as childbirth and menstruation. Apana vayu moves downward and outward.

Samana vayu is related to the element of fire and is seated in the small intestine. As the vayu of digestion, samana rules the space below the chest and above the navel. Samana vayu determines what is to be absorbed and kept by the body and what is to be excreted and eliminated. The liver, pancreas, spleen, and abdominal viscera are the main sites of movement for samana vayu, as it is concerned with digestion, absorption, and all movement of the gastrointestinal tract. Samana moves in a linear direction.

Udana vayu is related to the element of air and is seated in the diaphragm and throat. Udana moves through the nose, throat, and navel in an upward direction, although this subdosha can be thought of as mainly governing the chest region. Udana vayu rules the exhalation and represents the movement of energy, physical growth, ambition, strength, enlightenment, and enthusiasm.

Vyana vayu is related to the element of water. The seat of vyana vayu, which is in charge of circulation, heat distribution, walking, and the movement of the eyes, is in the heart as well as the whole body. Its sites of movement are from the heart to the periphery and from the periphery to the heart, encompassing the entire body. Vyana vayu moves in a circular direction.

Subtle Bodies: The Five Koshas, Three Shariras, and Three Subtle Essences

Ayurveda recognizes that humans are multidimensional beings; any change in any part of the body, gross or subtle, will change every other part of the body. The three doshas, five koshas, three shariras, and three subtle essences all exist within but not without each other. For example, consider the symbol for yin and yang: The dot of black in the white field and the white in the black part of the symbol represent that there is always a little bit of yin in the yang and vice versa. Although one element of the five may be assigned to each kosha, or two elements to each dosha, they all contain all of the elements. Also, no one being can exist without all of the doshas, koshas, and shariras alike. Therefore, even if one subtle energy is presenting in dominance or imbalance, all of the subtle energies are present. The five koshas (sheaths) move from gross to subtle and exist within the three shariras (bodies). (See Chapter 2 for the origins of the *panchamaya kosha* model.)

Although the koshas are often observed (and experienced) from gross to subtle, they are fed from subtle to gross. Each subtle kosha informs and supports the next in line, until *annamaya kosha*, the physical/food sheath, is reached. For this reason, observing and supporting all five koshas in a yoga therapy protocol is crucial.[11]

Annamaya kosha, the food sheath, is the most gross sheath and resides within the *sthula sharira*, or gross body. It contains the *pancha jnanedriya* and *pancha karmendriya*, the five sense organs and five action organs. Annamaya kosha is related to the element of earth. Part of *pranamaya kosha*, namely the part that physically breathes, lives in sthula sharira as well. *Sukshma sharira*, or the astral body, is home to the rest of pranamaya kosha (energetic or vital air sheath) and to *manomaya kosha* (mental/emotional sheath) and *vijanamaya kosha* (knowledge or wisdom sheath); these koshas are related to water, fire, and air elements, respectively. *Anandamaya kosha*, related to the element of ether and sometimes known as the bliss body, resides within the causal body, *karana sharira*.

The three doshas of vata, pitta, and kapha each have relative subtle essences called, respectively, *prana*, *tejas*, and *ojas*. (See Chapter 20 for more information on the subtle essences.) The doshas are considered more gross than the subtle essences, and although they are still not tangible, the doshas can be used to balance annamaya kosha; prana, tejas, and ojas are used to bring the remaining four, even more subtle, sheaths into balance. Two principles underpin the restoration of balance: Like increases like, and opposites balance. The doshas can be "used" to balance annamaya kosha through consideration of which qualities are exaggerated in the doshas. For example, if a client is feeling cold, mobile, rough, and dry in their body due to aggravated vata dosha, activities that bring heat, stillness, smoothness, and moisture to the body would be beneficial. The same two principles apply to the more subtle essences as well.[12]

In yoga therapy, working with the koshas is often viewed as a way to move from lower-self to higher-self using asana, pranayama, meditation, and more. Ayurveda recognizes a similar path of needing to heal the koshas and works with *manodosha*, the subtle essences of prana, tejas, and ojas (sometimes called the doshas of the mind). Ayurvedic therapy may use modalities such as *daivavyapasraya chikitsa* (divine therapy),[13] *yukthivyapasraya chikitsa* (rational treatment), and *satvavajaya chikitsa* (talk therapy) to balance prana, tejas, and ojas. Yoga chikitsa can be used to bring healing and balance into the subtle essences as well.[14]

Summary

Ayurveda, the medical system indigenous to India, is viewed as the "sister science" to yoga. This science of life is a five-elemental approach to etiology, pathology, healing, and existence; it seeks to manifest a physical body that is well enough to traverse the path of yoga. In the key Ayurvedic concept of tridosha, vata, pitta, and kapha determine the constitutional makeup of all people in both their balanced and unbalanced states. Each dosha represents a combination of the five elements, and each embodies the innate qualities of the gunas.

Dinacharya and *ritucharya* are, respectively, the clock that divides each day into 4-hour cycles corresponding with the three doshas and the three seasons of the calendar year (also corresponding as such). Recommending asana and pranayama in concert with these temporal concepts may be particularly useful in yoga therapy practice. The pranavayus—subdoshas of vata, the dosha concerned with movement of elements through the body—are also useful in yoga therapy, as aspects of assessment, as are the concepts of kosha, sharira, and the subtle essences.

Additional Resources

Bavadekar, S. (2011). Mimansa. *Journal of Ayurveda and Integrative Medicine, 2*(1), 37–41.

Karmananda, S. (2001). *Yogic management of common diseases.* Nesma Books India.

Lad, V. (2001). *Textbook of ayurveda: Fundamental principles*, Vol. 1. Ayurvedic Press.

Lad, V. (2007). *Textbook of ayurveda: A complete guide to clinical assessment*, Vol. 2. Ayurvedic Press.

Lad, V. (2012). *Textbook of ayurveda: General principles of management and treatment*, Vol. 3. Ayurvedic Press.

Panja, A. K., Upadhyaya, O. P., & Chattopadhyaya, A. (2011). A critical review of the philosophical concepts of Carakopaskara commentary. *Ayu, 32*(3), 422–426.

Endnotes

1 Fundamental principles of ayurveda and Samkhya philosophy are primarily sourced from classic texts representing thousands of pages of dense (often only roughly translated) material. This chapter therefore

generally references more accessible contemporary work for the benefit of the reader, as in this case: Lad, V. (2001). *Textbook of ayurveda: Fundamental principles*, Vol. 1 (pp. 4–10). Ayurvedic Press.

2 Lad, *Textbook of ayurveda*, Vol. 1 (pp. 5–8).

3 Lad, *Textbook of ayurveda*, Vol. 1 (pp. 8–10).

4 Lad, *Textbook of ayurveda*, Vol. 1 (pp. 5–10).

5 Lad, *Textbook of ayurveda*, Vol. 1 (pp. 29–30).

6 Srikantha Murthy, K. R. (2009). *Vagbhata's astanga hrdayam. Text, English translation, notes, appendix, and indices*, Vols. 1–3 (5th ed., p. 11). Chowkhamba Krishnadas Academy.

7 Lad, *Textbook of ayurveda*, Vol. 1 (pp. 45–78).

8 Lad, V. (2012). *Textbook of ayurveda: General principles of management and treatment*, Vol. 3 (pp. 98–106). Ayurvedic Press.

9 Lad, *Textbook of ayurveda*, Vol. 3 (pp. 106–130).

10 Dash, B., & Sharma, R. K. (2009). *Caraka samhiṭa. Text with English translation and critical exposition based on Cakrapani Datta's ayurveda dipika*, Vols. 1–7. Chowkhamba Sanskrit Series Office.
Lad, *Textbook of ayurveda*, Vol. 3 (pp. 46–53).
Srikantha Murthy, *Vagbhata's astanga hrdayam*.

11 Lad, *Textbook of ayurveda*, Vol. 3 (pp. 194–196).

12 Lad, *Textbook of ayurveda*, Vol. 1 (pp. 207–229).

13 Lad, *Textbook of ayurveda*, Vol. 3 (pp. 29, 303–304).

14 Lad, *Textbook of ayurveda*, Vol. 3 (pp. 303–304).

5

Spanda: The Fundamental Impulse of the Shaiva Tantra Tradition

LEIGH BLASHKI AND GINA MACAULEY

Spanda, the dynamism of consciousness and much more, is one of the most important foundational principles in the Shaiva Tantra tradition. An understanding of spanda can have wide-ranging applications in the practice of yoga therapy.

As a spiritual tradition, Tantra developed out of the Hindu religion of Shaivism (worship of Shiva) between the 6th and 7th centuries CE, at a time when Brahmanism was the predominant religion in what we now know as India.[1] (See Chapter 2 for an overview of Tantra.) Shaiva Tantra is the longest standing and most influential non-Vedic spiritual tradition in India. Initially, Shaiva Tantra was focused in Northern India, particularly in the area we know as Kashmir. Over the years, its influence and practices spread to other areas of the subcontinent, but its roots remain acknowledged by its more common name, Kashmir Shaivism.

Beginning in the 9th century CE, Shaiva Tantra (or Kashmir Shaivism) comprised two main sects, the Trika and the Krama.[2] This chapter focuses on the principles of the Trika tradition of Kashmir Shaiva Tantra, as this tradition is more widely practiced and its principles offer numerous benefits in the practice of yoga therapy.

Trika is a Sanskrit word meaning "triad," and the philosophy of Trika Shaiva Tantra is based on the triad of *shiva* (unqualified pure consciousness), *shakti* (flowing energy of power to manifest; see Chapter 15), and *nara* (bound or embodied soul).[3]

Shaiva Tantra Fundamentals

A detailed treatise on the principles of Trika Shaiva Tantra is beyond the scope of this chapter, but some of the more important fundamentals are instructive for the work of yoga therapists:

1. Consciousness, rather than matter or energy, is the "stuff of the universe."[4] All of manifestation is a vibration of consciousness at varying degrees of grossness, depending on the level of involution, or manifestation.

2. Shaiva Tantra is an "unqualified" non-dual philosophy. Unlike Advaita Vedanta, Shaiva Tantra does not regard manifestation as an illusion (*maya*). Advaita teaches a principle of *neti neti* (not this, not that) and that only Brahman is reality, whereas non-dual Shaiva Tantra teaches the principle of "all of this, all of that"—everything is an immanent expression of transcendent consciousness. Shaivism is considered unqualified non-dualism because the ultimate state of our true nature as pure consciousness is beyond nameable qualities.

3. Reality can be mapped into 36 principles, or *tattvas*, that indicate involution from pure consciousness to gross matter and the return evolution from matter to consciousness. The 36 tattvas of Shaiva Tantra include and build on the 25 tattvas expounded in Samkhya philosophy (see Chapter 2).[5]

4. The divine feminine principle, or shakti, is the operative power behind all levels and aspects of involution (manifestation) and evolution.

5. Spanda is the motive impulse of all aspects, actions, and experiences of all levels of involution and evolution. An understanding of the principles of spanda is fundamental to the work of a yoga therapist, and a more detailed exploration follows.

6. All of manifestation is subject to the five acts, or stages, of the Divine.

Spanda

Numerous words have been used to try to define spanda, but each is only an approximation of the felt experience of those who have offered their descriptions. Some of the more common definitions are

- creative tension[6]
- vibration

- pulse
- throb of absolute reality[7]
- sacred tremor[8]
- subtle movement
- subtle creative pulse[9]
- divine pulse of the universe
- great cosmic movement[10]

For the purpose of informing the work of a yoga therapist, the term *motive impulse* is especially useful, as it points toward how spanda can form part of yoga therapy practices.

A means of expression

According to the *Spanda Karika*, a 9th-century Tantra Yoga text of the Kashmir Shaivism tradition, all of life is imbued with spanda—something that is not quite physical, but more than only energetic.[11] The term is used to describe the pulsing or wave-like movement of consciousness within manifested life. Spanda can be regarded as a means by which Shiva consciousness moves into expression through the power of shakti (expressed as both cosmic and terrestrial nature).

Spanda is the creative tension between principles of Shiva and Shakti. This tension is the unending and ever-present process of actualization at the source of all there is.[12] The eternal motive impulse of spanda spans the domains of potentiality and actuality and is the fount of the processes of creative actualization, including the involution of the tattvas from pure consciousness to the physical elements and the evolution from physical elements back to consciousness.

Paradoxically, spanda is both the unmanifest field in which and out of which everything is experienced and the actual dynamic of all that is manifested. As philosopher Peter Wilberg[13] explained,

> The divine [feminine] dynamic of creation that is spanda is therefore also a simultaneous process of emergence of possibilities into actuality and their submergence or demergence into the realm of unmanifest potentiality as symbolized by the simultaneous opening and closing of the eye of [Shiva].

Spanda-shakti

Spanda is often referred to as *spanda-shakti* because it is a form of power that involves no depletion in activity as is seen in physical energy. Sociologist Anne Marie Walsh described spanda as

> the sea of all in which we and all things, arise as forms and subside back to formlessness from which we arose. We are entirely immersed in this sea of all, inseparable from it, formless in some conditions, with form (body) at others.[14]

Life is a dynamic interplay of expansion and contraction, pulsing backward and forward, sometimes subtly and imperceptibly and at other times on a gross and easily recognized level. This pulsing of expansion and contraction is one of the ways in which spanda underpins everything in life.

The *Spanda Karika* teaches that everything in the world is vibration, pulsing at different levels of frequency. More recently, physicists have proposed similar theories. From the work of Bohr, Schrödinger, and Heisenberg we have learnt about packets of a form of emanation that is paradoxically always in flux, yet in itself a singularity. Einstein called these packets quanta and his quantum theory reveals a basic oneness of the universe.[15] Basic chemistry teaches that atoms, the basis of all forms of life, are in a constant state of pulse-like flux.

According to yoga teacher trainer Julie Smerdon,

> The human body is a perfect repository for this never-ending throb of life force. Every time the heart beats, for example, it contracts, causing a wave of pressure that pushes fresh blood into the arteries. Between contractions the heart briefly expands to allow in more blood. As long as a person lives, this reliable pattern never changes. The breath also has a rhythm, and the organs and glands pulse—even the bones gently throb with the energy of life, known in yoga as prana.[16]

As photons are to light, in a similar way spanda can be regarded as the foundation of *prana*, or the impulse that creates pranic flow. Prana can only support life if it is flowing; prana that has become stagnant indicates a disease state, and life ends when it ceases to flow. As spanda provides the motive impulse for the flow of prana, spanda also is essential for life. Much has been written in yogic literature regarding the importance of removing obstacles to the free flow of prana, and this is indeed an important part of yoga for therapeutic purposes.

One might expect, however, that attuning to the spanda that *creates* the pranic flow would be much more effective. Tuning in to and moving with the pulsation of this energy in the body enables one to move closer to understanding one's true nature and the nature of life. At times, people naturally feel expanded, or "swollen with light." At other times people feel dull or agitated—contracted. Both states are normal, natural elements of the ebb and flow of life.

Perception and experience

From the spanda principle, the senses acquire their power of moving out toward their objects, holding the objects in perception for a while, and then withdrawing back toward the center of presence. It is more than the will or desire of the individual that moves the senses toward objects—the motive impulse of spanda (shakti) powers the process of sensory perception.

Spanda imbues both subject and object, but it is only objects that change, arising in and disappearing from perception. Changeless spanda constitutes the eternal subject.[17]

This principle is important for yoga therapists to understand. In a therapeutic yoga session, the yoga therapist generally casts themselves in the role of subject and the client in the role of object. Yet as the subject the yoga therapist certainly experiences a multitude of changes as they engage with the client (object). They have changing thoughts, perceptions, body sensations, etc., which can be regarded as "subjective objects." However, Shaiva Tantra teaches that behind or as a background to the changes one experiences as the subject (having objective experiences) is this unchanging presence, the eternal subject—spanda. Paradoxically, although spanda itself is unchanging, it is replete with motive impulse in potentiality and able to actualize this motive impulse at any time in any manner, without disturbing its own unchanging equanimity.

The same unchanging presence is also the background of all that the client (object) experiences. Therefore, the client is both object and subject—changing and changeless. Yoga therapy clients' self-agency may be increased by an understanding that behind the play of changing experiences is an unchanging presence imbued with the power to effect change.

In discussing movement and *asana*, physical therapist and yoga therapist Matthew Taylor suggested that yoga therapists are not the agents of this movement, but rather an openness to possibilities that can become actualized through some motive force.[18] Although Taylor does not directly mention spanda, his description fits well with its principles.

Spanda can be more easily experienced when mental activities are brought to quiescence. However, this mental quieting is easier to achieve if one is oriented toward and has developed a sensitivity to perceiving and experiencing spanda. For yoga therapists, it does not matter whether the chicken came before the egg or vice versa! Developing practices that both quiet the mind and increase sensitivity to spanda is an important part of the professional skill set.

As spanda is a mediator between consciousness and energy, sensitivity to spanda can be used to access the primal energetic of emotions and other affective mind states, assisting with the passage from agitation to greater quiescence. At a more gross level, sensitivity to spanda can be a powerful skill for accessing and better understanding the genesis of patterns of movement, breath, posture, and other somatic experiences. This skill is helpful, if not essential, for developing a more interoceptive approach to asana and *pranayama* as well as the more subtle yoga practices.

Yoga therapists can assist clients in discovering and attuning to the motive impulse of spanda to consciously sense the vibrations of the energies awakened by each posture and try to recognize, in those vibrations, the underlying motive impulse. This awareness, in turn, supports clients in reframing their relationships with new movements and postures, as they learn to start with an attunement to spanda and allow that motive impulse to establish the foundations for the new somatic patterns and actions.

An asana is more than a physical posture, pose, movement, or body position. Underpinning these somatics of *annamaya kosha* is an energetic blueprint in the *pranamaya kosha*, and underpinning this energetic blueprint is the motive impulse of spanda. Although Shaiva Tantra as a non-dual philosophy does not emphasize the *panchamaya* model, which comes from more dualistic traditions, Shaiva Tantra does not exclude these principles and accepts many apparently dualistic ideas into its non-dual inclusivity. (See Chapter 3 for an outline of panchamaya.) The very nature of unqualified non-dual philosophy is such that everything is regarded as part of a unitive whole; anything that appears as separate from anything else can be experienced both in its apparent separateness and its non-separate wholeness.

For the purpose of understanding spanda in the context of yoga practices often defined or described according to the koshas, spanda can be said to be beyond any kosha while being the motive impulse behind or within each.

Attuning to spanda

Developing sensitivity and attuning to spanda can occur in any activity. However, from a yoga therapy perspective there is possibly no better practice than *savasana* (corpse pose) for developing this skill. Savasana can be interpreted as simply resting in one's true nature, where all masks, armor, and veils can be released, allowing an experience of perfect wholeness. As people soften into savasana, they may begin to notice how vibrant and alive they are. The pulsing, vibrant, radiant sensation of spanda fills the body, enlivens the senses, and directs the thoughts.

As sensitivity to the play of spanda develops, a greater sense of aliveness can be felt in all areas of life, from resting to vigorous activity. Greater awareness of the initial motive impulse that momentarily precedes thoughts and actions allows those thoughts and actions to be more conscious and intentional while retaining an openness and spontaneity. One can start to live with greater trust in their essential nature of non-separation. This subtle, internalized awareness is a fundamental aspect of interoception, which involves receiving and appraising internal signals in the body (see Chapter 16). As an iterative process, interoception involves integrated mind-body awareness to inform the appropriate responses or actions. Without interoception, which, like spanda, is happening behind the scenes all the time, self-regulation and maintenance of homeostasis would be compromised.[19]

Spanda is at play as the motive impulse that underlies every aspect of a yoga therapist's work. Given an understanding that spanda has a pulsing quality and that knowledge and skills do not necessarily develop in a linear or straightforward way, one can accept that there will be bursts or pulses of understanding, intuition, and insight.

Yoga therapists sometimes report that while teaching or advising a client, an insight appears as if bursting onto the scene. There is a sense of wonder as to how that came about. This is spanda at play, expressing through *jnana-shakti*—the power of spontaneous, pure Knowing. Insight and intuition are pulses of spanda, underlying other thought processes. These bursts or pulses need not be rare occurrences; they can become more regular as one attunes to spanda, allowing the feeling of that motive impulse whether working with a client or simply feeling-knowing when it is time to have a cup of tea.

As spanda is the motive impulse behind the operation of the senses and the mind, yoga therapists can develop a greater trust in their faculties when sitting with a client and allowing what comes through the senses and mind to inform thoughts and decision-making (along with background information about the client and knowledge of the presenting condition). Such trust allows the yoga therapist to be more present with a client, with fewer preconceived ideas about what needs to be known and what needs to happen. This allows yoga therapists to both be open to the impulse of spanda and to develop a greater resonance with the client.

It can be equally helpful for clients to understand the concept of these spontaneous bursts or pulses of new insight. As with the physical symptoms of disease, what appears to be a turnaround for the better can seem to just happen.

Again, this is spanda. This is not to say that spanda's impulse occurs without all the other attendant actions that create the fertile ground for wellness to unfold, but what helps to create those attendant actions? The ubiquity of spanda is at the heart of all mental and physical activities of both therapist and client, regardless of whether they are aware of or sensitive to it. However, their work on bringing about greater well-being is certainly enhanced by developing sensitivity and attunement to this sometimes-arcane motive impulse.

The 36 Tattvas of Shaiva Tantra

The tattvas outline levels or principles of reality that form a map of conscious experience. A basic understanding of the tattvas and their interplay is helpful to inform the work of yoga therapists, particularly in terms of how matter and consciousness are related and how everyday experiences have the potential to point toward experiences of one's true nature. The tattvas can be considered from either top to bottom or bottom to top. Top-down describes the principles of involution, manifestation, or creation; bottom-up describes the principles of evolution or liberation.

The tattvas of essential nature

1. ***Shiva***, pure consciousness, or the ground of reality that is beyond qualities. The word *shiva* here does not refer to the aspect of the pantheon in which the god Shiva is associated with the processes of dissolution, but rather to a state without definable qualities. This undefinable state nevertheless represents a universal coherence of all potentials for manifestation (shaktis)—it holds space for their unfolding.[20] The word *shiva* can also be interpreted as "lying down in one's true nature," deriving from the Sanskrit word *śīvan*. The tattva of shiva is considered to be masculine.

2. ***Shakti***, power of action that is the essence and source of all energy.[21] Although shakti is separate from shiva for the purposes of mapping the tattvas, Shaiva Tantra teaches that shiva and shakti are never separate; rather, they carry different potentials. Shakti is understood as a power or potential for action, activity, and actualization, in contrast to the pure quiescent awareness that is shiva.[22] The tattva of shakti is considered to be feminine.

As a result of the self-generated motive impulse—spanda in and between shiva and shakti—a subtle patterning for manifestation establishes itself in the following three tattvas.

Tattvas that pattern manifestation

3. ***Sada shiva***, correlating with *iccha*, the power of willing. Sada shiva is the first subtle patterning or potential for manifestation. It brings forth the concept of the apparent subject (or Self), which at this stage remains quiescent.

4. ***Ishvara***, correlating with *jnana*, the power of knowing, is the subtle patterning for the sprouting of the manifest universe. It brings forth the concept of apparent objects (or the world), which are not yet fully differentiated from the subject. The word *ishvara* is often translated as the concept of a personal god. In this tattva, it refers to the nascent unfolding of knowable qualities that can both underpin the changing universe and act as pointers back to divine, unitive consciousness.

5. ***Shuddha vidya***, correlating with *kriya*, the power of action, is the stage at which subject (Self) and object (world) appear as distinct. Here, the concept of a changing universe is established. Abhinavagupta, the author of the *Spanda Karika*, suggests that the subjective and objective are convertible into each other, that they are two modes of awareness linked to the same experience.[23]

The tattva of differentiation

6. ***Maya*** represents the power of differentiation, wherein the one appears as many and "I" can be experienced as distinct from "this." Maya is the principle by which what is inseparable can appear as separate and changing parts.

Maya is also the power of Self-remembering, or revelation, and Self-forgetting, or concealment. It is at this stage of involution that misperceptions emerge, along with the potential for correct perceptions, as expounded in the next five tattvas. These five tattvas derive from maya and are known collectively as the *kanchukas*.[24] Each kanchuka can be both concealing and revealing, at times obscuring one's true nature and at other times pointing toward it.

In some yogic traditions, in particular Advaita Vedanta, maya is translated as "illusion." Another translation of maya is wisdom, and the Shaiva Tantra interpretation includes both the concept of wisdom and illusion. Maya is a good example of the paradox of something being both apparently separate (illusion) and non-separate (wisdom) simultaneously. As detailed in the following five tattvas, maya offers the opportunity to recognize that what conceals has the potential to develop the wisdom of revealing.

Tattvas of the kanchukas, or pointers to wholeness

7. ***Kalā*** (pronounced "kalar"), through the agency of spanda, animates the individual soul and is the capacity for doing. When it is concealing, it leads to feelings of limitation in relation to actions and a consequential belief that one needs to do more or something better to feel whole. In its revealing aspect, kalā points toward the omnipotence of one's true nature, leading to feelings of not needing to do anything particular to simply be whole, even as the functionality of doing may continue.

8. ***Vidya*** is related to knowledge. This tattva is the capacity to feel connected and complete. However, concealment results in feelings of disconnection and confusion; with them arise feelings of needing to know something more to feel complete. Vidya in its revealing aspect points toward an innate sense of knowing one's true nature, a familiar feeling wherein no extra knowing is needed to rest in one's completeness, even as knowledge supports functioning and the need for social connection continues. The concept of vidya and its opposite, *avidya*, also forms an important part of the teachings of Patanjali's yoga *darshana*: Avidya—ignorance (of our true nature) or incorrect knowledge—is the basis for all mental obstacles (*kleshas*).

9. ***Raga*** is related to desire, which in its concealing aspect creates a sense of being flawed and that something is lacking and needs to be gained or acquired. This sense of lack can lead to repetitive cycles of ever-greater desire when that which is acquired fails to create feelings of perfection or wholeness. This cycle is echoed in the kleshas espoused by Patanjali. In its revealing aspect, raga points toward the natural wholeness or perfection of one's innate being, wherein nothing extra is required; trying to acquire something takes one further from the experience of one's true nature (see Chapter 3).

10. ***Kāla*** (pronounced "karla") is related to perceptions of time. When it conceals the individual's true timeless nature, kāla creates a sense of being time-bound, wherein time rules the ability to be happy. In this concealment, people feel that they need more time to recover a sense of wholeness. However, kāla can point toward an experience beyond the usual perceptions of time, revealing a sense of timelessness that is beyond past, future, and even the present. In this state of simply being, time is irrelevant, although paradoxically the psychological need for time may continue. In this state beyond the time-bound, thoughts, like the perception of time itself, slow down and can come to a stop.

11. ***Niyati*** is related to spatial limitation. Through its aspect of concealment, niyati leads to a sense of contraction and restriction in relation to one's place within physical space. People feel diminished and limited in what is perceived as the smallness of physical presence. This brings about a belief that more space is needed to feel whole. In its revealing aspect, niyati points toward one's innate spaciousness, an indescribable and undeniable presence that is everywhere and nowhere in particular. Individuals can experience an omnipresence that does not have a distinct location with a defined center or boundary. One becomes more like a boundless field of presence that is spacious, unlimited, and whole, even as the functionality of maintaining healthy boundaries continues.[25]

An understanding of the workings of the kanchukas (numbers 7 to 11 above) is fundamental to the work of a yoga therapist. At any time, one or more of these pointers will be at play in clients' lives, creating feelings of limitation, lack of wholeness, and other psychological symptoms associated with living as though separate from the rest of the manifested world. Yoga therapists can assist clients to recognize the other side of the coin, the wholeness and non-separation toward which the kanchukas point. This flip from the concealing to the revealing aspects of the pointers primarily occurs through reflective self-inquiry and is mediated by the most subtle operation of spanda.

Tattvas underpinning Samkhya

The following 25 tattvas are essentially the same as those of the Samkhya tradition introduced in Chapter 2. As these tattvas form the basis of the dualistic philosophy of Samkhya and our focus in this chapter is on the non-dual philosophy of Shaiva Tantra, only a brief description is provided for some of them. However, those that form an important part of the underpinnings in Shaiva Tantra are expounded.

12. ***Purusha***, individual subject, is a contracted form of universal consciousness.

13. ***Prakriti*** is the matrix of all objectivity, including holding the *triguna* in balance (see Chapter 3).

14. ***Buddhi*** is ascertaining intelligence, including discernment (*viveka*).

15. ***Ahamkara***, derived from buddhi, is the I-making or self-appropriating principle.

16. ***Manas***, derived from ahamkara, cooperates with the senses to build perceptions and concepts.

Knowledge of these aspects of the *antahkarana* (internal mental processes) is important in informing the yoga therapist's understanding of not only how yoga regards the mind, but also for developing effective therapeutic relationships (see Chapter 13).

Tattvas of sense capabilities: Jnanendriyas or buddhindriyas

17. **Hearing**

18. **Touching**

19. **Seeing**

20. **Tasting**

21. **Smelling**

In the Shaiva Tantra tradition, the senses are regarded as important doorways or access points to an experience of the timeless present moment, through a variety of mindfulness-based practices. Although in Samkhya these senses correlate fully with their respective physical organs (ears, skin, eyes, mouth, nose), in Shaiva Tantra spanda is the primary and ultimate activator of sensing. Through development of sensitivity to spanda, the whole body has the potential for experiencing all sensations.

Tattvas of action capabilities: Karmendriyas

22. **Mouth**, speech

23. **Hands**, handling

24. **Feet**, locomotion

25. **Genitals**, reproduction

26. **Excretory organs**, evacuation

Tattvas of subtle elements: Tanmatras

27. **Sound**

28. **Tactility**

29. **Form**

30. **Taste**

31. **Odor**

In Shaiva Tantra, as with the *jnanendriyas*, the *tanmatras* form an important part of the mindfulness-based inquiry practices. Although directly related to the jnanendriyas, the tanmatras are also closely related to the *bhutas*, as briefly shown below.

Tattvas of materiality: Bhutas

Shaiva Tantra, along with Samkhya, proposes that bhutas are formed from the tanmatras, the latter creating a subtle potential for materiality. It may be tempting to regard materiality as less spiritually significant than the more subtle tattvas toward the top of the map. However, Shaiva Tantra regards every level as important, and many of its practices have a strong base in this materiality. Scholar Christopher Wallis suggests that "at the top of the tattva hierarchy (śiva-Tattva) all the principles are present in potential form, while at the bottom (earth-tattva) all those potentialities inherent in the Divine are fully expressed."[26]

32. **Space**, from sound

33. **Air/wind**, from tactility

34. **Fire**, from form

35. **Liquid**, from taste

36. **Earth/solidity**, from odor

The Five Acts or Stages of the Divine

The principle of the *pancha-krtya*, or five acts of the Divine, offers another model for understanding the manifested world and its innate connection with pure consciousness. These acts or stages are (1) manifestation or creation; (2) maintenance or stabilization of manifestation; (3) dissolution or withdrawal of manifestation; (4) concealment or forgetting (of Self); and (5) revelation, grace, or remembering (of Self).[27] Everything happening in the universe expresses one or more of these acts at any time. In other words, there is nothing that is not being created, sustained, or dissolved in any moment, and there is nothing that is not either helping to conceal or reveal one's true nature or Self. These acts occur on all scales from the macrocosmic to the atomic, in both outer and inner experiences of reality, whether that be the creation and dissolution of galaxies or the arising and falling away of thoughts.

All physical and mental manifestation is continually in a state of flux, even when some things appear to be fixed or static. This continual state of change is an expression of spanda, which itself remains changeless while being the pulse or motive impulse behind all change.

An understanding of the five acts is useful for yoga therapists. Helping clients to recognize that whatever they are experiencing physically and mentally is not only changeable but also follows a trajectory provides encouragement and can offer perspective on present circumstances.

Psychologist and yoga therapist Richard Miller offers an interpretation of the five acts that can provide a simplified approach in therapeutic settings.[28] Miller's five stages of birth, growth, stability, decay, and dissolution correlate closely with the five stages of disease. By recognizing phenomena as changing and discontinuous, one can start to release identification with them.

It is interesting to note that the first three of the five acts correlate with the Vedic triune of Brahma (creator), Vishnu (maintainer), and Shiva (destroyer).

Therapeutic Skills

The principles of Shaiva Tantra can help yoga therapists develop a number of useful skills and offer a range of tools (*upaya*) that can assist clients. In her exegesis of the *Pratyabhijnahrdayam*, a pivotal 11th-century text of Shaiva Tantra, Joan Ruvinsky advises that,

> Numerous methods (of inward self-reflection) may be employed. Practices abound. They may involve the interruption of the continuous flow of thought, the recognition of stillness behind movement, inward gazing even as the outward world is manifesting, or awareness in the gaps between the end of one perception or activity and the beginning of the next. Any means that promotes the recognition of the heart of being (or true nature) will suffice.[29]

Following are examples of simple skill-building practices. Suggestions to support these practices can be found in the Additional Resources.

Kanchuka self-inquiry

Taking time to regularly inquire into the interplay of the five pointers is one of the fundamental practices yoga therapists can undertake to build their therapeutic skills. Through these self-inquiries, practitioners can develop a deeper understanding of their own relationship to these pointers, which in turn better prepares them for guiding clients in their respective inquiries. An example of this self-inquiry can be found in Appendix 5A.

Engaging with spanda

Despite what the mind usually thinks, the body is multidimensional vibration, without center or periphery. Innocent, unconditioned welcoming of physical sensation restores the body to its innate ground of radiance.[30] Feeling the impulse that comes before movement, as in a practice of spanda engagement like that in Appendix 5B, can help to identify areas that are energetically or pranically blocked and is useful in recognizing and unraveling unhealthy or compensatory movement patterns.

Given a baseline awareness of spanda, a practice of body sensing can help to deepen the somatic experience with less involvement of thoughts. Body sensing (Appendix 5C) is a non-postural form of movement that develops the ability to sense into one's essential vibratory nature, or spanda. It helps to develop more refined levels of interoceptive perception, leading to the detection of more subtle levels of being. Body sensing can also be a segue into the Tantric spontaneous-movement dance of *tandava*, which, according to writer Daniel Odier, frees the body into a spaciousness where matter and consciousness are experienced as one.[31]

Spandana

Spandana provides a series of simple and effective tools that are applied at the physical level to gain a connection with one's subtle spanda. It uses a range of pulsing techniques that help the physical body better align with its subtle counterpart of spanda. These pulsing techniques can be self-applied or provided by another person.

Vijnana Bhairava Tantra

Another way of developing greater attunement with spanda as well as deepening the experience of non-separation is through many of the practices outlined in the *Vijnana Bhairava Tantra*, which dates to the beginnings of Shaivism.[32] Like many of the texts in the various yogic traditions, the *Vijnana Bhairava* is comprised of short, pithy *slokas* (verses) or sutras that can initially seem obscure. However, through meditation on the slokas and immersion in the suggested or implied practices, their fuller meaning unfolds. An example can be found in Appendix 5D.

Yoga nidra

Yoga nidra is probably the most commonly known and widely accessed practice from the non-dual Shaiva Tantra tradition. Although yoga nidra is occasionally referred to in pre-Tantric Vedic texts, its practice from the mid-20th century onward has been an expression of classical non-dual Shaiva Tantra. Its popularity grew from the teachings of Swami Satyananda Saraswati, a student of the Tantra scholar Swami Sivananda. Other teachers have continued to build the popularity of yoga nidra as an accessible and effective meditation practice. Notably, Miller's iRest yoga nidra meditation has become recognized as well-suited to contemporary life through its use of secular language and incorporation of understandings from neuroscience and psychology.

The Shaiva text *Cincinimatasarasamuccaya* describes yoga nidra as "peace beyond words."[33] According to Satyananda, during the practice of yoga nidra one appears to be asleep, but the consciousness is functioning at a deeper level of awareness. For this reason, yoga nidra is often referred to as psychic sleep or deep relaxation with inner awareness. Interestingly, another translation of the word *nidra* is "the budding of a new flower." It is possible that the early teachers were pointing toward yoga nidra's ability to help the flowering of the state of yoga within the practitioner.

Yoga therapists are encouraged to undertake a regular yoga nidra practice to build their skills of inner awareness and be better informed on how to include the practice as part of the toolkit for clients.

Pratyabhijnahrdayam

The *Pratyabhijnahrdayam* is one of the early non-dual texts in Shaiva Tantra and the primary text in the Pratyabhijna school of Shaivism.[34] The work's name has been variously translated or interpreted as *Recognition Sutras*, *Recognition of the Heart*, and *Recognition of Our Own Heart*. The 20 slokas outlined in the *Pratyabhijnahrdayam* emphasize apperception and direct immersion of the entire body-mind into the heart of one's true nature. Meditation on many of these slokas will be helpful to yoga therapists in further accessing the fullness of their true nature and developing tools for clients.

Summary

The Shaiva Tantra tradition includes many principles that provide valuable foundational knowledge for yoga therapists. In this chapter, the principles of the tattvas and spanda have been the primary focus. The 36 tattvas of Shaiva Tantra provide a useful model for understanding levels of reality, which can be helpful to inform the work of yoga therapists, particularly in terms of how matter and consciousness are related and how everyday experiences have the potential to point toward experiences of one's true nature.

Spanda is a subtle yet important principle within the Shaiva Tantra tradition. This motive impulse underpins every movement, emotion, and thought and is a bridge between consciousness and energy. Knowledge of and developing skills to work with spanda can enhance the effectiveness of the practice of yoga therapy, helping both yoga therapist and client to address the subtle energetics of the body-mind.

Additional Resources

Non-dual meditation

Miller, R. (2017). *Awakening to your essential nature* [audio CD]. iRest Institute.

Pratyabhijnahrdayam

Ruvinsky, J. (2019). *The recognition of our own heart* (p. 18). Babaji's Kriya Yoga and Publishing.

Spandana

Spindler, B. (n.d.) Shake it off: 3 short practices to do when you're angry. https://yogainternational.com/article/view/shake-it-off-3-short-practices-to-do-when-youre-angry

Spindler, B. (n.d.) *Spandana practice for yoga therapeutics* [online course]. Yoga International.

Vijnana Bhairava Tantra

Roche, L. (2014). *The radiance sutras: 112 gateways to wonder and delight.* Sounds True.

Appendix 5A: Kanchuka Self-Inquiry

Wholeness is your essential nature. But when you don't recognize your basic wholeness, you feel that something's amiss in your life. When you realize your wholeness, you recognize an indestructible resource that allows you to weather every challenge you'll face.

You discover wholeness through experiencing the simple feeling of being in your true nature, which is a universal felt sense, or non-verbal inner knowing, that we all experience. Being, or true nature, is a quiet background presence that's always with you but that can go unnoticed until it's directly pointed out. Take a few moments to notice where and how you experience simply being in your body.

When you forget your felt sense of being or true nature, you can easily lose touch with your non-separate wholeness.

When you forget your true nature or simply being, you believe you need more space to feel whole again. Ask yourself: "Where am I when I'm simply being?" Then, experience your basic feeling of being that reveals your spacious wholeness. When you're simply being, how would you describe your felt sense of location? Where are you when you're simply being?

When you forget your true nature or being, you believe you need more time to feel whole again. Ask yourself: "When am I when I'm simply being?" Then, experience your basic feeling of being that reveals your timeless wholeness. When you're simply being, what's your relationship to time? When are you when you're simply being?

When you forget your true nature or being, you believe you're lacking and need to acquire something to feel whole again. Ask yourself: "Do I need to add anything when I'm simply being?" Then, experience your basic feeling of being that reveals your perfect wholeness. When you're just being, is there anything you need to make you any better or more perfect than you already are, as being? Can you feel how trying to acquire something can take you away from the feeling of being?

When you forget your true nature or being, you feel confused and disconnected. You believe there's something you must understand to feel whole again. Ask yourself: "What more do I need to know when I'm simply being?" When you're just being, is there anything you need to know that would make you any more connected than you already are, as being? You don't need extra knowledge to recognize the familiar feeling of being.

When you forget your true nature or being, you believe there's something you need to do to feel complete and whole again. Ask yourself: "What more do I need to do when I'm simply being?" When you're just being, is there anything you need to do that, by doing it, would make you any more complete than you already are, as being? Can you feel how being doesn't need any particular doing to be what and how it is? It's complete and whole just as it is.

Appendix 5B: A Practice of Engaging with Spanda

Starting in any comfortable or stable posture such as savasana or simple sitting, set an intention to move into another posture or body position. Before moving, try to feel into the very throb, pulse, or radiance of life within you—the sensation that life is living itself in or through you. This might be felt in one or many parts of the body. Then, as you focus thoughts on the posture or position you wish to take, before moving at all, feel into the subtle motive impulse(s) that arise before any movement. Slowly follow those impulses, letting them gradually express themselves as movements toward the new posture or position, being in no hurry to reach the final position and feeling the motive impulses in the various parts of the body preceding each part of the movement.

Appendix 5C: A Practice of Body Sensing

Starting the same way as with the practice of spanda engagement, tune into the motive impulses within the body. Let go of any preconceived idea of where and how the body is to move and simply allow the motive impulses to gradually create movements, be they small or large. With each new position in which you find your body, again tune into the motive impulse of spanda, following along with its spontaneous directions for movements without analysis or thought commentary. Allow spanda to dictate when the practice comes to a finish.

Appendix 5D: *Vijnana Bhairava Tantra* Meditation

Lift your hands and with a gesture
Turn aside all the forces of the outer world.
Attend to the vibrancy within.

Let the fingers lightly touch and bless
Eyes, ears, nostrils, mouth,
All the entrances to the head.
Invite attention to be within the skin, and
Cherish the quiet shimmer of vital energies.

When you notice an inner gateway,
Enter with love, as one coming home.

As the surge of light-substance rises
Follow it up into the space between the eyebrows
Where it breaks out as an orgasm of light.[35]

Endnotes

1 Wallis, C. (2014). *Tantra illuminated.* Mattamayura Press.

2 Rustogi, N. (1979). *The krama tantricism of Kashmir.* Motilal Banarsidass.

3 Singh, J. (1979). *Śiva sutras.* Motilal Banarsidass.

4 Ruvinsky, J. (2019). *The recognition of our own heart* (p. 18). Babaji's Kriya Yoga and Publishing.

5 Wallis, *Tantra illuminated.*

6 Wilberg, P. (2011). *The new spanda kārikās.* New Yoga Publications.

7 Singh, J. (1991). *Spanda kārikā.* Motilal Banarsidass.

8 Odier, D. (2004). *Yoga spandakārikā.* Inner Traditions.

9 Blashki, L. (2016, June). Spandana—Exploring healing pulsations [Conference session]. Symposium on Yoga Therapy and Research, Reston, Virginia. Handout. https://cdn.ymaws.com/www.iayt.org/resource/resmgr/Docs_SYTAR2016_General/2016_Handouts/Blashki_SYTAR2016.pdf

10 Odier, *Yoga spandakārikā.*

11 Singh, *Spanda kārikā.*

12 Wilberg, *New spanda kārikās.*

13 Wilberg, *New spanda kārikās* (p. 12).

14 Walsh, A. (2009). The resonant body: Preliminary considerations for social work practice. *Critical Social Work, 10*(1), 48–58 (p. 50).

15 Gaikwad, S., Jetli, P., Bapat, D., & Gaikwad, R. (2015). A study of parallels between modern physics and concept of spanda śāstra. *IJCA Proceedings on National Conference on Role of Engineers in Nation Building, 2015*(2), 19–23.

16 Smerdon, J. (2015). Contraction and expansion: The rhythm of life. *Shri Yoga.* www.shriyoga.com.au/contraction-and-expansion-the-rhythm-of-life

17 Singh, *Spanda kārikā.*

18 Taylor, M. J. (2018). *Yoga therapy as a creative response to pain.* Singing Dragon.

19 Farb, N., Daubenmier, J., Price, C. J., Gard, T., et al. (2015). Interoception, contemplative practice, and health. *Frontiers in Psychology, 6*, 763.

20 Wallis, *Tantra illuminated.*

21 Wilberg, *New spanda kārikās* (p. 14).

22 Wilberg, *New spanda kārikās* (p. 15).

23 Biernacki, L. (2014). A cognitive science view of Abhinavagupta's understanding of consciousness. *Religions, 5*(3), 767–779.

24 Singh, *Śiva sutras.*

25 Miller, R. (2015). When self falls away: Exploring key aspects of self and non-self. https://vimeo.com/ondemand/whenselffallsaway

26 Wallis, *Tantra illuminated* (p. 125).

27 Wallis, *Tantra illuminated* (p. 125).

28 Miller, R. (2019). *Integrative Restoration (iRest) yoga nidra meditation level 2 training manual.* iRest Institute.

29 Ruvinsky, J. (2019). *Recognition* (p. 20).

30 Miller, *Integrative Restoration.*

31 Odier, D. (2004). *Yoga spandakārikā.*

32 See, e.g., Roche, L. (2014). *The radiance sutras: 112 gateways to wonder and delight.* Sounds True.

33 Birch, J., & Hargreaves, J. (2015). Yoganidrā: An understanding of the history and context. *The Luminescent.* www.academia.edu/10140963/Yoganidr%C4%81_History_and_Context

34 See, e.g., Ruvinsky, *Recognition.*

35 Roche, *The radiance sutras* (p. 48) © 2014 excerpted with permission from the publisher, Sounds True, Inc.

Section II

BIOMEDICAL AND PSYCHOLOGICAL FOUNDATIONS

The most effective clinical work weaves together multiple threads to create a therapeutic relationship and plan tailored to the individual client. A working understanding of human physiology and psychology serves as a key thread for yoga therapists to use in clinical work.

It is not uncommon in yogic texts and philosophy to understand the human body by conceptualizing smaller parts or sections, which together make up the whole being (e.g., the *chakras* or the *panchamaya koshas*). Similarly, in human physiology, function is often understood through the systems model, in which groups of organs and tissues that work together (e.g., the digestive system, the cardiovascular system) are studied individually. These distinctions are helpful for educational purposes, and it is important to remember that these systems interconnect to form a complex human organism.

Knowing how physiological systems function through the biomedical lens allows the practitioner a deeper understanding of how yoga therapy may support clients. This knowledge opens the possibility of working in a truly integrative model and provides the opportunity for the yoga therapist to contextualize information about how the body works through the lens of yogic tradition.

This section emphasizes the role of evidence-informed practice, which some have misinterpreted to mean a centering of biomedical perspectives and a dismissal or marginalization of yogic principles. In fact, however, evidence-informed practice highlights the practitioner's role in combining an understanding of the extant biomedical evidence with their training and clinical experience, while considering the client's needs, values, and circumstances. Working within this model, yoga therapists may use their deep understanding of yogic values and philosophy as a lens through which to examine and interpret biomedical information.

Camille Freeman

6

Research Literacy: A Critical Skill for Yoga Therapists

CRYSTAL L. PARK

Research literacy is an essential skill set for yoga therapists, as it involves abilities to access, interpret, and critically evaluate scientific literature. These skills are not inherently intuitive, but they can be learned, practiced, and refined to enable yoga therapists to appropriately use the available literature. Successful research literacy requires that yoga therapists know how to formulate their clinical questions in a way that is searchable. When reading specific research articles, an ability to understand the basics of each study and evaluate the soundness of its findings is essential. Finally, yoga therapists must be skilled at determining how clinically meaningful and applicable the results are to their own work.

Research literacy is important for client care, for collaboration with colleagues, and for advancing the field of yoga therapy. Accessing and understanding research are essential for yoga therapists to implement evidence-informed practice. For these reasons, the International Association of Yoga Therapists (IAYT) considers research literacy a necessary competency. This chapter presents some basics on research literacy, which should help yoga therapists to find and evaluate information on the science of yoga.

Accessing Scientific Evidence

Many yoga practitioners and yoga therapists are highly committed to yogic practices and, through their personal experiences, have become convinced of their many benefits. This kind of intuitive knowing is highly meaningful to the practitioners themselves, but on its own is of limited utility for informing clinical practice or communicating with other healthcare professionals, clients, or the public.

Science has evolved as a set of philosophies and techniques (methods) to produce information that is "empirical"—knowable by others and replicable (i.e., repeatable by other scientists). The first step in using science to inform yoga therapy practice is to appropriately frame the question, to identify clearly the specific knowledge being sought.

Framing a research question

A research question is simply what one wants to know. A potentially infinite number of questions could be posed about yoga. How common is yoga practice? Who practices yoga? How much? What types? What are the barriers and facilitators to practicing yoga? What motivates practice? Does yoga help with a particular condition? What types of yoga practices are most effective for a particular condition? Are particular aspects of yoga (e.g., *asana*, *pranayama*, *yamas* and *niyamas*) more or less helpful—or even essential—for benefits to be manifested? How frequently or how long does one need to practice yoga to experience benefits? What happens to the benefits if one stops practicing yoga?

Some questions might arise out of curiosity or a desire to learn more about a study mentioned in the news. Or perhaps a client with a specific condition prompts a need for input on how to approach a treatment plan. When consulting the research literature in any of these cases, it is important to frame the question well to enable the location of the necessary information. Well-framed questions are clear, focused, and precise. For example, a yoga therapist might begin with a general question like, "How can I help a client with lower back pain?" A more useful research question would be, "What types of integrative medicine techniques have been shown to be effective in reducing pain in people with low back pain?"

Locating scientific information

Scientific information can come from many sources, sometimes classified as primary, secondary, and tertiary. "Primary sources" most often refers to original research reports based on data collected by the authors, although information obtained directly from an expert (in, e.g., ayurveda) may be considered primary in some cases.[1] Primary source articles are found in scientific journals, usually available online.

Articles published in journals that use peer review are typically of much higher quality than those in other publications. When an article has been reviewed by other expert scientists and returned to the authors for revisions, the final version of a peer-reviewed primary source often represents multiple iterations and more trustworthy findings. Beginning in the first decade of the 21st century, many predatory journals have appeared; these journals seldom use rigorous peer review and are driven by financial profit. It is increasingly difficult to determine the quality of a journal with which one is not familiar, and predatory journals often adopt titles that sound credible (and sometimes even quite similar to highly regarded journals). Thus, the onus of evaluating the quality of studies is increasingly falling on the reader, heightening the importance of sharp research literacy skills.

"Secondary sources" are summaries, descriptions, or reviews of original works. Secondary sources are usually written by someone other than the author of the original works. "Tertiary sources" are works produced by a writer or reporter who may reference the results of a study in a news report, blog, website, or magazine article. Tertiary reports are usually cursory and often overgeneralize or distort the findings of a study by shaping them to meet a particular editorial aim. Tertiary sources should thus be interpreted with skepticism; the best approach is to get the citation for the study (e.g., author[s], journal title) and locate the original primary source article.

Academic libraries can be tremendously helpful in locating journal articles. Even without access to an academic library, abstracts (brief summaries of journal articles) are easily available, but locating the full text of articles can sometimes be challenging. Academic libraries subscribe to search engines such as Scopus, PsychInfo, Cumulative Index of Nursing and Allied Health (CINAHL), and Web of Science, all of which may help locate articles relevant to a research question. The US federal government maintains PubMed, which is freely available (pubmed.ncbi.nlm.nih.gov). Another useful tool is Google Scholar (scholar.google.com). Both of these search engines will help in the location of relevant research articles. Often only the abstract of the article is available, but sometimes links direct readers to the final or penultimate version of the full text. Members of IAYT have access to articles published in the peer-reviewed *International Journal of Yoga Therapy.*

Understanding Yoga Research

Publications reporting on scientific studies of yoga are accumulating at an accelerating rate,[2] and making sense of the findings can seem overwhelming. However, the more familiar yoga therapists become with research issues, the more comfortable they will be with this literature.

There are two basic types of primary source research: descriptive studies and interventional studies. Within each of these types are many different specific methods, some of which are reviewed in this section. The research design of any particular study depends on the specific questions it is addressing. When evaluating a study, it is helpful to identify the key questions posed by the researchers and the rationale for the design employed.

Empirical studies measure "variables," factors that differ between people or within people over time. Variables correspond to the concepts of interest in the study. The process of mapping study variables onto the concepts of interest is called *operationalization*. The quality of operationalization should always be evaluated because operationalization can be a weak point in studies if researchers select variables that are not a good match to the concepts they are interested in measuring (Table 6.1).

Table 6.1 Evaluating study quality

Study Aspect	Questions to Help Determine Quality
Research question	Was the study clear in informing the reader of its overall purpose and specific aims? Was the study rationale clear and logical? Did the study rely on any theoretical base? Would another theoretical perspective have been more effective or appropriate? Did the study make specific hypotheses?
Background	Did the researcher thoroughly evaluate the relevant literature?
Study design	What method did the researchers employ? Were there alternative study designs that might better address the study question(s)?
Population and sample	Who were the study participants? How well does the sample represent the population to which it aims to generalize?
Sample size	How many participants were included in the study? Is the sample large enough to allow reasonable representation of the population and appropriate statistical analyses? Was a power analysis conducted to determine adequate sample size?
Response and attrition rate	What proportion of the selected sample completed the study? In longitudinal studies (those that measure the same variable[s] over time), what proportion of sample members participated in follow-up studies?
Main concepts and variables	Are each of the main variables or concepts of interest described fully? Are descriptions comprehensive, or are important aspects missing?
Operationalization of concepts	Did the authors choose variables that serve as good measures of the main concepts in the study? Have these variables been used in previous studies?
Study design	Was the design of the study appropriate to answer the research questions laid out in the introduction?
Missing data	Is the number of cases with missing data specified? Is the statistical procedure(s) for handling missing data described?
Appropriateness of statistical techniques	Does the study describe the statistical technique used? Does the study explain why the statistical technique was chosen? Does the study include caveats about the conclusions that are based on the statistical technique?

Control of confounding variables	Extraneous variation can influence research findings, so were methods to control relevant confounding variables applied?
Conclusions	What were the study's conclusions? Were these conclusions justified? Are there logical weaknesses in the argumentation? Does the study allow generalization? Does the study make a significant contribution to knowledge or understanding in the field?
Limitations and alternative explanations	Did the study discuss findings that were not consistent with expectations as well as those that were? Were limitations of the study mentioned? Could the results of the study be due to alternative explanations?

Descriptive studies

"Descriptive" studies are those in which no interventions or manipulations are made. These can be simple observational studies of behavior. For example, one could count how many people sign up for different types of yoga classes at a particular yoga studio. Most descriptive studies, however, go beyond simple observations and involve directly asking participants questions, either through interviews or surveys. An example of a simple descriptive study is shown in Box 6.1. The researchers in that study asked the participants some simple questions about themselves and their motivations for practicing yoga.

BOX 6.1 SIMPLE DESCRIPTIVE STUDY OF YOGA

Park, C. L., Quinker, D., Dubos, G., & Cramer, H. (2019). Motivations for adopting and maintaining a yoga practice: A national cross-sectional survey. *Journal of Alternative and Complementary Medicine*, 25(10), 1009–1014.

Background: Yoga practice is becoming increasingly popular around the world, yet little is known regarding *why* people adopt the practice of yoga or how their reasons for practice change with continued practice. Furthermore, whether those who practice different types of yoga have different motives remains unknown. **Methods:** To address these issues, the authors conducted a national cross-sectional online survey of 1,702 yoga practitioners in Germany, asking about demographic information and motives for initiating and continuing yoga practice. **Results:** The most common primary reasons for starting yoga were relaxation (26.6%) and prevention (25.5%), which were also the most common secondary reasons. Nine hundred and forty-one (55.3%) reported a different primary reason for maintaining than for adopting yoga practice. Prevention (38.4%) and spirituality (26.4%) were the most commonly reported primary reasons for maintaining yoga practice. More highly educated participants and those practicing longer than 5 years at the time of the survey were more likely to have reported a different current primary reason for yoga practice than that for which they started practicing. **Conclusions:** These results shed light on yoga's appeal to novices and regular practitioners, with important implications for making yoga appealing to beginners as well as promoting the practice as a long-term lifestyle behavior.

Some descriptive research is a detailed report of a single person, or "case," or of several cases. These case reports can be very useful for describing a new or unusual phenomenon, but their results generate hypotheses rather than conclusions. A "cohort study" follows a group of people over time to study associations among variables within the group. Descriptive research often uses standardized questionnaires to measure concepts that are of widespread interest, such as health-related quality of life or depression. Because these standardized scales are used in many different studies, they provide useful data for comparing the scores obtained in a study with those of other groups. An important component of questionnaires is their "validity," the extent to which the questionnaire measures what it purports to measure. In addition to self-report measures, yoga studies commonly include performance measures (e.g., of joint movement) or biomarkers (measurable indicators of biological states, e.g., interleukins or cortisol). Box 6.2 shows an example of a descriptive study that included standardized questionnaires of well-being.

BOX 6.2 DESCRIPTIVE STUDY INCLUDING STANDARDIZED QUESTIONNAIRES OF WELL-BEING

Park, C. L., Cho, D., & Wortmann, J. H. (2013). The impact of yoga upon young adult cancer survivors. *Complementary Therapies in Clinical Practice*, 19(2), 77–82.

This study explored the use of Yoga by using a cross-sectional analysis of 286 young adult cancer survivors. The aim was to explore yoga practice, reasons for using this therapy[,] predictors of yoga use and any potential relationship between yoga use and well-being. Ninety one participants (32.82%) reported practicing yoga from their initial diagnosis. Practitioners reported a relatively high intensity (mean: 7.46 h/month) and length (25.88 months) of practice.

The most common reasons given for undertaking yoga were to maintain flexibility and promote relaxation. Sociodemographic predictors of yoga use included gender [and] higher education. Greater use of yoga (overall amount of yoga practiced) was generally associated with better quality of life and positive states of mind. Results suggest that yoga...is more commonly used by cancer survivors with greater resources. Understanding more about the use of yoga by cancer survivors may facilitate the development and promotion of yoga-based interventions.

Observational studies are always open to multiple interpretations. These studies will be at best "correlational" in their approach to the data, meaning they assess whether two variables are related (as one variable increases, the other increases, or as one variable increases, the other decreases; see Figure 6.1).

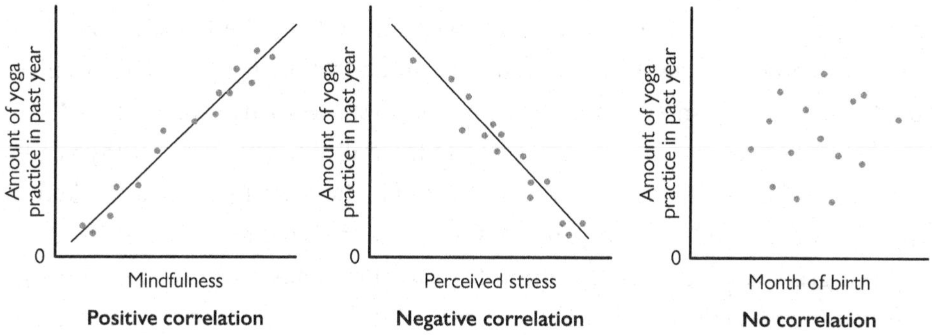

FIGURE 6.1 CORRELATIONS INDICATE RELATEDNESS BUT NOT CAUSALITY

Correlations indicate relatedness but should *never* be interpreted as indicating causality. It is always possible that another variable accounts for the relationship between any two variables. For example, in the study described in Box 6.2, it might be that the more yoga one does, the higher is one's health-related quality of life, or it could be that yoga leads to better mental and physical health, or that better health allows one to do yoga more frequently. Another possibility is that a third variable, such as financial resources or education, accounts for both more yoga practice and better health. Observational studies often try to account for ("control for") potential "confounding" third variables, effectively removing that confounding variable's influence, but it is impossible to identify every potential confound.

Interventional studies

"Interventional" studies involve manipulations. Some manipulations can be made in the context of a laboratory-based experiment (e.g., assigning yoga practitioners to two types of stressful encounters, such as an interpersonal argument versus loud intermittent noise, to see if they are better at handling one or the other type of stress). However, in the context of yoga therapy, most interventional research is designed to examine whether a yoga intervention is effective or to determine the mechanisms through which the yoga operates. These types of studies are termed "clinical trials." Some clinical trials include a single condition, or "arm"; other clinical trials include multiple conditions or arms. Measurements of the target health or well-being variable are taken at baseline, before the intervention starts, and at the end of the intervention. Sometimes additional follow-up measurement points are included to determine the extent to which the intervention effects last beyond its end.

A single-arm yoga trial typically measures the targeted health or well-being measure before and after the yoga intervention to test whether scores on the measure changed across the intervention period. Most often conducted to collect "pilot" (preliminary, small-scale) data, single-arm studies usually include relatively small sample sizes and aim to demonstrate feasibility (i.e., that the study is able to be carried out) rather than effectiveness (i.e., how well the yoga worked to influence the desired outcome). Box 6.3 illustrates a single-arm clinical trial.

Changes observed after the study (pre-to-post) may suggest that the yoga intervention was effective, but changes may have been observed for many other reasons. For example, the mere passage of time may have allowed improvements in health or symptom remission; the transition of season from winter to spring or a political or cultural shift might explain the changes in the targeted health or well-being variable. In addition, non-specific factors, such as the attention and expectancies of the participants, are always at play in intervention studies and can produce strong "placebo" effects.[3] These powerful non-specific factors are usually part of the reason individuals experience improvement in any behavioral or mind-body intervention and need to be considered as potential confounds (alternative explanations for the findings). Thus, single-arm trials can at best support therapeutic benefits of yoga; they are far from conclusive.

BOX 6.3 SINGLE-ARM CLINICAL TRIAL

Orsey, A., Park, C. L., Shankar, N., Pulaski, R., Popp, J. M., & Wakefield, D. (2017). Results of a pilot yoga intervention to improve pediatric cancer patients' quality of life and physical activity and parents' well-being. *Rehabilitation Oncology, 35*(1), 15–23.

Background and Purpose: Yoga is increasingly proving beneficial in improving distress, pain, physical activity, and health-related quality of life (QOL) in adult patients with cancer, but few studies have examined the efficacy of yoga therapy for pediatric patients with cancer. We aimed to study the feasibility and preliminary efficacy of a yoga intervention for pediatric cancer patients in active treatment and for their families. **Methods:** We conducted 2 separate studies: (1) a survey of 20 patients and parents regarding preferences (eg, convenient days and times), experiences, and expectations regarding yoga (including barriers and positive expectancies); and (2) an 8-week single-arm clinical trial of a yoga intervention in 10 children and their family members. Targeted outcomes of the clinical trial were patients' fatigue, QOL, and physical activity. Secondary outcomes were caregivers' well-being (QOL and burden). **Results:** Study 1 demonstrated fairly high levels of interest from patients and family members. Study 2 demonstrated improved patients' and parents' QOL pre- to post-yoga intervention. **Conclusions:** Parents and patients found the intervention highly acceptable. Conducting the intervention in the context of active cancer treatment proved feasible. Despite limited statistical power, QOL of patients doing yoga improved. Our findings support the notion that yoga for pediatric cancer patients during active treatment is feasible and potentially helpful in improving both patients' and parents' well-being.

Multiple-arm clinical trials of yoga are important to determine how well yoga works relative to a comparison condition. A true experimental design in a yoga intervention study—a "randomized controlled trial" (RCT)—is considered the gold standard in terms of evidence regarding the effects of the intervention (Figure 6.2).

In an RCT, participants are randomly assigned to one of two or more arms of a study, meaning that they have an equal chance of being in any condition. Pre-post measures are taken. One source of potential bias[4] in multiple-arm studies is the investigators' knowledge of the conditions to which specific participants are assigned (thus potentially exerting subtle influence over how the participants fare in the intervention). This potential problem can be overcome by blinding or masking evaluators in an intervention, although instructors may still subtly exert bias and blinding them is impossible. Interventions should report the extent to which the intervention showed "fidelity" to the treatment protocol or manual to ensure that the intervention was delivered as it was supposed to be.

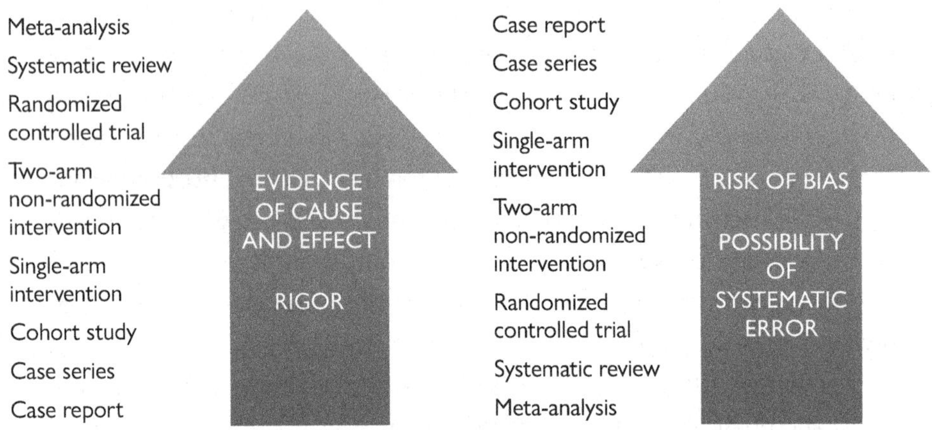

FIGURE 6.2 DIFFERENT TYPES OF CLINICAL RESEARCH VARY IN RIGOR AND RISK OF BIAS

Evaluating the results of RCTs requires close scrutiny of the adequacy of the comparison condition.[5] Sometimes the comparison condition is quite weak, such as a no-treatment control group for which pre–post measures are taken. The advantage of this study design over a single-arm trial is that it at least takes into account some of the potential confounds noted above, such as a change in the season or historical or cultural events (e.g., terrorist attacks, political elections) that might account for any noted changes in health or well-being. However, the powerful non-specific factors described above, such as participants' expectations for improvement rather than anything about the yoga intervention itself, cannot be ruled out as accounting for any observed pre-to-post changes.

A much stronger RCT design is to also control for non-specific factors by using an appropriate active comparison condition. This design requires the researchers to implement a comparison condition that matches yoga in terms of time, effort, attention, expectancies, instructor enthusiasm, plausibility, and other factors to help isolate the specific effects of the yoga relative to the control intervention. Box 6.4 offers an example of an RCT that employed an active comparator condition. Depending on the theory underlying the RCT, the active control might consist of, among other interventions, exercise, supportive counseling, cognitive therapy, health education, or physical therapy.[6]

BOX 6.4 RCT WITH AN ACTIVE COMPARATOR ARM

Riley, K. E., Park, C. L., Wilson, A., Sabo, A. N., et al. (2017). Improving physical and mental health in frontline mental healthcare providers: Yoga-based stress management versus cognitive behavioral stress management. *Journal of Workplace Behavioral Health*, 32(1), 26–48.

The need for brief, low-cost, easily disseminable, and effective interventions to promote healthy lifestyles is high. This is especially true for mental health providers. The authors developed two studies to compare the impacts of Cognitive Behavioral Stress Management (CBSM) and Yoga-Based Stress Management (YBSM) interventions for health care professionals. Study 1 offered an 8-week YBSM intervention to 37 mental health care participants and collected health data pre- and post. Study 2 offered YBSM and CBSM classes to 40 randomly assigned mental health care providers and collected mental and physical health data at four time points. In Study 1, using t tests, the YBSM intervention affected a number of mental and physical well-being indices pre to post. In Study 2, using linear mixed modeling, YBSM and CBSM groups both improved significantly ($p<.05$) in fruit and vegetable intake, heart rate, alcohol consumption, relaxation and awareness, professional quality of life, compassion satisfaction, burnout, depression, and stress levels. There was a group by time effect for coping confidence (CBSM increased more, $p<.05$, $F=4.34$), physical activity (YBSM increased more, $p<.05$, $F=3.47$), overall mental health (YBSM increased more, $p<.10$, $F=5.32$), and secondary traumatic stress (YBSM decreased more, $p<.10$, $F=4.89$). YBSM and CBSM appear to be useful for health care professionals' mental and physical health. YBSM demonstrates some benefit above and beyond the extremely well studied and empirically supported CBSM, including increased physical activity, overall mental health, and decreased secondary traumatic stress benefits.

Some clinical trials include multiple arms but do not assign participants randomly, a "quasiexperimental design" that precludes a demonstration of true causality. The lack of randomization is a serious limitation because it introduces the possibility that some factor besides the intervention led to any observed change in health or well-being. For example, if a study implemented two different intervention arms targeting depressive symptoms, a yoga class held in the morning and an exercise class at night, and allowed participants to choose to attend in the morning or evening, any differences between the groups could be due to the fact that the "morning people" and "night owls" who self-selected into the two conditions differ in the rates at which they recover from depression, among other possibilities.

Systematic reviews and meta-analyses

In addition to the two types of primary research described above, some researchers aggregate the results of many single studies by systematically reviewing the literature. Some of these reviews are simply narrative, describing the various findings, whereas others, such as meta-analysis, rely on formal statistical methods of aggregating and summarizing the findings of multiple studies.

These summaries can be useful in smoothing over some of the differences across studies (e.g., type or dosage of yoga) and allowing the bigger picture to emerge. Box 6.5 gives an example of a meta-analysis. In general, findings that have been replicated across many studies conducted in different places in different populations by different research groups tend to be more reliable than those with a narrower evidence base. However, interpreting results of reviews requires caution because limitations are always present. For example, the criteria used to determine which studies are included and which are left out should be scrutinized because these decisions will influence the conclusions drawn.

BOX 6.5 META-ANALYSIS

Wu, Y., Johnson, B. T., Acabchuk, R. L., Chen, S., et al. (2019). Yoga as antihypertensive lifestyle therapy: A systematic review and meta-analysis. *Mayo Clinic Proceedings*, 94(3), 432–446.

Objective: To investigate the efficacy of yoga as antihypertensive lifestyle therapy and identify moderators that account for variability in the blood pressure (BP) response to yoga. **Methods:** We systematically searched 6 electronic databases from inception through June 4, 2018, for articles published in English language journals on trials of yoga interventions that involved adult participants, reported preintervention and postintervention BP, and had a nonexercise/nondiet control group. Our search yielded 49 qualifying controlled trials (56 interventions). We (1) evaluated the risk of bias and methodological study quality, (2) performed meta-regression analysis following random-effects assumptions, and (3) generated additive models that represented the largest possible clinically relevant BP reductions. **Results:**

On average, the 3517 trial participants were middle-aged (49.2±19.5 years), overweight (27.9±3.6 kg/m²) adults with high BP (systolic BP, 129.3±13.3 mm Hg; diastolic BP, 80.7±8.4 mm Hg). Yoga was practiced 4.8±3.4 sessions per week for 59.2±25.0 minutes per session for 13.2±7.5 weeks. On average, yoga elicited moderate reductions in systolic BP (weighted mean effect size, -0.47; 95% CI, -0.62 to -0.32; -5.0 mm Hg) and diastolic BP (weighted mean effect size, -0.47; 95% CI, -0.61 to -0.32; -3.9 mm Hg) compared with controls (P<.001 for both systolic BP and diastolic BP). Controlling for publication bias and methodological study quality, when yoga was practiced 3 sessions per week among samples with hypertension, yoga interventions that included breathing techniques and meditation/mental relaxation elicited BP reductions of 11/6 mm Hg compared with those that did not (ie, 6/3 mm Hg). **Conclusion:** Our results indicate that yoga is a viable antihypertensive lifestyle therapy that produces the greatest BP benefits when breathing techniques and meditation/mental relaxation are included.

Evaluating studies: Factors to consider

Many useful resources and tools are available to evaluate the quality of a given study. Some of the key issues to consider are shown in Table 6.1; more detailed sources are listed in the Additional Resources.

Summary

This chapter provides a brief overview of research issues relevant to the scientific study of yoga. Yoga therapists are strongly encouraged to read more about how studies are conceived, conducted, and interpreted. When reading scientific literature, maintain an attitude of healthy skepticism. Because science advances by building on the current evidence base and pushing forward the boundaries of knowledge, the soundness of prior work is an essential foundation.

Being skeptical does not mean rejecting science, but rather evaluating it and looking at each study's strengths and weaknesses, ensuring that strong methods were used and interpretation of results was in accordance with the findings. In studies that claim causal connections, in particular, skepticism will help to determine whether any plausible alternative explanations might underlie the findings and suggest future research to better understand causal relationships.

As savvy consumers of the scientific literature on yoga, yoga therapists will enhance their professional credibility and advance yoga's therapeutic applications.

Research literacy allows yoga therapists to partake in larger conversations about which studies are needed to further the credibility and adoption of therapy practices. Research is a common language among medical professionals, and actively participating in these conversations can increase collaboration across professions and further yoga's inclusion in healthcare delivery systems.

Additional Resources

Erb, S., & Sullivan, M. (2017). I shall please—Placebo & yoga therapy. *Yoga Therapy Today*, Spring, 32–35.

Guthrie, S., Wamae, W., Diepeveen, S., Wooding, S., & Grant, J. (2013). Measuring research: A guide to research evaluation frameworks and tools. RAND Corporation. www.rand.org/pubs/monographs/MG1217.html

Menard, M. B. (2009). *Making sense of research* (2nd ed.). Curties-Overzet Publications, Inc.

Pain, E. (2016). How to (seriously) read a scientific paper. *Science*, March 21. http://dx.doi.org/10.1126/science.caredit.a1600047

Pyrczak, F., & Tcherni-Buzzeo, M. (2019). *Evaluating research in academic journals: A practical guide to realistic evaluation.* Routledge.

Subramanyam, R. V. (2013). Art of reading a journal article: Methodically and effectively. *Journal of Oral and Maxillofacial Pathology, 17*(1), 65–70.

US Centers for Disease Control and Prevention. (n.d.) Understanding scientific research. www.cdc.gov/des/consumers/research/understanding_scientific.html

Endnotes

1 For a discussion of evidence-based medicine, evidence-informed practice, and valid sources in clinical yoga therapy practice, see Sullivan, M., Finlayson, D., & Moonaz, S. (2017). Understanding yoga's roots in evidence-informed practice. *Yoga Therapy Today*, Summer, 40–42.

2 Park, C. L., Groessl, E., Maiya, M., Sarkin, A., et al. (2014). Comparison groups in yoga research: A systematic review and critical evaluation of the literature. *Complementary Therapies in Medicine, 22*(5), 920–929.
Wu, Y., Johnson, B. T., Acabchuk, R. L., Chen, S., et al. (2019). Yoga as antihypertensive lifestyle therapy: A systematic review and meta-analysis. *Mayo Clinic Proceedings, 94*(3), 432–446.

3 Kaptchuk, T. J., & Miller, F. G. (2015). Placebo effects in medicine. *New England Journal of Medicine, 373*(1), 8–9.

4 Bias in research occurs when "systematic error [is] introduced into sampling or testing by selecting or encouraging one outcome or answer over others" (Merriam-Webster, s.v. "bias," merriam-webster.com/dictionary/bias).

5 Park et al., Comparison groups.

6 For a review, see Park et al., Comparison groups.

7

Physiological Systems Foundations

ROBYN TIGER

The human body is composed of approximately 37 trillion cells, each with its own innate intelligence, structure, and function.[1] The cells can be thought of as players divided among body systems or teams. These teams simultaneously work together to maintain proper physiological function. (Chapter 4 discusses the systems from an ayurvedic perspective.)

A builder must first develop a strong structural foundation prior to constructing a house. Similarly, it is imperative that yoga therapists develop a foundational understanding of the body's systems to create and teach safe and effective client programs. This summary offers that foundational knowledge as viewed through the eyes of a yoga therapist and physician.

Circulatory System

The circulatory system includes three main components: (1) the heart, or the pump; (2) the hollow channels of the blood vessels; and (3) blood, the liquid medium carrying nutrients and waste within these channels throughout the body.

The heart

The heart, about the size of a fist, sits in the center left chest protected by the surrounding ribcage. The heart pumps blood to the body via the aorta and simultaneously to the lungs via the pulmonary artery. In the lungs, carbon dioxide is released and oxygen supplies restored. Once replenished, the oxygen-rich blood from the lungs returns to the heart, and the heart's muscular pumping mechanism sends the blood through increasingly smaller blood vessels to feed all of the body's cells.

The heart is divided into four main chambers: two atria and two ventricles. The chambers are separated by tissue walls called *septa*. One-way cardiac valves prevent blood from moving in the wrong direction. The atria and ventricles receive blood when their muscles are relaxed (*diastole*) and pump blood when their muscles contract (*systole*).

The heart contains two types of cells: cardiomyocytes (contractile cells; *myo* means muscle), which make up most of the heart, and a small percentage of pacemaker (electrical impulse) cells. Single cardiac cells placed outside the body can actually beat independently even when separated from the heart.

Blood vessels

Vessels of varying sizes and functions create a branching network of highways through which blood travels. Blood vessels are largest in diameter the closer they are to the heart. There are three types of blood vessels: arteries, veins, and capillaries.

Arteries carry blood away from the heart and are muscular, thick-walled vessels that contract and relax in response to signals in the body. Veins carry blood toward the heart and are thin-walled vessels composed predominantly of connective tissue with valves directing the flow of blood. Capillaries are tiny, permeable, even thinner walled vessels that form an intricate connection between arteries and veins for nutrient and waste exchange. There are between 60,000 and 100,000 miles of blood vessels in the human body (from child to adult), equivalent to 2.5 to 4 trips around the earth.[2]

Blood

Blood is composed of both liquid and solid components. Plasma, the liquid component, is the medium of transport for nutrients, waste, hormones, antibodies, enzymes, and cholesterol. Blood cells, the solid component, are made in the bone marrow. There are three main types of blood cells: Red cells (erythrocytes) carry oxygen, white cells (leukocytes) provide protection through immune function, and platelets (thrombocytes) are for clotting.

Systemic function

There is a specific continuous circuit by which blood flows through two simultaneous circulations: systemic (body) and pulmonary (lungs). In general, arteries carry oxygenated blood away from the heart and veins carry deoxygenated blood toward the heart. There is one exception: In the pulmonary system, the pulmonary arteries carry deoxygenated blood and pulmonary veins carry oxygenated blood.

It takes less than 1 minute for a single blood cell to make a complete cycle from heart to body and back. The heart contracts an average of 80 beats per minute, averaging 100,000 beats per day, and pumps 2,000 gallons of blood per day.[3]

The Respiratory System

The respiratory system is composed of three main components: the airway, lungs, and muscles of respiration. Its primary function is the exchange of oxygen (inhalation) and carbon dioxide (exhalation) within the lungs with each breath. A normal respiratory rate for adults is roughly 12 to 18 breaths per minute. (See Box 7.1 for more detail and a yogic perspective.)

BOX 7.1 RESPIRATORY PHYSIOLOGY FOR YOGA THERAPY PRACTICE

SUNDAR BALASUBRAMANIAN

Regardless of the form it takes, respiration is an essential physiological process for all living beings, from single-cell organisms to large animals. The human system is equipped to use oxygen, which makes up 21 percent of atmospheric air, through breathing.

At rest under normal conditions, the process of oxygen entering the body (Figure 7.1) requires 6 to 8 liters of air per minute (minute ventilation or minute volume) and can be altered by physiological conditions including physical and emotional status or exercise. Involuntary breathing normally is shallow and exchanges about half a liter of air (tidal volume), whereas the inhalation and exhalation can be forced voluntarily to a maximum possible extent. The maximum forced inspiration plus maximum forced expiration constitutes the vital capacity (Figure 7.2), and studies have indicated that certain types of *pranayama* could improve vital capacity when practiced over time.[4]

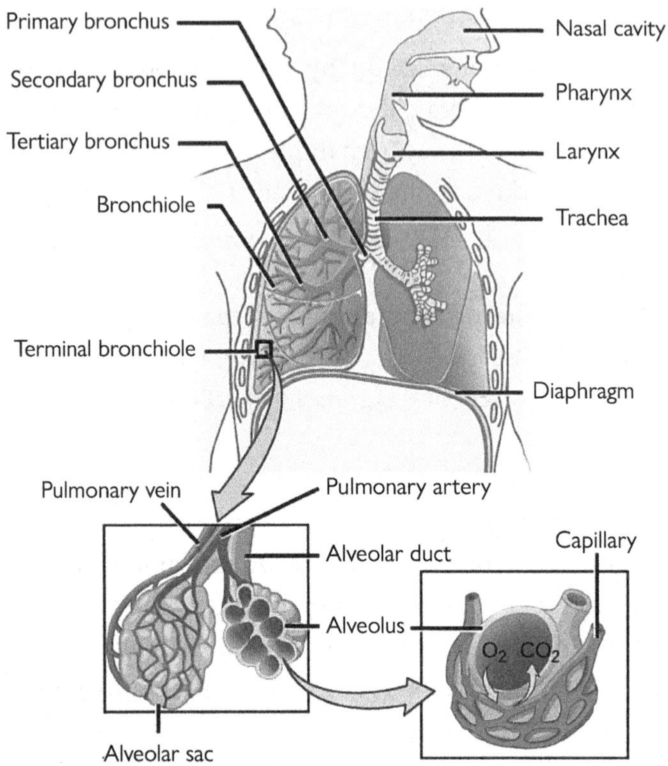

FIGURE 7.1 OVERVIEW OF THE RESPIRATORY SYSTEM

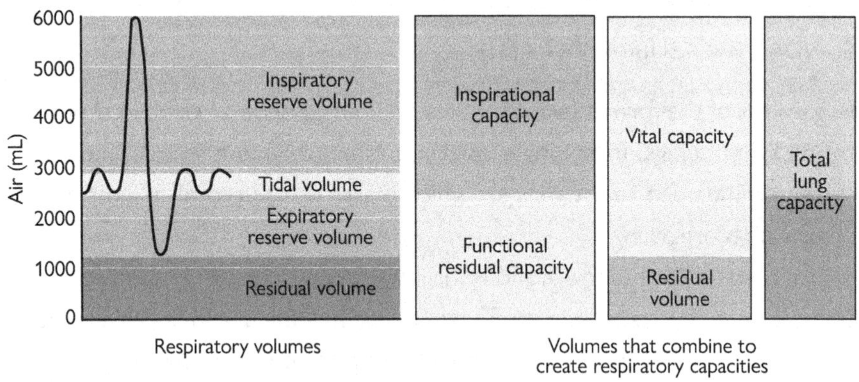

FIGURE 7.2 RESPIRATORY VOLUMES AND THE COMBINATION OF VOLUMES THAT RESULTS IN RESPIRATORY CAPACITIES

The key feature in the process of oxygen diffusion from alveoli (the final destination, or functional subunit of the respiratory system) into capillaries is that the distance between these two entities is less than 100 microns. This thin barrier is not only found in the alveoli but also in nasal and oral airway capillary linings.

Breathing and the chakras

As noted in the main chapter, the respiratory system can be classified into the upper and lower respiratory tracts. This classification is also helpful for understanding pranayama. The lower respiratory tract is mainly the lungs and encompasses the *anahata* (cardiac plexus) and *manipura* (solar plexus) chakras. The upper respiratory tract is related to the *ajna* and *sahasrara* chakras (both part of the carotid plexus). *Vishuddha* (pharyngeal plexus) acts as the bridge between the upper and lower respiratory tracts.[5]

The lower respiratory tract is involved in the primary alveolar gas exchange, facilitated by contraction of the diaphragm, intercostal, and accessory muscles of the shoulders and the chest. Activation of the cardiac and solar plexi stimulates deeper and slower breathing or ease in breathing. This also could activate vagal afferents to contribute to a relaxation response and could improve heart rate variability (HRV), the ability of the heart to better adapt to changes in physiological demand by altering the beat-to-beat intervals.[6] Abdominal involvement through activation of the diaphragm helps with deep breathing to reach total lung capacity of 4.5 to 6 liters.

Exhalation to the fullest possible extent (forced expiratory capacity) activates the lower plexi, *svadhisthana* (pelvic plexus) and *muladhara* (coccygeal plexus). Although both muladhara and svadhisthana can be activated through physical means like asana, extended exhalation is an important way to connect the chakras and may increase awareness of the lower chakras and their functions.

The upper respiratory tract and the nasal cycle

While the lower respiratory tract is key to the physical process of breathing, the upper respiratory tract connects the breath to the conscious state and ultimately the spiritual level. The upper respiratory tract, which houses the nostrils, oropharynx and nasopharynx, sinuses, and olfactory bulbs, physically conditions the air and provides mucosal immunity.

Air enters the nostrils and moves through the sinuses, setting the optimum physiological temperature and moisture. During this process, information is also sent to the olfactory bulb, making the nostrils a major information source for the brain. The olfactory bulb neurons are the most exposed central nervous system neurons, connecting an external organ directly to the central nervous system. It is through the nostrils that environmental cues are sent to the brain hemispheres contralaterally.

The nasal cycle, an ultradian rhythm that changes every 2 to 4 hours, alters this neural input. The right nostril (also referred to as *pingala* or *surya nadi*) is linked to increasing heart rate and blood pressure, whereas the opposite is true with the left nostril (also called the *ida* or *chandra nadi*).[7] An exercise such as alternate-nostril breathing facilitates the passage of air through both nostrils equally and thus would be expected to balance the heart rate and blood pressure. Research suggests that this exercise improves attention and reduces errors in hand-eye coordination tasks.[8]

According to the Siddha tradition (see Chapter 19), the nasal cycle follows a pattern throughout the week: Mondays, Wednesdays, and Fridays are left-nostril dominant; and Saturdays, Sundays, and Tuesdays are right-nostril dominant. Thursdays are an exception, as the left nostril is dominant during the waxing moon phase, and the right nostril is dominant during the waning moon phase.[9] Siddha tradition values entraining the nasal cycle as a way to attain higher consciousness.

It can be hypothesized that changes in nostril dominance regulate the individual olfactory bulbs, which, in turn, could connect to the piriform cortex and individual hippocampal areas, leading to altered hemispheric dominance; thus, the nasal cycle may be not only a way to keep the airways moist or a cleaning cycle as is commonly perceived.[10] The nasal cycle may also change according to the state of mind and external cues such as physical posture, age, etc.

The sinuses

The sinuses are yet another important component of the upper airway. The four pairs of sinuses on each side of the face—frontal, ethmoidal, sphenoid, and maxillary sinuses—are key areas where immune cells are activated by external information (e.g., an allergen).

The sinuses, innervated by branches of the trigeminal nerve, stimulate the secretion of several types of neurohormones. The sinuses drain into the nasal passage, thereby connecting to the oral cavity and the gut. Slow breathing practices may remove stale air in the sinuses by efficiently circulating air through them.

Preliminary animal research suggests that spontaneously occurring low-frequency vasomotion (contraction and dilation of blood vessels) allows the removal of waste products from the brain.[11] Studies in humans have found a link between respiration and the way the non-neuronal (glial) cells organize to function as the lymphatic system of the brain (known as the glymphatic system) to help circulate cerebrospinal fluid, removing metabolic waste from the brain.[12] Glymphatic circulation is promoted by sleep, and meditative/relaxation practices including pranayama could promote glymphatic flow to maintain the health of the central nervous system. Because slow breathing in particular may improve vasomotion,[13] this is a potential pathway to clear metabolic waste such as amyloid plaques, a hallmark of Alzheimer's disease.

The sinuses open to the airway through small *ostia*. These small openings allow gas exchange between the sinuses and airway. During sinusitis (nasal congestion), the ostia are blocked by mucus or air-pressure changes. Pranayama such as *bhramari* (humming bee breathing) could help with breaking up sinus congestion.

Connecting awareness of ajna chakra at the middle of the eyebrows to respiration allows fine sensation of the movement of the breath through the upper respiratory tract. In the Siddha tradition, this is considered an important step toward attaining higher consciousness through awareness of the central channel of *sushumna (suzhumunai) nadi*.[14]

Other significant upper respiratory tract areas related to pranayama are the salivary glands, soft palate, and tongue. Activation of the salivary glands through the relaxation response evoked by pranayama could lead to the secretion of biomolecules with significant physiological activities and implications for immunity and digestive function (see Chapter 19). Awareness of the soft palate during breathing exercises (e.g., *ujjayi*) could connect the lower and upper respiratory tracts toward the activation of sushumna nadi.

The bridge between upper and lower airways

Vishuddha, the throat chakra, also bridges the upper and lower respiratory tracts. Breathing, speech, and swallowing are finely coordinated here. This includes the pause in breathing when swallowing, altering air flow to change the pitch and volume of the voice, and regulating the volume of breath during oral breathing. Several minor salivary glands located in the throat region could also be activated through pranayama.

In summary, the lower respiratory tract provides a mechanism for gas exchange through the lungs. The upper respiratory tract is associated with connecting the breathing, via environmental cues, to the functioning of the brain. Both the lower and upper respiratory tracts could be activated and utilized for overall well-being through pranayama practice.

The airway

The airway is the passageway by which the breath travels to and from the lungs. It is divided into the upper and lower respiratory tracts.

Upper respiratory tract

Air enters the body through either the nose or mouth, collects in the pharynx (back of the throat), and continues downward into the larynx (voice box). The nostrils contain cilia (small hairs) that prevent unwanted particles from entering. Mucus is secreted to eliminate any trapped particles. The mucous membranes within the nostrils warm the incoming air before it travels deeper into the body.

Lower respiratory tract

Air continues downward from the larynx to the trachea (windpipe), which extends through the neck to the mid-chest. The trachea can be imagined as the trunk of an upside-down tree with two main branches: The right and left main stem bronchi each enter a lung. These bronchi further branch into smaller bronchi, which divide into even smaller bronchioles that terminate in tiny air sacs called alveoli. It is here in the alveoli where gas exchange takes place. Each alveolus is only about 0.2 mm in diameter; each lung has more than 400 million alveoli.[15]

The lungs

Filling the space within the rib cage are two lungs surrounding the centrally placed heart. The lungs are divided into sections, or lobes. The right lung has three lobes, and the left has two. The lungs are triangular, narrowest at the top and widest at the bottom. The lower, widest part of each lung is where the highest concentration of alveoli and blood vessels resides and the largest amount of gas exchange takes place.

Alveoli can be thought of as tiny, thin-walled balloons with numerous capillaries filling the walls. Gas exchange between the alveoli and capillaries occurs within these walls. Inhaled oxygen molecules cross the alveolar wall and enter the capillary blood to be transported to the body. Carbon dioxide leaves the capillary blood by crossing the alveolar wall, entering the alveoli to be exhaled.[16]

Breath also plays a role in maintaining the body's correct pH levels, which occur within a narrow, tightly regulated range. The amount of carbon dioxide exhaled affects the pH of the blood; if insufficient CO_2 is released, the blood becomes more acidic (pH decreases). The brain and lungs are able to regulate blood pH by adjusting the speed and depth of the breath.

Oxygen makes up 21 percent of the air that we breathe and is the key ingredient required by the body's cells to burn sugars and fats to make energy. Cells require a steady flow of oxygen to function properly.

The muscles of respiration

The pumping force that moves air in and out of the lungs is predominantly created by the diaphragm, a dome-shaped muscle that separates the thorax from the abdomen. It is assisted by the intercostal muscles between the ribs. On inhalation, the diaphragm flattens and lowers, the intercostal muscles contract and expand the ribcage, and air is drawn inward. On exhalation, the diaphragm, intercostal muscles, and ribcage relax and air is pressed out.

Accessory muscles of respiration include the scalenes and sternocleidomastoids in the neck, the pectorals, and the abdominals.[17] These muscles become more involved in respiration as a result of exertion and stress, so yoga therapy assessment might include visualization of which muscles a client habitually engages during breathing. The diaphragm is the only muscle in the body that contains both smooth and striated muscle. It can function under involuntary and voluntary control. Voluntarily controlling the breath is a key yoga therapy tool.

The Nervous System

The nervous system is divided into two main systems: central and peripheral.

Central nervous system

The central nervous system (CNS) is composed of the brain and spinal cord. The cells of the nervous system (neurons) communicate with one another through electrical signals (impulses) and chemical signals (neurotransmitters). The CNS contains billions of neurons. Nerves, which are projections of neurons, contain bundles of fibers (tracts) and can be only sensory (afferent), only motor (efferent), or mixed. Neurons conduct nerve impulses: Dendrites receive impulses from within the CNS and project toward the soma (cell body), whereas the single axon carries information away from the soma (either within the CNS or toward the peripheral nervous system).

Protected by the skull, the brain analyzes, processes, and responds to information received from the body. The brain is divided into the cortex, cerebellum, and brainstem and made up of gray matter (neurons), white matter (axons), and supporting cells (glia). The axons are thin neural extensions by which signals travel between neurons. Twelve pairs of cranial nerves with sensory, motor, and combined functions derive from the brain or brainstem.

The cortex is divided into the right and left hemispheres, each of which contains four lobes. The frontal lobe, located in the anterior cortex, controls cognition, decision-making, problem-solving, and movement. The parietal lobe, in the mid-cortex, processes sensory information and interprets body position, movement, language, and mathematics. The temporal lobe, in the lateral (side) cortex, is responsible for hearing, memory, emotions, and speech. The occipital lobe, in the posterior (back) cortex, governs vision.

The cerebellum, below and behind the cortex, controls motor movement and balance. The brainstem connects the brain and spinal cord and controls basic body functions including breath, heart rate, blood pressure, sleep, temperature, and swallowing.

The spinal cord is protected by the vertebral column and travels through the vertebral canal. It provides the two-way information path between brain and body. The spinal cord and the body communicate through 31 pairs of spinal nerves. The spinal cord is also responsible for reflex movements.

Figure 7.3 illustrates specific regions of the brain.

Peripheral nervous system

The peripheral nervous system is divided into sensory and motor branches. The sensory (afferent) division detects sensory information from the body and sends that information to the CNS. The motor (efferent) division sends processed and reflex information from the CNS to the body. The motor branch divides further into the somatic motor system, responsible for voluntary skeletal muscle movement, and the autonomic ("automatic") nervous system (ANS), responsible for involuntary visceral functions. The enteric nervous system is the largest portion of the ANS and governs gastrointestinal function primarily independently of the CNS; the "gut-brain axis" represents the significant bidirectional communication between the CNS and enteric nervous system. Yoga therapy often focuses on decreasing the stress response via the ANS.

The ANS is an essential control panel that maintains internal balance (homeostasis). It regulates crucial body functions including heart and respiratory rate, blood pressure, digestion, and hormone levels. The vagus nerve, cranial nerve 10, is an integral component in this regulation. (See Chapter 16 for a discussion of polyvagal theory.)

The **cerebrum**, which contains several deep structures that have essential central nervous system functions, consists primarily of the two hemispheres/four lobes, along with subcortical structures including the hippocampus and olfactory bulb.

The **somatomotor cortex** is housed in the distal (back) portion of the frontal lobe.

The **somatosensory cortex** is distal to the somatomotor cortex, in the parietal lobe.

The homunculi mentioned in Chapter 21 are located in these cortices. Each cerebral hemisphere contains sensory and motor representations of the contralateral side of the body; specific areas of the body send neural signals to defined areas of the cortex.

Behavior, emotions, judgment, planning, problem-solving, speaking and writing, movement, concentration, self-awareness, and intelligence are housed in the **frontal lobes** of the brain.[a]

The **parietal lobe** is responsible for interpreting language, vision, sensory information, memory, and hearing. This area of the brain interprets touch, pain, and temperature. Visual and spatial perception are also housed here.

The primary goal of the **temporal lobe** (not shown) is auditory processing. It is responsible for understanding language, long-term memory, sequencing, and organization. This area processes information from the senses of smell, taste, and sound.

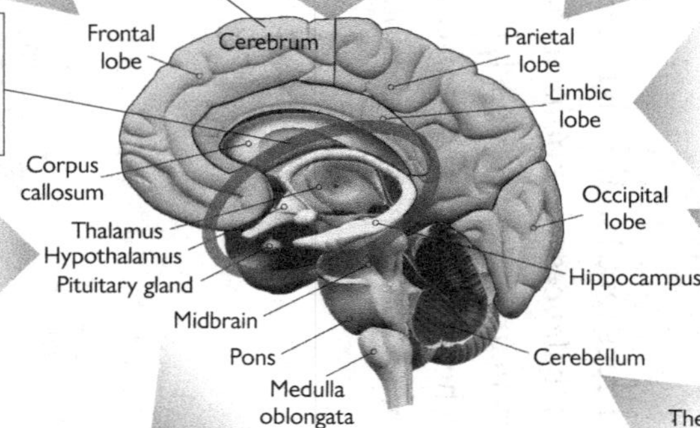

The limbic system contains the **limbic cortex**, **hypothalamus**, **amygdala**, **hippocampus**, and **septal area.** This system is involved with emotional state and the formation of memories.

The **hypothalamus** links the nervous and endocrine systems and is responsible for maintaining homeostasis by affecting blood pressure, heart rate, sleep, temperature, hormones, weight, appetite, and thirst.

The **occipital lobe** interprets vision; color, light, and movement are processed here.

The **cerebellum**, under the **cerebrum**, coordinates movement, maintaining posture and balance.

The **brainstem** includes **midbrain**, **pons**, and **medulla.** This relay center connects the **cerebrum** and **cerebellum** to the **spinal cord** and controls autonomic functions (e.g., respiration, heart rate, body temperature, sleep cycles, digestion, sneezing, coughing, vomiting, swallowing). Ten of the 12 cranial nerves originate in the **brainstem**.

FIGURE 7.3 SAGITTAL VIEW OF BRAIN REGIONS AND KEY STRUCTURES

[a]The frontal lobe, which is vital in moderating social behavior, arousal, cognition, and mood, is often the area damaged in traumatic brain injury. McAllister, T. W. (2011). Neurobiological consequences of traumatic brain injury. *Dialogues in Clinical Neuroscience*, *13*(3), 287–300.

Figure developed with assistance from Kelli Bethel.

The ANS is divided into the sympathetic nervous system (SNS) and parasympathetic nervous system (PNS), which work together to maintain homeostasis. One mechanism for yoga therapy's effects is thought to be improved balance in the SNS and PNS.

The SNS activates the human system in response to a demand or threat (real or imagined). This activation, like pressing on the gas pedal in a car, is called the fight/flight/freeze, or stress, response. Its neurotransmitters, epinephrine (adrenaline) and norepinephrine (noradrenaline), work to dilate pupils, increase heart rate, increase blood pressure, dilate bronchi, and divert blood flow to the brain and large muscles to ready the body for action. The SNS shuts down or impairs non-urgent functions such as the digestive and immune systems to redirect resources to emergency needs.

The PNS allows for regeneration through the rest and digest, or relaxation, response (Figure 7.4). It balances the actions of the SNS, like pressing on the car's brake pedal. Its primary neurotransmitter, acetylcholine, works to constrict pupils and bronchi, decrease heart rate and blood pressure, stimulate digestion, store energy, and allow for proper immune system function.

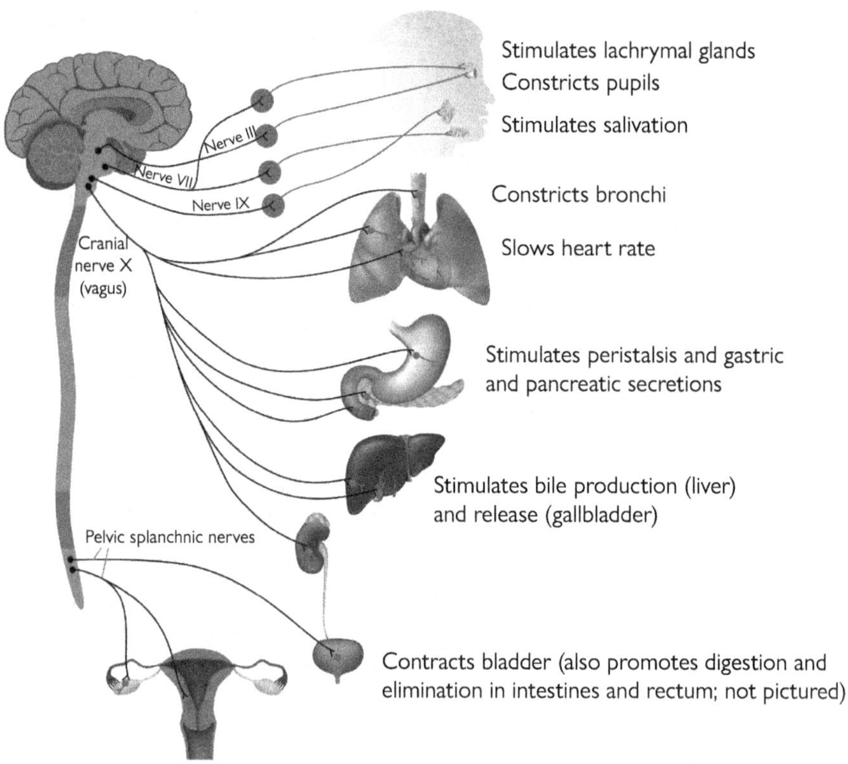

FIGURE 7.4 MAJOR PARASYMPATHETIC NERVOUS SYSTEM FUNCTIONS

With chronic stress comes loss of homeostasis. The SNS works overtime, pressing the gas pedal to the floor. The resulting overproduction of the stress hormone cortisol significantly damages the body's cells and tissues and is responsible for many types of illnesses.

The Endocrine System

The endocrine system is a complex integrated network of four main components: glands, hormones, bloodstream, and target organs. Like the nervous system, the endocrine system is integrally involved in body system communication. Endocrine glands secrete hormones (chemical messengers) that circulate through the bloodstream, attach to specific cell receptors on target organs, and communicate a needed function in that organ to maintain homeostasis in the body. The endocrine system works primarily through negative feedback loops. Some glands act as internal thermostats, sensing the amounts of circulating hormones to determine the need for increased or decreased hormone secretion.

Pituitary gland and hypothalamus

The pea-sized pituitary gland is located below the center of the base of the brain and connected to the brain by the hypothalamus. Known as the "master gland," the pituitary secretes many hormones that communicate with other glands, which in turn release hormones that deliver instructions to cells and organs throughout the body. The hypothalamus secretes many hormones, most of which communicate directly with the pituitary gland.

Adrenal glands

The adrenal glands sit on top of each kidney like a hat. The adrenals are known as the "stress glands," as they play an integral role in the SNS and stress response. The outer cortex is part of the hypothalamic-pituitary-adrenal (HPA) axis and secretes cortisol in response to pituitary adrenocorticotropic hormone (ACTH), which regulates the chronic stress response. The cortex also secretes aldosterone for water balance. The inner medulla of the adrenal gland secretes epinephrine and norepinephrine (catecholamines) through direct neural stimulation by hypothalamic signals that communicate by way of the thoracic spinal cord.

Thyroid gland

The thyroid gland, shaped like a butterfly, sits in front of the trachea below the larynx. The thyroid gland secretes thyroid hormones to regulate metabolism.

Parathyroid glands

The four parathyroid glands are located behind the thyroid. These glands secrete parathyroid hormone, which targets the bones, kidneys, and intestines to regulate calcium levels.

Thymus gland

The thymus gland, part of both the endocrine and immune systems, is located behind the sternum between the lungs. It is most active from birth to puberty and is responsible for differentiating T-cells, white blood cells important for the adaptive immune response.

Pancreas

The pancreas is located in the central left abdomen behind the stomach. Its islet cells secrete hormones to both raise and lower blood sugar (glucose) levels. Insulin lowers blood sugar by stimulating blood sugar transport into cells for energy storage as glycogen. Glucagon increases blood sugar by breaking down glycogen to make glucose for energy use (see Box 7.2).

Pineal gland

The pineal gland is a pea-sized, cone-shaped gland located in the central brain between the thalami. It secretes melatonin, which modulates the circadian rhythm and sleep cycle.

Gonads

The gonads—ovaries and testes—secrete hormones including estrogen and testosterone that stimulate the development of eggs and sperm. They are also responsible for determining secondary sex characteristics such as hair growth, muscular size, and voice depth.

BOX 7.2 CLINICAL APPLICATION OF YOGA THERAPY IN DIABETES CARE

JUDI BAR

The endocrine system is complicated, regulating directly or indirectly all other body systems. Although yoga must be considered a complementary therapy for the care of diabetes and other endocrine conditions, it can have a significant effect on the endocrine system and on symptomatology, contributing to the healing process.

To regulate glucose (blood sugar) levels, which are implicated in diabetes development, the body primarily uses the hormone insulin. Physical movement, including *asana*, engages skeletal muscle, which can also aid in glucose use (and process the molecule directly, independent of insulin); particularly when larger skeletal muscles such as the quadriceps or latissimus dorsi are involved, physical exercise is an excellent glucose-regulation technique.[18] The lifestyle modifications that are within a yoga therapist's purview may be particularly helpful for downregulating the sympathetic response, supporting better balance in body systems and working toward homeostasis.

Stress response

Diabetes is one of the most prevalent endocrine disease processes faced by contemporary society. In the United States, 34.2 million adults have type 1 or 2 diabetes; 26.9 million of these cases are diagnosed, leaving 7.3 million undiagnosed. Eighty-eight million people over the age of 18 have prediabetes, and 24.2 million people who are 65 or older have prediabetes.[19]

During a stress response, the hypothalamus sends a signal to the pituitary gland to produce a hormone that signals the adrenal glands, via the process of the hypothalamic-pituitary-adrenal (HPA) axis, to increase the production of epinephrine (adrenaline), norepinephrine (noradrenaline), and cortisol. Epinephrine stimulates the sympathetic nervous system's fight/flight response (increasing heart rate, respiratory rate, blood flow to skeletal muscle, etc.), whereas norepinephrine suppresses the parasympathetic system's rest-and-digest functions (including digestion, reproductive-hormone release, melatonin production for sleep, and detoxification processes). Cortisol eventually suppresses insulin's functions, increasing levels of sugar, or glucose, in the bloodstream. Cortisol, although extremely helpful and necessary in an acute stressful situation, is detrimental when constantly present.

Many people live in a state of chronic stress in which cortisol and other stress-related hormones are being continually secreted. This ongoing barrage can be harmful over the long term and impacts many of the body's systems. Stress hormones affect the way the body metabolizes sugars and fats, potentially leading to diabetes. A diagnosis of type 2 diabetes represents the end stage of metabolic syndrome, a cluster of conditions that occur together and include heart disease, high blood sugar (hyperglycemia), excess body fat around the waist, and usually abnormal cholesterol and triglyceride levels.

The diagnosis

The mechanism of type 1 diabetes (previously known as juvenile diabetes), in which the body does not produce sufficient insulin, differs from that of type 2 diabetes. Type 2 diabetes (previously known as adult-onset diabetes) can be differentiated into insulin-dependent and non-insulin-dependent types. In both cases, the body's cells are unable to use the glucose in the bloodstream and it builds to harmful levels.

Yoga therapists need to be aware of clients' diagnoses and, if at all possible, remain in contact with their healthcare providers, as glucose levels have important effects on physical and mental function. Reducing stress may reduce cortisol, lowering glucose and potentially decreasing the need for medication; in this case, a client could experience symptoms of *hypo*glycemia (low blood sugar), including dizziness/light-headedness or weakness, so it is important that clients and their doctors understand these possible effects.

This background information is important to understanding stress-management techniques, which overlap with lifestyle and behavioral changes for the client.

Client considerations

When meeting with a new client it is vital to get a better understanding of their overall health and lifestyle. An in-depth intake should include information on sleep patterns, mood, eating habits, work/life balance, exercise, stress, spiritual practices if any, and overall well-being.

Yoga therapists who can support clients to calm the stress response with practices based in self-observation and presence will be better able to help them, affecting their overall health and well-being. The way the client takes these principles off the mat to make mindful lifestyle choices is as important as the daily practice itself. As an adjunct to accessible asana, pranayama, and meditation techniques, writing in a journal can boost accountability and provide a means for the client to review progress.

As one of the main purposes of yoga therapy for clients with diabetes will likely be to provide coping tools to help curtail the stress response, which can help to regulate glycemic control, mindfulness practice can be a useful basis for the plan of care. The mindful client can make conscious decisions about health and well-being.

Using the breath can bring clients into the moment to assist in conscious decision-making. One possibility is the introduction of 10-second practices using the five senses. Consider beginning with twice a day and gradually expand to ten times a day. Such a practice slows the client down, cultivating gratitude and appreciation of the simple pleasures in life. This, in turn, begins to change thought patterns. A lower stress burden creates the possibility to begin making more conscious choices about food and other aspects of health. It may be useful to refer to a dietician if the client is unsure of dietary choices and their impact.

When the client is ready for asana practice, consider seated and standing chair-assisted poses consisting of range of motion (ROM; primarily stretching major muscle groups), core strengthening, and balancing. Negative self-talk may well be part of a client's story, especially if they have type 2 diabetes, and this kind of practice offers accomplishment in a simple way. Include basic belly breathing, a foundational breath practice that humans do from birth but is bypassed by the stress response. This pranayama can be carried into the client's day as they learn to stay "in the moment."

Slow and easy cueing is important, with mindfulness and gratitude woven throughout the session. Introduce any appropriate *yamas* or *niyamas*.

Techniques to avoid, particularly early on, include

- complex, multilayered practices
- breath retention or complicated pranayama
- intentionally or specifically attempting to stimulate organs or glands—less is more

A general practice will be more than sufficient and safer. The motion of asana and breathwork stimulates circulation, important for nerve health in diabetes because circulating oxygen-rich blood helps to prevent peripheral artery disease (PAD).[20] Yoga's capacity to improve stress management supports the normalization of biomarkers like HbA1c (a measure of glucose levels over time).[21]

Case example

In addition to type 2 diabetes, "Jayne," who is 55 years old, has obesity, anxiety, unspecified lower back pain, generalized achy joints, and knee pain. She is postmenopausal (an important consideration because a decrease in sex hormones predisposes females to osteoporosis). Jayne does not get much exercise and reports no spiritual or relaxation practices. She has lethargy and likely untreated depression (which she denies). Yogic assessment (not detailed here) suggests excess *tamas*.

Practice goals: more ease in joints, relax excess muscular tension, and improve core awareness and strength in mindful seated and standing postures. Establish a relaxed diaphragmatic breath.

Contraindications and considerations:

- **Diabetes:** dizziness
- **Obesity:** excess tissue potentially obstructing movement
- **Anxiety:** shortness of breath
- **Joint aches:** joint pain; avoid extensive pressure, employ gentle ROM[22]
- **Lower back pain:** no specific diagnosis, so begin slowly, depend on Jayne's ability to move; focus on relaxing tension and on alignment during core strengthening
- **Knee pain:** avoid floor work, stretch gently, eventually strengthen leg muscles (especially quadriceps and adductors)

Sample trajectory of sessions:

- The first session includes intake, basic gentle ROM exercises, easy breathwork and a meditation to do at home, co-creating goals, and explaining the logistics of a home practice.
- Incorporating client feedback, the next session gives Jayne more specific content with which to practice:
  - **body awareness** (posture and how the body feels in the present moment): begin to teach "being in the body" through mindfulness, demonstrating that the client can make conscious choices about how the body feels

  - **breath awareness** (and avoiding breath holding): cultivating a more relaxed and conscious breath through mindful attention
- Daily home yoga therapy practice, as co-developed with Jayne, includes 20 minutes of asana and pranayama and
  - **mindful walking:** start with 5 minutes and add 5 minutes each week (goals of getting out in nature and building activity)
  - **relaxation practice** (e.g., listening to a meditation recording; whatever works best for her)
  - **gratitude journal with intentions and affirmations**—eventually orienting thoughts to a more positive and hopeful way of looking at life
- Add **mudras** when Jayne exhibits being ready (through openness to something she is not familiar with).
- Build and expand the program according to feedback from and observation of the client throughout sessions.

The Digestive System

The digestive system is a complex highway of anatomic parts and accessory organs by which food enters; food is deconstructed, processed into nutrients, and absorbed, and waste products are eliminated. These processes occur through both chemical and mechanical digestion.

Mouth

Mechanical digestion begins in the mouth with the teeth grinding food into smaller particles to increase surface area and improve the efficiency of chemical digestion. Salivary glands act as accessory organs by secreting saliva into the mouth to moisten food particles; the salivary enzyme amylase chemically digests carbohydrates. This first step in digestion forms a food bolus, or mass.

Esophagus

Swallowing moves the bolus to the back of the mouth (oropharynx) and into the esophagus "food tube" located behind and parallel to the trachea.

Muscular contractions (peristalsis) propel the bolus through the esophagus into the stomach. Esophageal secretions lubricate the bolus to assist in its passage. The muscular opening of the gastroesophageal sphincter connects the esophagus and stomach to prevent reflux (backward movement) of stomach contents into the esophagus.

Stomach

The muscular action of the stomach continues mechanical digestion of the bolus by its churning motion, which mixes the bolus with digestive enzymes including pepsin and acids for further chemical digestion. This takes place over several hours, liquifying the bolus into chyme.

Small intestine

The chyme passes from the stomach to the small intestine, which is about 20 feet long. The small intestine is the primary site of chemical digestion and nutrient absorption. Chemical digestion is facilitated here by three accessory organs. Bile made in the liver is sent to the gallbladder for concentration and eventual release into the small bowel through the bile duct to digest fats. The pancreas releases enzymes such as protease, amylase, and lipase into the small intestine through the pancreatic duct to digest, respectively, proteins, sugars, and fats. Aided by a multitude of microorganisms (the microbiome), nutrients are absorbed through the walls of the small intestine into the bloodstream, leaving predominantly water and undigested materials as residual chyme.

Large intestine

The remaining chyme passes into the large intestine, or colon, which is about 5 feet long. The intestines are named for their diameter, not their length: The small intestine is only 1 inch in diameter, compared to the 3-inch diameter of the colon. Water, vitamins, and minerals are absorbed through the walls of the large intestine into the bloodstream, and some bacterial digestion forms important vitamins, such as vitamin K (important for blood clotting). The residual concentrated waste material forms feces.

Rectum and anus

Feces moves from the large intestine into the rectum and is eliminated from the body through the anus in the process of defecation.

The Genitourinary System

The genitourinary system includes the reproductive and urinary systems. They are grouped together because they form simultaneously from the same embryologic origin, are close together in the body, and share some common anatomic components. For these reasons, many syndromes and illnesses involve both systems.

The reproductive system

The reproductive system is composed of male and female sex organs responsible for the development, storage, and release of sex cells (eggs and sperm) that contain genetic material for the creation of offspring.

Female reproductive system

Within the pelvis are two ovaries of up to 5 cm in length (a little larger than a golf ball). At birth, each ovary houses 1 to 2 million eggs that carry the maternal genetic contribution; no additional eggs are made over a female's lifetime. Connected to the ovaries by two fallopian tubes is the uterus, a muscular organ within the mid-pelvis where the fetus develops. The lower part of the uterus is called the cervix, which then connects to the vagina (birth canal).

The mammary glands (breasts) create and supply milk to feed offspring.

Male reproductive system

Two testicles, similar in size to the ovaries, are housed outside the lower body within the scrotal sac. The testes create and store the sperm that carry the paternal genetic contribution. Billions of sperm are present within each testicle; because of their short lifespan, millions are produced each day at a rate of over 1,000 per hour. The prostate gland and seminal vesicles within the pelvis create a liquid substance that mixes with the sperm for transport through the penis via the channel of the urethra.

Putting it together

During the fertile years, one egg is typically released each month, traveling to the uterus through a fallopian tube. Throughout the month, the uterine lining thickens. If a sperm fertilizes the egg, a zygote is formed and implants within this cushion to develop into a fetus. If no fertilization takes place, menses occurs and the blood lining is shed through the vagina. This entire process is monitored by the endocrine system and communicated through hormones secreted by the sex glands, hypothalamus, and pituitary gland.

The urinary system

The urinary system comprises the kidneys, ureters, bladder, and urethra. Like the colon, this system is responsible for eliminating waste from the body. In addition, it regulates blood volume and blood pressure and monitors electrolyte and pH levels.

Elimination

The two kidneys are located in the posterior abdomen at the level of the navel. They are each about the size of a fist and contain millions of nephrons (filtration stations) that return necessary elements such as electrolytes and water to the bloodstream. The residual liquid waste (urine) travels down hollow muscular tubes (ureters) to the urinary bladder within the pelvis. The bladder stores the urine and releases it through the urethra to exit the body. The male and female urinary anatomy is similar, except the male urethra is longer.

Blood volume and pressure

The kidneys control blood volume and blood pressure through a complex series of hormonal interactions called the renin-angiotensin-aldosterone system (RAAS). This system works by controlling the amount of sodium, potassium, water, and vascular constriction throughout the body.

pH

The kidneys regulate pH by maintaining an acid-base balance through control of the quantity of hydrogen ions and bicarbonate in the bloodstream and urine. An overabundance of hydrogen ions creates an acidic environment—low pH—which weakens the body's systems and is associated with several types of illness including bone resorption, infection, and cancer. Unwanted bacteria and cancer cells thrive in an acidic environment, allowing for infections as well as cancer growth.[23]

Figure 7.5 shows the placement of the previously discussed major organs in the body.

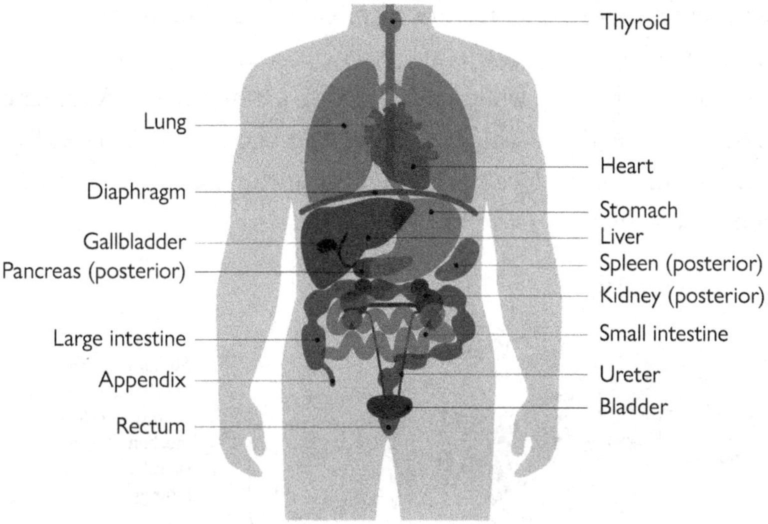

FIGURE 7.5 GENERAL LOCATIONS OF MAJOR ORGANS

The Musculoskeletal System

The musculoskeletal system provides bodily support, protection, shape, and movement.

Muscular system

The type of muscle within this system, skeletal muscle, is controlled by the somatic motor division of the peripheral nervous system. This muscle type differs from both the involuntary smooth muscle found in blood vessels and organs and the cardiac muscle found in the heart because it allows for voluntary control of the body through conscious contraction.

Skeletal muscles create mechanical movement and stabilization of the body when contracting. These muscle fibers are composed of contractile units, sarcomeres, which contain actin and myosin protein filaments. Muscle cells and muscle bodies are surrounded by connective tissue called fascia, which supports and protects the muscle, blood vessels, and nerves. Fascia extends beyond the muscle body to form tendons (dense connective tissue that connect muscles to bone). Each skeletal muscle crosses a joint and partners with an opposing muscle or group of muscles to balance function; when one muscle contracts (agonist), the opposite muscle (antagonist) must neurologically relax for joint movement to occur.

Skeletal muscle (Figure 7.6) contraction differs based on the function being performed. With *isometric contraction*, a muscle creates a supportive force without changing its length (or moving a joint), as when the biceps isometrically contracts (against the force of gravity) while a person holds a heavy object. Another example of isometric contraction—this one involving agonist/antagonist forces—is the simultaneous triceps/biceps contraction of the grounded arm possible in *vasisthasana* (side plank).

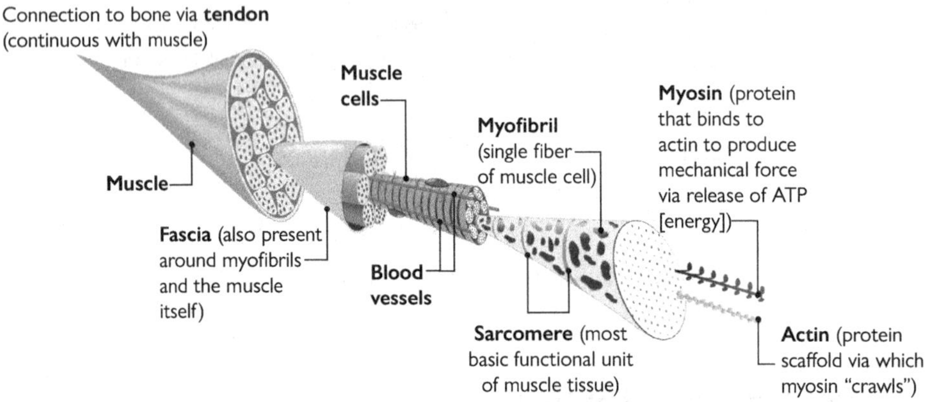

FIGURE 7.6 STRUCTURE OF SKELETAL MUSCLE

Note that the structure of smooth muscle fibers (e.g., within organs and blood vessels) and cardiac muscle fibers differs from skeletal muscle.

With *isotonic contraction*, muscles may shorten (*concentric* contraction) or lengthen (*eccentric* contraction) with movement. Lifting that heavy object up would result in concentric contraction, shortening the biceps; lowering it back down would result in eccentric contraction, lengthening the biceps. Moving from *tadasana* (mountain) to *uttanasana* (standing forward fold), for example, the spinal erector muscles are in eccentric contraction, lengthening under tension as the upper body folds over the hips; lifting from forward fold to standing concentrically contracts the spinal erectors.

Additional skeletal muscle functions include pumping blood and lymph from the body tissues back to the heart, providing postural support, creating facial expressions, and producing heat by shivering.

The skeletal system

Like a wood framework that supports a house, the bones of the skeletal system form the infrastructure to support the body. Tissues and organs are protected by and attach to the skeletal system, which is divided into two main components: the axial skeleton (skull, spine, sternum, and ribs) and the appendicular skeleton (arms, hands, feet, shoulders, and pelvis). There are 206 bones that form the adult skeleton in five shapes:

1. short (e.g., most carpals and tarsals in the hands and feet, respectively)
2. long (e.g., humerus and femur)
3. flat (e.g., ribs, sternum, and cranium)
4. irregular (e.g., vertebrae, sacrum, and pelvic bones)
5. sesamoid (e.g., patella)

Connective tissue forms ligaments to connect bones to each other, cartilage to protect the ends of bones, and periosteum, which covers the bones' surfaces to supply nutrients and blood and provide sensation.

Bones connect to one another at joints that allow for different types and degrees of movement. Classified according to their structure, the basic joint types are

- **synovial joints** (e.g., hip), which provide the greatest amount of movement and are formed by bones with cartilage caps, a surrounding fibrous capsule, and a joint space filled with lubricating synovial fluid (Figure 7.7)
- **cartilaginous joints** (e.g., intervertebral discs and growth plates), which connect bones by cartilage with little to no movement
- **fibrous joints** (e.g., skull sutures), which attach bones by dense fibrous connective tissue

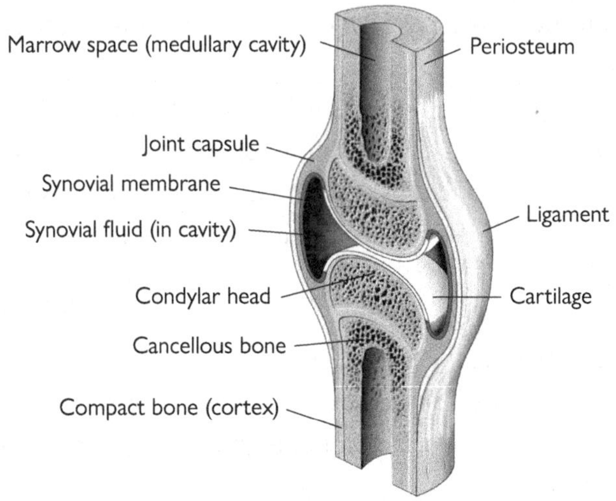

FIGURE 7.7 BASIC LONG BONE/SYNOVIAL JOINT STRUCTURE

Figure 7.8 illustrates functional joint types.

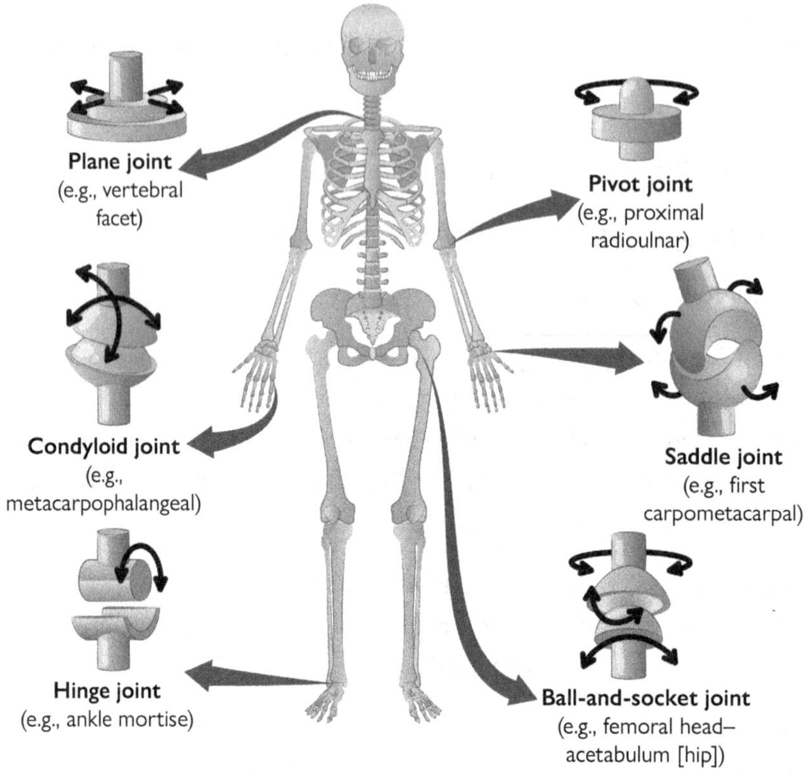

FIGURE 7.8 FUNCTIONAL JOINT TYPES

Bones have an outer thick supportive cortex made of compact bone that stores calcium and phosphorus, and a thin inner matrix made of cancellous bone (marrow) that forms the medullary cavity where red and white blood cells develop (Figure 7.7).

Two main cells work together for bone health: osteoblasts form new bone, and osteoclasts remove old bone. This balance is monitored by endocrine hormones. Bone growth may also be stimulated by compressive forces, such as in weight-bearing exercises, and tensile forces that lengthen muscles, as in yoga asana.[24]

The Lymphatic and Immune Systems

The immune system protects the body against illness and disease. The lymphatic system makes up a large component of the immune system and provides additional important body functions.

The lymphatic system

The lymphatic system is composed of a clear fluid called lymph, ducts through which lymph travels, the filtering stations of the lymph nodes, organs, and tissues.

Lymphatic fluid is similar to plasma, the liquid part of the blood. Lymphatic vessels travel parallel to blood vessels. Each time the heart pumps, plasma leaks out of the blood vessels within the capillary beds. Cellular waste products, bacteria, damaged cells, and large fatty acids in this interstitial fluid are too large to enter nearby blood vessels. Instead, these substances are collected into small lymphatic vessels, which drain into the larger ductal system that transports the lymph back to the circulatory system.

Along its path, lymph travels through many lymph nodes, filtration stations containing white blood cells that remove or sequester the waste, bacteria, and damaged cells. The body's more than 400 lymph nodes are predominantly located centrally within the trunk and each measures approximately 1 cm in diameter. The thoracic duct is the largest channel in which the lymph travels. It starts within the abdomen at the level of the upper lumbar spine, travels upward through the diaphragm, and drains into the left subclavian vein. A smaller duct on the right side of the body drains into the right subclavian vein.

Unlike the blood, which the heart pumps throughout the body, lymph does not have its own pump and must depend on other means for circulation. Lymph movement occurs both actively and passively. Active movement results from two pumping mechanisms: skeletal muscular contraction and diaphragmatic contraction with breath (the thoracic duct travels through the diaphragm). Passive lymph movement occurs by gravity, such as when the extremities are resting higher than the heart (e.g., in inverted-leg pose). Valves within the lymphatic vessels prevent backward flow of lymph.

There are two important organs within the lymphatic system: the thymus and spleen. The thymus gland, which typically atrophies by adulthood, is in the upper chest, behind the sternum and between the lungs. It transforms lymphocytes, white blood cells made in bone marrow, into T-cells that kill bacteria and other invaders. The spleen is located in the back of the left upper abdomen. It filters out old or damaged red blood cells, stores white blood cells and platelets, and makes specialized protective proteins called antibodies. Additional lymphoid tissue is located in the tonsils, skin, gut, and respiratory tract.

The immune system

The immune system uses the lymphatic system in addition to several types of white blood cells (and multiple chemical defenses) to protect the body from disease and clean up debris. Each type of white blood cell has specific important tasks, including identification and destruction of invaders. Only a small percentage of white blood cells are circulating at a time; most are stored in the lymph nodes, spleen, and lymphoid tissue, ready for action when needed.

The immune system provides multilevel responses, with physical and chemical defenses to repel invaders. When a pathogen bypasses these barriers, which include the skin, mucus, etc., the body's inner defenses are divided into two main subsystems, the innate system (broad-spectrum, immediate response that does not confer long-lasting immunity) and the adaptive system (which continuously develops, maintaining a non-chemical "memory" of invaders in the form of antibodies and other molecular substances). Both innate and adaptive immunity use the following protective mechanisms:

- Humoral-mediated immunity protects against external invaders or pathogens (e.g., bacteria, fungus, virus, parasites, foreign matter) through antibodies created by B-cells made in the bone marrow.
- Cell-mediated immunity protects against internal invaders or non-normal cells (e.g., cancer; see Box 7.4) through recognition of abnormal substances (e.g., proteins). This response triggers white blood cells, including cytotoxic T-lymphocytes (T-cells), and usually involves the release of cytokines (inflammatory signalers).

Inflammation

When the immune system identifies an acute or immediate need to protect and repair the body, it sets up a cascade of events that create an inflammatory response. For example, it may sense an injury to the skin causing bleeding, or an inhaled allergen such as pollen causing sneezing. With inflammation, the blood vessels dilate, increasing blood flow to quickly bring the necessary cells and nutrients needed to prevent infection, induce clotting, and remove pathogens. This acute inflammatory response may include symptoms of redness, swelling, pain, and warmth in the area involved; these signs resolve when the injury has healed or the threat has been mitigated. A strong acute inflammatory response is important to keep the body healthy and protected.

Problems arise with chronic or ongoing inflammation in the body, which can be caused by a prolonged stress response and SNS activation that keep the HPA axis on overdrive, continuously circulating the stress hormone cortisol—essentially like pressing on the gas pedal without release. With chronic inflammation, markers called proinflammatory cytokines are elevated, as are free-radicals that damage cells and tissues throughout the body. Many illnesses and conditions are associated with chronic inflammation and elevated cytokine levels, including

- atherosclerosis[25] and cardiovascular disease (heart attack and stroke)[26]
- type 2 diabetes[27]
- obesity[28]
- depression[29]
- muscle loss[30]
- cancer[31]
- ulcerative colitis and Crohn's disease[32]
- gastric ulcers[33]
- autoimmune diseases[34]
- arthritis[35]

Summary

This chapter provides a simple overview of the body's systems to offer yoga therapists a foundational understanding. Although Western biomedicine divides the human organism into these systems for study and convenience, they truly form an integrated whole akin to yoga's *panchamaya kosha* model. Readers are encouraged to explore sources like those listed in the Additional Resources for further understanding of the body's complex physiological processes.

Additional Resources

Karmananda, S. (2005). *Yogic management of common diseases*. Yoga Publications Trust.
Marieb, E. N., & Hoehn, K. (2019). *Human anatomy & physiology* (11th ed.). Pearson.
OpenStax. (2013). *Anatomy and physiology*. XanEdu Publishing Inc.
Story, L. (2017). *Pathophysiology: A practical approach* (3rd ed.). Jones & Bartlett Learning.

BOX 7.3 CLINICAL APPLICATION OF YOGA THERAPY IN CARDIAC REHABILITATION

COURTNEY D. BUTLER-ROBINSON

An essential purpose of incorporating yoga therapy into cardiac rehabilitation is to help decrease inflammation to facilitate healing. Hyperactivity of the sympathetic nervous system, involved in the stress response, is linked to heart failure.[36] Self-directed, readily available techniques like *pranayama*, gentle *asana*, meditation, visualization, and progressive relaxation may improve the stress response[37] and physiological signs of inflammation.[38] When combined with other lifestyle changes like a balanced and healthy diet, proper exercise, and love and support, the outcomes of such interventions may be life changing.

Comorbidities are common in cardiac care. Yoga therapy clients in these settings may also have muscle or joint issues such as sciatica or arthritis, many will also have diabetes, and some will have cancer or autoimmune conditions.[39] Work must therefore adapt to accommodate walkers, oxygen tanks, and wheelchairs.

An intensive cardiac rehab program might take place over 2 months or more, with two meetings per week. Each session might include

- an hour of exercise, which could include asana practice, modified to each person's ability
- an hour of love and support through a group discussion led by a social worker or other mental health professional
- an hour of stress management, which could be the yoga therapy component
- a shared meal, with a lesson on preparing and maintaining a healthy diet or on one of the other program elements

When delivered in an integrative medicine setting, yoga therapy for stress management would generally be by prescription and follow a strict research-based plan.[40] A session could involve elements such as the following.

- **Centering the body-mind:** This component might include basic diaphragmatic or two-part breathing, noticing the rhythm of the breath; simple body scanning (e.g., noticing points of contact); and basic visualization techniques such as leaving one's to-do list at the door.

- **Pranayama:** Two-part breathing can be done with a focus on expansion and contraction of the lungs, diaphragm, and organs with inhalation and exhalation. A count such as "breathe in for four, breathe out for four to six" may help to establish a slower respiratory rhythm. The session might continue with three-part breath with a focus on lengthened exhalations.
- **Progressive relaxation:** Similar to a body scan, this technique encourages noticing and releasing tension via the peripheral nervous system (legs and arms), then working toward the spinal column and brain. This type of relaxation follows the *panchamaya* model's inward journey and, especially for beginners, can involve "breathing awareness into" and releasing each body part in turn.
- **Meditation:** Single-pointed focus is one type of meditation that might be included. Other potential practices are candle-flame gazing (*trataka*), focus on a real or imagined place of peace and comfort, mantra to incite a peaceful reaction, or focus on the breath. Affirmation is an important part of successful outcomes for many, so focus on an individualized, positive, present-oriented statement is another option.
- **Asana:** Physical postures may increase circulation, decrease lymphatic congestion, reduce muscular tension, and improve mobility and range of motion. Lifting the chest in a seated cobra pose, for instance, may increase flexibility in the arteries and overall circulation while gently mobilizing tender surgical sites. Other common postures include seated spinal twist, modified forward folds with the head above the heart (to mitigate blood pressure-related risks), legs on a chair (possibly with the head and shoulders slightly elevated), and joint movements that employ the joint's normal range of function. Each mindful posture would have a specific intention and be adapted to the client's needs.
- **Final meditation and/or visualization:** A variety of techniques could be appropriate, including a check-in (e.g., "How am I today?") to build awareness, followed by self-inquiry (e.g., "What do I need today for peace, for joy, for health?") to promote self-agency. Although formal data are preliminary,[41] a gratitude practice may be especially transformational in such settings.
- **Closing the practice:** Continuing to loosely follow the panchamaya

model, a return to everyday awareness can be guided outward to the spine and extremities. Possible action steps might be offered at this point for a home practice or incorporation into a daily routine, such as noticing the feet as a reminder of one's connection to nature.

Ongoing communication with other caregivers is essential in cardiac rehab, and routines may need to be adapted frequently as a result of fatigue, back pain, or the tingling and discomfort of peripheral neuropathy. As with any major illness, depression and anxiety are also often seen in these populations, underscoring the importance of the stress-relieving effects of yoga therapy.

BOX 7.4 CLINICAL APPLICATION OF YOGA THERAPY IN THE CANCER CARE CONTINUUM

LEIGH LEIBEL

Cancer is complex and affects all ages and populations, impacting each individual and their loved ones in unique and profound ways physically, psychologically, and spiritually. In its basic definition, this group of diseases is caused by the proliferation of abnormal cells that have the potential to spread to other areas of the body.

The word *cancer* often carries with it a stigma that confounds an already-complicated medical condition that runs the gamut from non-threatening localized skin cancer to life-limiting widespread metastatic disease. The number of cancer survivors is increasing due to early detection and improved therapies, and many individuals who have been diagnosed with cancer are thriving and managing the disease as a chronic condition. This underscores the necessity of lifelong supportive care and healthy lifestyle behaviors to help manage lingering, late, and long-term effects of treatment.

A growing body of research shows that yogic practices can mitigate physical and psychological side-effects of cancer and its treatment, affect clinical outcome, and support patients, survivors, families, and healthcare providers through each stage of care.[42] As a mind-body science, yoga is uniquely positioned to address the biopsychosocial-spiritual aspects of patient-centered care while respecting the individual and cultural diversity of the human experience throughout the lifespan and across the care continuum (Figure 7.9).

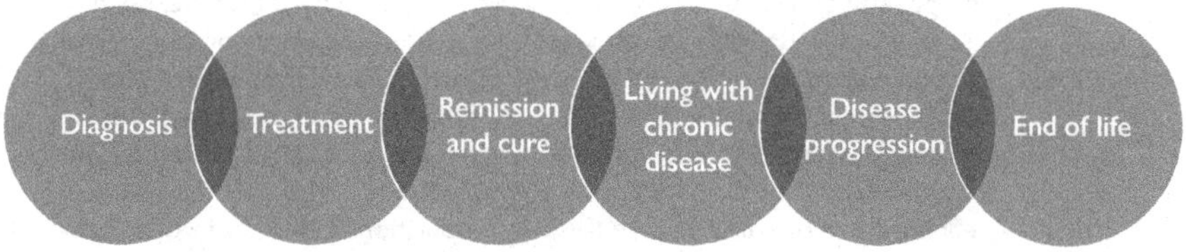

FIGURE 7.9 THE CANCER CARE CONTINUUM ILLUSTRATES A DYNAMIC JOURNEY, WHICH MAY NOT OCCUR IN A STRAIGHT LINE AND CAN INCLUDE MULTIPLE VISITS TO SOME STAGES

Integration with conventional care

Western oncology treatment planning is based on several factors: the type and stage of cancer; previous cancer treatments; and the individual's overall health, goals, and preferences. Many different conventional therapies are available to treat cancer, including those listed in Table 7.1. Although several experiences (fatigue, anxiety, depression, sleep disturbance, fear of recurrence, decreased quality of life) are commonly seen across all treatment modalities, each particular protocol comes with unique side-effects (Table 7.1).

Table 7.1 Common cancer therapies and side-effects

Treatment	Description	Possible Side-Effects
Surgery	The goal of surgery is to remove a malignant tumor (or as much of it as possible). Surgeries may be complex and require removal of organs/limbs.	Hernia, lymphedema, axillary webbing, fibrosis, scarring and adhesions, range of motion limitations, blood clots, amputations, anesthesia effects, pain, impact on body systems of removed organs.
Chemotherapy	Chemotherapy is a drug treatment that uses chemicals to kill growing cells in the body. Many different chemotherapeutic agents are available; they can be used alone or in combination. Treatment is *primary* (cure the cancer without other treatments); *adjuvant* (given after other treatments to kill hidden cancer cells); *neoadjuvant* (to shrink a tumor so that other treatments, e.g., radiation and surgery, are possible); or *palliative* (ease signs and symptoms).	Some side-effects are mild, whereas others cause serious complications. Acute: nausea, vomiting, diarrhea, constipation, loss of appetite, hair loss, weight gain or loss, fatigue, fever, mouth sores, pain (including joint), easy bruising, low white blood cell count (nadir is average 7–12 days postinfusion, posing high risk of infection). Long-lasting and/or late developing: cognitive dysfunction ("chemo brain"), lung damage, heart problems, infertility, kidney problems, nerve damage (peripheral neuropathy), osteoporosis, persistent fatigue, risk of second cancer.

Radiation	Radiation therapy uses high-powered energy beams, such as photons, to kill cancer cells. Radiation treatment can come from a machine outside the body (*external beam radiation*), or it can be placed inside (*brachytherapy*). Indications for radiation therapy: definitive cure or palliative care (i.e., rapid and durable symptom relief; partial to complete pain control in majority of patients; improvement in quality of life, function, and possibly overall survival; may obviate need for escalating opioid doses and avoid unwanted sedative effects).	Effects are cumulative. Acute: fatigue; burns and dermatitis. Late: bone fractures; vertebral collapse; fibrosis/scarring; spinal cord myelopathy; "radiation recall" skin reactions; trauma from diagnostic and treatment procedures, especially in at-risk populations with history of sexual or domestic abuse; "scan anxiety."
Hormone therapy	Some cancers (e.g., subtypes of breast cancer and ovarian, endometrial, testicular, or prostate cancers) are fueled by hormones. Removing those hormones from the body by blocking the ability to produce them or interfering with how they behave may halt cancer cell growth.	Both women and men can receive hormone therapy, with effects including osteoporosis from aging or secondary to surgery or drugs, hot flashes, urinary or fecal incontinence, erectile dysfunction, vaginal dryness, weight gain, sleep disturbance. For women, tamoxifen and aromatase inhibitors (AI) have different side-effects (e.g., AI can cause osteoporosis and joint pain; tamoxifen is bone protective but increases risk of clots). Also consider pelvic floor, fertility, and menopausal symptoms.
Immunotherapy	Immunotherapy uses the immune system to fight cancer, helping the body recognize and attack the cancer. There are three types of immunotherapy: monoclonal antibody therapies, immune checkpoint inhibitors, and adoptive T-cell modulators such as CAR-T cell interventions.	Two types of immunotherapy (immune checkpoint inhibitor therapy and CAR-T cell therapies) can trigger a hyperimmune response that targets non-involved organs, causing inflammation to normal tissue such as lungs, liver, colon, skin, and joints.
Targeted therapy	Targeted drug treatments focus on specific abnormalities within cancer cells that allow them to accumulate; these drugs may inhibit signals that stimulate proliferation, or they may reactivate cell-death pathways.	Skin rash, fluid retention, diarrhea, easy bruising (platelet dysfunction), fatigue.
Bone marrow transplant	Bone marrow transplant (stem cell transplant) can use an individual's own cells or cells from a donor. This treatment allows doctors to use higher doses of chemotherapy to treat cancer and can also be used to replace diseased bone marrow.	Immune issues, graft vs. host disease, side-effects from long-term steroids, patient isolation, deconditioning, fascial inflammation leading to lack of function.

Table 7.2 describes common physical considerations related to cancer treatment, although important emotional and psychological considerations also affect mental health and well-being during active treatment and beyond; yoga therapists must be aware of both the physical and emotional impact of the various cancer treatments to design safe and comprehensive plans—whether delivering the interventions in person or remotely via telehealth. Given the breadth of possible adverse physical events described above, it is understandable and well-documented that cancer-related distress is common at pivotal periods in the trajectory of care and ranges from normal, "situation-appropriate" responses that may comprise initial fear postdiagnosis, to more severe chronic stress reactions that adversely affect functionality and general well-being.[43]

Table 7.2 Common physical problems related to cancer treatment (listed alphabetically)

Issue or Area	Cause	Considerations
Bones	Metastatic cancer to the bones, multiple myeloma, hormonal therapy (aromatase inhibitors), osteoporosis (age or treatment related), radiation therapy, steroids, some chemotherapy.	High risk of bone fracture. Avoid dangerous movements of the spine, rapid movements, excessive weight bearing, and excessive weight-bearing twists.
Cardiotoxicity	Certain cancer drugs and radiation therapy to the chest may cause heart problems, including weakening of the heart muscle (congestive heart failure), causing shortness of breath, dizziness, and swollen hands or feet. Coronary artery disease (when vessels that supply blood and oxygen to the heart narrow) can cause chest pain or shortness of breath.	Shortness of breath, fatigue, swelling, weight gain. Anthracycline chemotherapies can cause heart arrhythmias (some oncologists recommend no exertion on the day of or day following infusion). Prior to radiation therapy, yoga therapists can work with the radiology team to teach patients how to safely breathe and hold breath while receiving radiation to the chest area (to better protect the heart).
Cognitive dysfunction	Chemotherapy, radiation therapy to brain or head, immunotherapy, anxiety, brain cancers, older age, comorbid dementia, anesthesia, pain medications, postmenopausal estrogen decrease, emotional distress, being frail or weak, insufficient nutrition, marijuana use, pain syndromes, fatigue, insomnia. Geriatric population metabolizes drugs differently; pain medications can cause cognitive issues, headache, seizures, language and motor impairments.	Difficulty following instructions or understanding; trouble focusing (give contralateral practices as "brain teasers"). Addressing anxiety, depression, fatigue, and insomnia can help, as can exercise, learning new movements, pranayama, chanting, simple meditations for focus and concentration, and present-moment mindfulness. Ensure that clients have a sense of where objects are around them, and be prepared to repeat activities.

Issue or Area	Cause	Considerations
Comorbidities	Chronic health conditions such as type 2 diabetes, obesity, cardiovascular disease, hypertension, osteoporosis, and arthritis are often comorbid conditions with cancer.	Consider comorbidities. Proceed with yoga therapy guidelines for these conditions while observing best practices for cancer patient safety.
External appliances or devices	Surgery, treatment interventions.	Know how to accommodate ports, PICC lines, exterior bags (ostomy/colostomy), tracheotomies, pacemakers, oxygen tanks, hearing aids, therapy animals, walking assists (walkers, canes), wheelchairs. Provide modifications and accessible alternatives for patients who cannot get on the floor or need assistance standing from seated.
Gastrointestinal	Surgery, pain medications, tumor blockages, antinausea medications, dehydration, lack of movement.	Consider abdominal movements that may be painful because of nausea, constipation, diarrhea, bloating; pain as the bowels move; no appetite; inability to eat; burned throat; colitis; reflux. Prone poses are contraindicated with gastrointestinal blockages.
Immune system	Chemotherapy, immunotherapy, steroids, graft vs. host disease.	Be conscious of infectious complications due to compromised immune system/neutropenia. If applicable, follow best practices for social distancing. Yoga therapists who are sick should not work with patients in person; do not expose patients who are sick to others or work with a patient who has a fever. Employ frequent hand washing. After each client, disinfect (and use barriers with) mat, bolsters, blanket, blocks, straps, the floor, etc. Patients treated with chemotherapy are very sensitive to odors; do not put patients on props/floor with chemical smells. Some cancer centers double-flush toilets (chemo products are excreted by urine for 24–36 hours; toxic agents excreted are conceivably toxic to others); shut the lid. For patients in isolation who are missing human touch, *abhyanga* self-massage (with non-allergic lotions/oils), acupressure, and self-hugs/gentle self-rocking may be useful.

Lymphedema	Lymphedema is the abnormal buildup of lymph fluid in the soft tissues just under the skin. Lymph node removal and/or regional lymph node radiation in the underarm, chest, groin, pelvis, or neck can cause lymphedema (which is distinct from transient fluid retention/edema). Lymphedema is a serious, under-recognized condition that is chronic, progressive, and may significantly affect an individual's function and quality of life. It may appear any time after treatment; the risk is lifelong. Symptoms include swelling, feelings of heaviness or tightness, restricted range of motion, recurring infections, and discomfort. At risk: breast cancer patients who have had all or part of their breast and/or axillary lymph nodes removed, and/or radiation. Lymphedema in the legs or abdomen may occur after surgery for uterine, ovarian, vulvar, and prostate cancers; lymphoma; or melanoma (or in individuals who have undergone inguinal or pelvic node resection). It occurs in patients with cancers of the head and neck due to combined radiation therapy and surgery.	As a holistic practice, yoga may be of benefit by reducing both the physical and psychosocial effects of lymphedema; however, to better understand the benefits/risks of yoga, further research is needed. Yoga therapists should work with a certified lymphedema specialist to coordinate care, safe movements, and whether compression garments should be worn during yoga. If axial lymph nodes have been affected, it is not known whether asana that require weight bearing on the arms will aggravate the condition. All individuals at risk for lymphedema should have medical approval before beginning any exercise or yoga, particularly in the presence of obesity or cardiovascular, pulmonary, or metabolic disease. Carefully controlled exercise is safe for patients with breast cancer-induced lymphedema; however, be cognizant of early signs of potential injury or symptom flareup (e.g., increased muscle soreness, joint pain, excessive fatigue, redness, or heaviness in the involved arm). Research suggests these individuals should begin with light upper-body exercise and increase it slowly under the supervision of a lymphedema therapist. If exercise is stopped for a week or longer, it should be started again at a low level and increased slowly. Exercising at a low level and slowly increasing again over time is likely better for the affected limb than stopping the exercise completely.[a] General advice: Keep blood and fluid from pooling in the affected limb. With upper limbs, keep the limb with lymphedema raised higher than the heart when possible. Do not swing the limb quickly in circles or let the limb hang down. Do not apply heat to the limb (no hot yoga). Avoid seated crossed-leg poses, change positions every 30 minutes, and avoid tight elastic bands on at-risk limbs.[b]
Neurological	Chemotherapy-induced peripheral neuropathy; whole brain or localized radiation to brain/head; stroke.	Peripheral neuropathy, balance problems (fall risk), tinnitus, hearing loss. Consider soft music during meditation/practice to mask tinnitus; chanting or *bhramari* may be helpful.

Issue or Area	Cause	Considerations
Ocular	Some chemotherapy drugs can cause dry eye syndrome and sensitivity to light. Brain, central nervous system, and ocular tumors can cause vision disturbance.	Know how to work with patients who are blind or have reduced sight. Fall risks (sensitivity to light; blurred, cloudy, or double vision). No *trataka* (fixed gazing) or inversions (glaucoma risk). Ask if patient is comfortable with visualization practices and engaging the sense of sight.
Oral	Radiation to head/neck, some chemotherapies, no saliva, dry mouth.	Exercise jaw (e.g., open and close mouth); practices to stimulate saliva; keep water available. Excess saliva due to inability to swallow requires a "spit bucket." Chanting and humming, cooling breaths, and cooling guided imagery may be welcome.
Pain	Surgery, radiation, ports, bruising from needles, tingling fingers and toes, headache, adhesions, constipation, tumor pressure.	Identify source of pain and proceed with interventions accordingly. Consider the multidimensional nature of pain and its relationship to the five *koshas*.
Respiratory	Primary cancer or metastasis to lung, COPD, surgical lung removal, radiation to lung or chest area, bleomycin, pneumonias/interstitial lung disease, chemotherapy (shortness of breath, wheezing, dry cough), steroids.	Breathing practices contraindicated during radiation for primary lung lesion or lung metastases include *kapalabhati, bhastrika*, and *ujjayi* (pneumothorax risk). Decreased stamina. Essential oils, incense, and candles can be harmful to compromised lungs, as are chemical smells from disinfectants to clean mats/floors. Know how to work with oxygen tanks. Follow COPD/asthma protocols. "Deep" breaths may not be possible, and relationship with breath may not be positive (caution with cues/language).
Rheumatology	Disease- or treatment-induced arthritis and arthralgias; rheumatologic issues from immunotherapy; joint pain, stiffness, swelling in large and small joints; muscle weakness; decrease in functional status; radiation therapy; some chemotherapy drugs; steroids (scar tissue, weakness, and bone loss). These problems can lead to loss of motion in joints (e.g., jaw, shoulders, hips, knees). Adverse effects from radiation therapy occur only in the treated area, whereas systemic treatments (chemotherapy, hormone therapy, immunotherapy) can cause global effects.	Consider pain and movement limitations; joint-loosening practices may feel good. Patients may prefer moving joints with the breath in lieu of prolonged poses. Consider breathing, mindfulness, and meditation practices. Can move the body in the imagination if not physically.
Sarcopenia or cachexia	Hospitalizations, bed rest, fatigue/lack of movement, disease, failure to thrive.	May have difficulty doing previously easy movements (e.g., getting up from the ground, certain asana).

Steroids	Prophylaxis for radiation-induced pain, palliative radiotherapy for bone metastasis, immunotherapy. Steroid-induced hyperglycemia, hypertension, cataract formation, thinning of skin, peptic ulcer disease.	Bone issues (bone loss, osteoporosis, fractures), fragile skin, proximal myopathy (steroids can weaken thigh muscles), tendonitis (tendons can rupture; avoid flexibility stretches). Variables: dosing, type, time since stopping.
Surgical complications	Pain, postoperative infections, deep vein thrombosis, loss of range of motion, swelling, altered bowel habits, permanent changes in vital organ functions, effects of anesthesia.	Consider surgical location and systems impacted. Range of motion: scapulothoracic motion, axillary webbing, lymphedema, frozen shoulder, hernia, postoperative muscular imbalance, surgical sites (and harvest sites for grafts for reconstruction), impingement syndrome, postsurgical reconstruction. Anesthesia effects.
Thromboembolic disorders	Cancer is a prothrombotic condition. Surgery, immobility, and some hormonal therapies increase clot risk. Stroke.	A blood clot can be life-threatening and must be managed medically. Do not recommend movement to a patient with a fresh clot; however, with medical approval, meditation and breath awareness may be appropriate depending on clot location. In at-risk cancer populations, avoid prolonged periods of asana that slow blood circulation to limbs (e.g., lotus, *vajrasana*). For at-risk stroke populations, consider prophylactic gentle movement for those who are bed-bound and immobile.

[a]There is limited research on exercise safety and lymphedema in lower limbs and other parts of the body.

[b]These statements are based on the limited currently available research. Always follow the most current evidence-based principles of care.

PICC = peripherally inserted central catheter; COPD = chronic obstructive pulmonary disease.

Among the most commonly reported problems is fear of cancer recurrence, often identified as one of the most prevalent unaddressed areas for cancer survivors and their carers. Those who survive cancer may face many other psychosocial challenges, including persistent fatigue; anxiety and depression; chronic stress; impaired cognitive function; multifaceted pain syndromes; sleep disturbance and insomnia; medical trauma/posttraumatic stress disorder (PTSD); body image, fertility, and sexuality issues; altered personal and professional relationships; financial concerns; decreased quality of life; and increased suicide risk.[44] All of these issues are often experienced through the lens of difficult emotions such as anger, guilt, sadness, and grief.

Yoga therapy is well-positioned to help quiet the minds of cancer patients, survivors, and their loved ones. As a mind-body science, yoga has the potential to foster wellness, improve well-being, enhance coping skills, and promote resilience so that everyone affected by a cancer diagnosis may navigate the experience with greater presence and compassion.

The information here highlights the challenges inherent in the management of a cancer diagnosis and the importance of intake, assessment, and individual yoga therapy plans reviewed at each session. Yoga therapists should have a working knowledge of the biology of cancer, its natural history, consequences and toxicities of therapeutic interventions, and client expectations in the framework of a holistic management plan. Given such a foundation, yoga therapy can become an essential intervention for helping clients toward a place of wellness, regardless of condition or prognosis.

Additional Resources

Brant, J. M. (2020). *Core curriculum for oncology nursing.* Saunders.
Eggert, J. (2017). *Cancer basics.* Oncology Nursing Society.

BOX 7.5 YOGA THERAPY AND PHARMACEUTICALS: A CAUTIOUS APPROACH TO INTERACTION

MARYBETH MISSENDA

Clear research does not yet link interactions between the practice of yoga and pharmaceuticals. As a result, the evidence-informed practitioner must bring together the best evidence available in a conscientious, explicit, and judicious way.[45] This intention includes careful consideration of the evidence supporting physiological changes seen with the practice of yoga and understanding the pharmacodynamics of modern medicine to assess the risk-benefits of combining these therapeutic approaches.

As more patients using pharmaceuticals seek to integrate yoga into their care plans, yoga therapists need to recognize, in collaboration with the client's prescribing healthcare provider or pharmacist, the potential risks associated with drug-yoga interactions. This section outlines considerations for several commonly encountered drug classes, including those prescribed for depression and antibiotics. Additional pharmaceutical categories are described in Boxes 7.6 and 7.7.

Antidepressants

A number of classes of antidepressants present different challenges in relation to yoga therapy. Tricyclic antidepressants like amitriptyline have anticholinergic effects (i.e., they block action of the neurotransmitter acetylcholine, potentially causing dry mouth, urine retention, blurred vision, dizziness, vomiting, etc.). These medications are also prescribed off-label for peripheral neuropathy, obsessive compulsive disorders, migraines, insomnia, and chronic pain. Clients who combine these with hot yoga may have difficulty cooling down the body because of decreased ability to sweat and increased core body temperature.[46] Common over-the-counter allergy medications such as diphenhydramine and asthma inhalers like ipratropium bromide have similar anticholinergic effects and also warrant caution.

Selective serotonin reuptake inhibitors (SSRI) like fluoxetine are associated with increased drowsiness and low energy levels, potentially affecting adherence to practice. Some patients find it helpful to take these medications in the evening to decrease the effect on daily function.

Fluoroquinolones and corticosteroids

Yoga therapists may also need to consider common adverse effects of some medications that may affect a client's care plan. One example is the adverse event reports associated with fluoroquinolone antibiotics (e.g., ciprofloxacin, levofloxacin) and intra-articular corticosteroids (e.g., hydrocortisone, beclomethasone) resulting in drug-induced tendon rupture.[47] *Asana* that load the Achilles tendon while taking these medications could increase the risk of tendinopathy. Shoulder tendinopathy has also been reported with these medications.

Although no research to date has specifically examined the interaction between these medications and the practice of yoga, one case report of a common flexor tendon tear following corticosteroid injections and continuation of the patient's yoga practice has been published.[48] Tzaveas and colleagues reported on another case of tendon rupture associated with yoga alone.[49] This suggests that combining these medications with a yoga practice may negatively affect client safety.

Future research may provide greater insights into the safety of yoga and yoga therapy for these patients and suggest when yoga can be restarted after finishing a course of fluoroquinolones or receiving corticosteroids.

BOX 7.6 CARDIORESPIRATORY MEDICATIONS

MARYBETH MISSENDA

Antihypertensives

Several studies show that yoga therapy may improve systolic blood pressure, heart rate, and serum cholesterol, which may reduce the risk of cardiovascular disease.[50] Physiological changes that contribute to yoga therapy's effect on cardiovascular risk include vagus nerve stimulation, musculoskeletal massage, and changes in perceived stress leading to parasympathetic activation.[51] When combining medications that lower blood pressure (e.g., angiotensin-converting-enzyme [ACE] inhibitors, diuretics, and calcium-channel blockers) with a yoga practice, clients may experience improvements in their blood pressure, requiring prescribing healthcare providers to adjust their medications to prevent hypotensive events that could lead to falls.

The initiation of antihypertensive medications is also associated with increased risk of orthostatic hypotension (OH). This risk increases with age and manifests as dizziness, fainting, and/or changes in vision with shifts in posture (e.g., lying to sitting, sitting to standing). Gangavati and colleagues noted an increased risk in falls with severe OH.[52] The potassium-sparing diuretic spironolactone appears to have the highest risk of OH. This adverse event typically occurs when patients first start these medications or when they change dosing. This suggests that yoga therapists, when developing the yoga care plan, should ask how long clients have been taking antihypertensive medications and whether they have experienced signs of OH. Increased care in monitoring transitions between postures or initiating postures contraindicated in patients with hypotension may be needed. As cardiovascular fitness increases, clients may see improvements in OH.

Beta-blockers as antihypertensive agents present potentially unique challenges when combined with therapeutic yoga, as both appear to regulate cardiovascular homeostasis through sympathetic nerve modulation and stimulation of cardiac baroreceptors. Beta-blockers may play an important role in reducing cardiovascular mortality and morbidity when combined with ACE inhibitors, antiplatelet drugs, and statins.[53] This class of medications works by altering the body's response to autonomic function that impacts heart rate and blood pressure, but not all beta-blockers have the same effect on intrinsic sympathetic activity. Selective beta-blockers like metoprolol seem to produce a greater decrease in parasympathetic activity over time, an effect not seen with non-selective beta-blockers.[54] The mechanisms of the selective beta-blockers may also differ in early versus late heart failure, making a thorough medical history relevant to the yoga care plan.[55]

Beta-blockers may also impair exercise endurance initially, as they can increase perceived exertion, lower VO_{2max} (maximal oxygen consumption, a measure of aerobic fitness), and lower heart rate variability. Non-selective beta-blockers like propranolol have also been associated with increases in lactate levels during exercise, which may be associated with a burning or painful sensation in working muscles.[56] This may affect clients' initial adherence to a yoga therapy plan. This category of medications has also been associated with more falls in older women than other antihypertensive medications.[57] Over time, however, the use of beta-blockers has been shown to increase exercise capacity in patients with heart failure.[58]

Non-selective beta-blockers like propranolol are also prescribed for non-cardiovascular indications like migraine, glaucoma, hyperthyroidism, fibromyalgia, generalized anxiety disorder, parkinsonian tremors, and stage fright. Given the variations in pharmacology of different beta-blockers, diverse indications for these medications, effects of yogic practice on the autonomic nervous system, and variations in response to sympathetic activity at different stages of cardiovascular disease, more focused research on how these variables affect the safety of those who combine these therapeutic modalities is still needed.

Cholesterol-lowering medications

Cholesterol-lowering medications like the 3-hydroxy-3-methylglutaryl coenzyme A (HMG-CoA) reductase inhibitors, commonly referred to as statins, may affect a client's ability to adhere to a yoga care plan due to decreases in energy level, exertional fatigue, reduced exercise capacity, and statin-induced myopathies ("muscle diseases").[59] Some drugs in this class (e.g., atorvastatin and simvastatin) may have higher incidence of myotoxicity due to their greater accumulation in skeletal muscle. Research on marathon runners showed that physical exercise can trigger exacerbations of statin-related myotoxicity, with the most-reported muscular symptoms being muscle pain, heaviness, stiffness, and cramps, with some experiencing muscle weakness.[60] These findings suggest a potential impact on adherence to a yoga care plan.

Beta-agonists

Beta-agonists such as albuterol and salbutamol are commonly used to treat asthma. These medications can increase heart rate and sympathetic activity: In healthy volunteers, a standard dose of inhaled salbutamol increased sympathetic nerve activity by 23 percent, independent of physiological mechanisms to maintain blood pressure. This increase in sympathetic outflow was similar to that observed with mental stress.[61] Edgell and colleagues concluded that this increase may be "physiologically and/or clinically important" and may reflect "altered central sympathetic regulation" or the direct activation of sympathetic nerves.[62]

De and Mondal observed that 15 to 22.5 minutes of yoga asana practice increased parasympathetic activity, which may counter the increase in sympathetic nerve activation of beta-agonists, resulting in a return to homeostasis. In contrast, they noted that 30 minutes of practice increased sympathetic activity.[63] More research is needed to determine how the combination of yoga and beta-agonists may improve overall treatment of asthma by reducing adverse effects and long-term consequences of sympathetic dominance caused by the medications used. Use of a beta-agonist before a yoga practice may also increase lung capacity to improve oxygenation of tissue during exercise in those with exercise-induced asthma. The routine use of short-acting inhaled beta-agonists, however, has been shown to increase tolerance to the beta-blocker and is not currently recommended.[64]

BOX 7.7 DIABETES MEDICATIONS

MARYBETH MISSENDA

Antihyperglycemics

Two key groups of medications used in the treatment of diabetes require increased monitoring and awareness on the part of yoga therapists: the sulfonylureas and insulin.

The research is inconclusive as to the relationship between yoga practices and fasting glucose, a key metric of diabetes control. Although a meta-analysis of randomized placebo-controlled trials did not show a significant decrease, other studies have suggested that combining asana and pranayama practices produces significant improvements in insulin resistance and fasting blood glucose levels.[65] The potential effects of decreased blood glucose should be part of the yoga therapist's care plan.

Some pharmaceuticals may be more likely to result in sudden drops in serum glucose levels, leading to potential adverse consequences. Gangji and colleagues demonstrated that the drug glyburide, when used in elderly people, has a higher risk of hypoglycemic episodes than other sulfonylureas.[66] Combining this medication with a practice of yoga may have an additive effect leading to dizziness, weakness, poor balance, anxiety, falls, and even loss of consciousness.

As blood glucose levels improve, more diligent monitoring for hypoglycemia is needed for patients taking any of the antidiabetic medications or dietary supplements that affect glucose metabolism, insulin secretion, or insulin resistance. Clients who take insulin injections may also need to be monitored for sudden drops in blood glucose levels following a yoga practice. The additive effect of a practice of yoga with insulin may lead to hypoglycemic events due to increased insulin sensitivity or the ability of working skeletal muscle to lower glucose levels independent of insulin. Research combining asana, pranayama, and chanting with standard pharmacological care for patients with type 2 diabetes showed significant improvement in insulin resistance, fasting blood glucose, and postprandial glucose levels.[67] Careful monitoring of glucose fluctuations associated with yoga practice may require adjustments in insulin dosing by the prescribing healthcare provider.

Endnotes

1 Bianconi, E., Piovesan, A., Facchin, F., Beraudi, A., et al. (2013). An estimation of the number of cells in the human body. *Annals of Human Biology*, *40*(6), 463–471.

2 Eckel, C. M. (2017). *Human anatomy lab manual* (3rd ed.). McGraw-Hill Education.

3 Eckel, *Human anatomy lab manual.*

4 Bal, B. S. (2010). Effect of anulom vilom and bhastrika pranayama on the vital capacity and maximal ventilatory volume. *Journal of Physical Education and Sports Management*, *1*(1), 11–15.
Singh, S., Gaurav, V., & Parkash, V. (2010). Effects of a 6-week nadi-shodhana pranayama training on cardio-pulmonary parameters. *Journal of Physical Education and Sports Management*, *2*(4), 44–47.

5 A nerve plexus is a control center where networks of afferent and efferent nerve fibers intersect and branch out. See Chapter 2 for more information on the chakras, part of yoga's system of the subtle body. Some contemporary interpretations place the six lower chakras (usually not including the seventh center of *sahasrara* at or above the crown of the head) anatomically at nerve plexi, as discussed here, or align them with glands. Others regard these areas of energetic focus solely as aids to meditation.

6 Gerritsen, R. J. S., & Band, G. P. H. (2018). Breath of life: The respiratory vagal stimulation model of contemplative activity. *Frontiers in Human Neuroscience*, *12*, 397.
Jerath, R., Edry, J. W., Barnes, V. A., & Jerath, V. (2006). Physiology of long pranayamic breathing: Neural respiratory elements may provide a mechanism that explains how slow deep breathing shifts the autonomic nervous system. *Medical Hypotheses*, *67*(3), 566–571.

7 Bhavanani, A. B., Madanmohan, & Sanjay, Z. (2012). Immediate effect of chandra nadi pranayama (left unilateral forced nostril breathing) on cardiovascular parameters in hypertensive patients. *International Journal of Yoga*, *5*(2), 108–111.

Bhavanani, A. B., Ramanathan, M., Balaji, R., & Pushpa, D. (2014). Differential effects of uninostril and alternate nostril pranayamas on cardiovascular parameters and reaction time. *International Journal of Yoga*, *7*(1), 60–65.

Telles, S., Nagarathna, R., & Nagendra, H. R. (1996). Physiological measures of right nostril breathing. *Journal of Alternative and Complementary Medicine*, *2*(4), 479–484.

8 Telles, S., Yadav, A., Kumar, N., Sharma, S., Visweshwaraiah, N. K., & Balkrishna, A. (2013). Blood pressure and Purdue pegboard scores in individuals with hypertension after alternate nostril breathing, breath awareness, and no intervention. *Medical Science Monitor: International Medical Journal of Experimental and Clinical Research*, *19*, 61–66.

9 Known as Swara Yoga in tantric and ayurvedic traditions. See, e.g., Muktibodhananda, S. (1984). *Swara yoga: The tantric science of brain breathing*. Bihar School of Yoga.

10 Schiff, B. B., & Rump, S. A. (1995). Asymmetrical hemispheric activation and emotion: The effects of unilateral forced nostril breathing. *Brain and Cognition*, *29*(3), 217–231.

Singh, K., Bhargav, H., & Srinivasan, T. M. (2016). Effect of uninostril yoga breathing on brain hemodynamics: A functional near-infrared spectroscopy study. *International Journal of Yoga*, *9*(1), 12–19.

11 van Veluw, S. J., Hou, S. S., Calvo-Rodriguez, M., Arbel-Ornath, M., et al. (2020). Vasomotion as a driving force for paravascular clearance in the awake mouse brain. *Neuron*, *105*(3), 549–561.

12 Jessen, N. A., Munk, A. S., Lundgaard, I., & Nedergaard, M. (2015). The glymphatic system: A beginner's guide. *Neurochemical Research*, *40*(12), 2583–2599.

13 Ovadia-Blechman, Z., Gavish, B., Levy-Aharoni, D., Shashar, D., & Aharonson, V. (2017). The coupling between peripheral microcirculation and slow breathing. *Medical Engineering & Physics*, *39*, 49–56.

14 For an explanation of some of these exercises, see Balasubramanian, S. (2019). *Mind your breathing: The yogi's handbook with 37 pranayama exercises*. Notion Press.

15 Angus, G. E., & Thurlbeck, W. M. (1972). Number of alveoli in the human lung. *Journal of Applied Physiology*, *32*(4), 483–485.

16 The common instruction to "empty the lungs" is neither helpful nor possible, partly because of the "residual lung volume" that prevents the lungs from collapsing, even with the most forceful exhalation. See, e.g., Freeman, C. (2018). Don't empty your lungs! *Yoga Therapy Today*, Summer, 22–23.

17 For more information on diaphragmatic versus chest breathing, see, e.g., Rama, S., Ballentine, R., & Hymes, A. (2007). *Science of breath*. The Himalayan Institute Press.

18 Evans, P. L., McMillin, S. L., Weyrauch, L. A., & Witczak, C. A. (2019). Regulation of skeletal muscle glucose transport and glucose metabolism by exercise training. *Nutrients*, *11*(10), 2432.

19 US Department of Health and Human Services, Centers for Disease Control and Prevention. (2020). National diabetes statistics report 2020: Estimates of diabetes and its burden in the United States. www.cdc.gov/diabetes/pdfs/data/statistics/national-diabetes-statistics-report.pdf

20 Raveendran, A. V., Deshpandae, A., & Joshi, S. R. (2018). Therapeutic role of yoga in type 2 diabetes. *Endocrinology and Metabolism*, *33*(3), 307–317.

21 Innes, K. E., & Selfe, T. K. (2016). Yoga for adults with type 2 diabetes: A systematic review of controlled trials. *Journal of Diabetes Research*, *2016*, 6979370.

Ramamoorthi, R., Gahreman, D., Skinner, T., & Moss, S. (2019). The effect of yoga practice on glycemic control and other health parameters in the prediabetic state: A systematic review and meta-analysis. *PLoS ONE*, *14*(10), e0221067.

Thind, H., Lantini, R., Balletto, B. L., Donahue, M. L., Salmoirago-Blotcher, E., et al. (2017). The effects of yoga among adults with type 2 diabetes: A systematic review and meta-analysis. *Preventive Medicine*, *105*, 116–126.

22 Note that teaching to simply "avoid pain" may not be in the client's best long-term interest. A well-balanced yoga practice supports proprioceptive and interoceptive awareness (see Chapter 16); as clients learn the nuances of the links among physical sensation, emotion, and controlled response they are able to better adjust their responses and fortify their practices. See, e.g., Pearson, N., Prosko, S., & Sullivan, M. (Eds.). (2019). *Yoga and science in pain care: Treating the person in pain*. Singing Dragon.

23 Riemann, A., Schneider, B., Gündel, D., Stock, C., Thews, O., & Gekle, M. (2014). Acidic priming enhances metastatic potential of cancer cells. *Pflügers Archiv—European Journal of Physiology*, *466*(11), 2127–2138.

24 Lu, Y. H., Rosner, B., Chang, G., & Fishman, L. M. (2016). Twelve-minute daily yoga regimen reverses osteoporotic bone loss. *Topics in Geriatric Rehabilitation, 32*(2), 81–87.

25 Libby, P. (2002). Inflammation in atherosclerosis. *Nature, 420*(6917), 868–874.

26 Black, P. H., & Garbutt, L. D. (2002). Stress, inflammation and cardiovascular disease. *Journal of Psychosomatic Research, 52*(1), 1–23.
Libby, Inflammation in atherosclerosis.

27 Dandona, P., Aljada, A., Chaudhuri, A., Mohanty, P., & Garg, R. (2005). Metabolic syndrome: A comprehensive perspective based on interactions between obesity, diabetes, and inflammation. *Circulation, 111*(11), 1448–1454.

28 Dandona et al., Metabolic syndrome.
Mohamed-Ali, V., Flower, L., Sethi, J., Hotamisligil, G., et al. (2001). Beta-adrenergic regulation of IL-6 release from adipose tissue: In vivo and in vitro studies. *Journal of Clinical Endocrinology and Metabolism, 86*(12), 5864–5869.
Parimisetty, A., Dorsemans, A. C., Awada, R., Ravanan, P., Diotel, N., & Lefebvre d'Hellencourt, C. (2016). Secret talk between adipose tissue and central nervous system via secreted factors—An emerging frontier in the neurodegenerative research. *Journal of Neuroinflammation, 13*(1), 67.

29 Berk, M., Williams, L. J., Jacka, F. N., O'Neil, A., et al. (2013). So depression is an inflammatory disease, but where does the inflammation come from? *BMC Medicine, 11*, 200.
Kiecolt-Glaser, J. K., Derry, H. M., & Fagundes, C. P. (2015). Inflammation: Depression fans the flames and feasts on the heat. *American Journal of Psychiatry, 172*(11), 1075–1091.

30 Toth, M. J., Matthews, D. E., Tracy, R. P., & Previs, M. J. (2005). Age-related differences in skeletal muscle protein synthesis: Relation to markers of immune activation. *American Journal of Physiology. Endocrinology and Metabolism, 288*(5), E883–E891.
Visser, M., Pahor, M., Taaffe, D. R., Goodpaster, B. H., et al. (2002). Relationship of interleukin-6 and tumor necrosis factor-alpha with muscle mass and muscle strength in elderly men and women: The Health ABC Study. *Journals of Gerontology, 57*(5), M326–M332.

31 Lutgendorf, S. K., & Sood, A. K. (2011). Biobehavioral factors and cancer progression: Physiological pathways and mechanisms. *Psychosomatic Medicine, 73*(9), 724–730.
Wu, Y., Antony, S., Meitzler, J. L., & Doroshow, J. H. (2014). Molecular mechanisms underlying chronic inflammation-associated cancers. *Cancer Letters, 345*, 164–173.
Khansari, N., Shakiba, Y., & Mahmoudi, M. (2009). Chronic inflammation and oxidative stress as a major cause of age-related diseases and cancer. *Recent Patents on Inflammation and Allergy Drug Discovery, 3*(1), 73–80.

32 Breit, S., Kupferberg, A., Rogler, G., & Hasler, G. (2018). Vagus nerve as modulator of the brain-gut axis in psychiatric and inflammatory disorders. *Frontiers in Psychiatry, 9*, 44.

33 Arakawa, T., Watanabe, T., Fukuda, T., Higuchi, K., et al. (1998). Ulcer recurrence: Cytokines and inflammatory response-dependent process. *Digestive Diseases and Sciences, 43*(9 Suppl.), 61S–66S.
Katagiri, M., Asaka, M., Kobayashi, M., Kudo, M., Kato, M., & Takeda, H. (1997). Increased cytokine production by gastric mucosa in patients with Helicobacter pylori infection. *Journal of Clinical Gastroenterology, 25*(Suppl. 1), S211–S214.

34 Moudgil, K. D., & Choubey, D. (2011). Cytokines in autoimmunity: Role in induction, regulation, and treatment. *Journal of Interferon and Cytokine Research, 31*(10), 695–703.

35 Lubberts, E. (2010). Th17 cytokines and arthritis. *Seminars in Immunopathology, 32*, 43–53.

36 Zhang, D. Y., & Anderson, A. S. (2014). The sympathetic nervous system and heart failure. *Cardiology Clinics, 32*(1), 33–45.

37 Djalilova, D. M., Schulz, P. S., Berger, A. M., Case, A. J., Kupzyk, K. A., & Ross, A. C. (2019). Impact of yoga on inflammatory biomarkers: A systematic review. *Biological Research for Nursing, 21*(2), 198–209.

38 Pascoe, M. C., Thompson, D. R., & Ski, C. F. (2017). Yoga, mindfulness-based stress reduction and stress-related physiological measures: A meta-analysis. *Psychoneuroendocrinology, 86*, 152–168.

39 As noted in the main chapter, inflammation is a common root of many diseases. Diabetes is a frequent comorbidity with heart conditions because it can damage blood vessels and cardiac nerves. The longer a person has diabetes, the greater the chance of comorbid heart disease. See, e.g., National Institute of Diabetes and Digestive and Kidney Diseases, National Institutes of Health, US Department of Health and

Human Services. (2017). Diabetes, heart disease, and stroke. www.niddk.nih.gov/health-information/diabetes/overview/preventing-problems/heart-disease-stroke

40 See, e.g., Chu, P., Gotink, R. A., Yeh, G. Y., Goldie, S. J., & Hunink, M. G. (2016). The effectiveness of yoga in modifying risk factors for cardiovascular disease and metabolic syndrome: A systematic review and meta-analysis of randomized controlled trials. *European Journal of Preventive Cardiology, 23*(3), 291–307.

41 See, e.g., Kreitzer, M. J., Telke, S., Hanson, L., Leininger, B., & Evans, R. (2019). Outcomes of a gratitude practice in an online community of caring. *Journal of Alternative and Complementary Medicine, 25*(4), 385–391.

42 Bhasin, M. K., Dusek, J. A., Chang, B., Joseph, M. G., et al. (2013). Relaxation response induces temporal transcriptome changes in energy metabolism, insulin secretion and inflammatory pathways. *PLoS ONE, 8*(5), e62817.

Carlson, L. E., Tamagawa, R., Stephen, J., Drysdale, E., Zhong, L., & Speca, M. (2016). Randomized-controlled trial of mindfulness-based cancer recovery versus supportive expressive group therapy among distressed breast cancer survivors (MINDSET): Long-term follow-up results. *Psycho-Oncology, 25*(7), 750–759.

Chandwani, K. D., Perkins, G., Nagendra, H. R., Raghuram, N. V., et al. (2014). Randomized, controlled trial of yoga in women with breast cancer undergoing radiotherapy. *Journal of Clinical Oncology, 32*(10), 1058–1065.

Cramer, H., Lange, S., Klose, P., Paul, A., & Dobos, G. (2012). Yoga for breast cancer patients and survivors: A systematic review and meta-analysis. *BMC Cancer, 12*(1), 412.

Kiecolt-Glaser, J. K., Bennett, J. M., Andridge, R., Peng, J., et al. (2014). Yoga's impact on inflammation, mood, and fatigue in breast cancer survivors: A randomized controlled trial. *Journal of Clinical Oncology, 32*(10), 1040–1049.

Lyman, G. H., Bohlke, K., & Cohen, L. (2018). Integrative therapies during and after breast cancer treatment: ASCO endorsement of the SIO clinical practice guideline summary. *Journal of Oncology Practice, 14*(8), 495–499.

Moadel, A. B., Shah, C., Wylie-Rosett, J., Harris, M. S., et al. (2007). Randomized controlled trial of yoga among a multiethnic sample of breast cancer patients: Effects on quality of life. *Journal of Clinical Oncology, 25*(28), 4387–4395.

Mustian, K. M., Sprod, L. K., Janelsins, M., Peppone, L. J., et al. (2013). Multicenter, randomized controlled trial of yoga for sleep quality among cancer survivors. *Journal of Clinical Oncology, 31*(26), 3233–3241.

43 Buffart, L. M., Uffelen, J. G., Riphagen, I. I., Brug, J., et al. (2012). Physical and psychosocial benefits of yoga in cancer patients and survivors, a systematic review and meta-analysis of randomized controlled trials. *BMC Cancer, 12*(1), 559.

Carlson et al., Randomized-controlled trial.

Dhruva, A., Miaskowski, C., Abrams, D., Acree, M., et al. (2012). Yoga breathing for cancer chemotherapy—associated symptoms and quality of life: Results of a pilot randomized controlled trial. *Journal of Alternative and Complementary Medicine, 18*(5), 473–479.

Lundt, A., & Jentschke, E. (2019). Long-term changes of symptoms of anxiety, depression, and fatigue in cancer patients 6 months after the end of yoga therapy. *Integrative Cancer Therapies, 18*, 153473541882209.

Moadel et al., Randomized controlled trial.

Mustian et al., Multicenter, randomized controlled trial.

Raghuram, N., Rao, R., Nagendra, H., Kodaganur, G., et al. (2017). Effects of a yoga program on mood states, quality of life, and toxicity in breast cancer patients receiving conventional treatment: A randomized controlled trial. *Indian Journal of Palliative Care, 23*(3), 237.

44 Bower, J. E., Greendale, G., Crosswell, A. D., Garet, D., et al. (2014). Yoga reduces inflammatory signaling in fatigued breast cancer survivors: A randomized controlled trial. *Psychoneuroendocrinology, 43*, 20–29.

Buffart et al., Physical and psychosocial benefits.

Carlson et al., Randomized-controlled trial.

Chakrabarty, J., Fernandes, D., Joisa, G., Varghese, P., Mayya, S., & Vidyasagar, M. (2015). Effectiveness of pranayama on cancer-related fatigue in breast cancer patients undergoing radiation therapy: A randomized controlled trial. *International Journal of Yoga, 8*(1), 47–53.

Cramer, H., Rabsilber, S., Lauche, R., Kümmel, S., & Dobos, G. (2015). Yoga and meditation for menopausal symptoms in breast cancer survivors—A randomized controlled trial. *Cancer, 121*(13), 2175–2184.

Cramer et al., Yoga for breast cancer.
Derry, H. M., Jaremka, L. M., Bennett, J. M., Peng, J., et al. (2014). Yoga and self-reported cognitive problems in breast cancer survivors: A randomized controlled trial. *Psycho-Oncology, 24*(8), 958–966.
Dhruva et al., Yoga breathing.
Kiecolt-Glaser et al., Yoga's impact.
Lin, P., Kleckner, I. R., Loh, K. P., Inglis, J. E., et al. (2019). Influence of yoga on cancer-related fatigue and on mediational relationships between changes in sleep and cancer-related fatigue: A nationwide, multicenter randomized controlled trial of yoga in cancer survivors. *Integrative Cancer Therapies, 18*, 153473541985513.
Lundt & Jentschke, Long-term changes.
Lyman et al., Integrative therapies.
Moadel et al., Randomized controlled trial.
Mustian et al., Multicenter, randomized controlled trial.
Raghuram et al., Effects of a yoga program.
Rao, R., Raghuram, N., Nagendra, H., Usharani, M., et al. (2015). Effects of an integrated yoga program on self-reported depression scores in breast cancer patients undergoing conventional treatment: A randomized controlled trial. *Indian Journal of Palliative Care, 21*(2), 174.
Vadiraja, H., Rao, M. R., Nagarathna, R., Nagendra, H., et al. (2009). Effects of yoga program on quality of life and affect in early breast cancer patients undergoing adjuvant radiotherapy: A randomized controlled trial. *Complementary Therapies in Medicine, 17*(5–6), 274–280.

45 Duke University. (2020). EBP tutorial interactive: Module 1: Intro to EBP. https://guides.mclibrary.duke.edu/ebptutorialinteractive/module1
Telles, S., Sharma, S. K., Kala, N., & Balkrishna, A. (2019). Yoga as a holistic treatment for chronic illnesses: Minimizing adverse events and safety concerns. *Frontiers in Psychology, 10*, 661.

46 Jamshidi, N., & Dawson, A. (2019). The hot patient: Acute drug-induced hyperthermia. *Australian Prescriber, 42*(1), 24.

47 van der Linden, P. D., Sturkenboom, M. C., Herings, R. M., Leufkens, H. M., Rowlands, S., & Stricker, B. H. C. (2003). Increased risk of Achilles tendon rupture with quinolone antibacterial use, especially in elderly patients taking oral corticosteroids. *Archives of Internal Medicine, 163*(15), 1801–1807.

48 Yeh, T. S., Chang, K. V., & Wang, T. G. (2011). Common flexor tendon tear following yoga and local corticosteroid injections: A case report. *Journal of Medical Ultrasound, 19*(3), 91–94.

49 Tzaveas, A., Anastasopoulos, N., Paraskevas, G., & Natsis, K. (2016). A rare case of quadratus femoris muscle rupture after yoga exercises. *Clinical Journal of Sport Medicine, 26*(5), e105–e107.

50 Cramer, H., Langhorst, J., Dobos, G., & Lauche, R. (2016). Yoga for metabolic syndrome: A systematic review and meta-analysis. *European Journal of Preventive Cardiology, 23*(18), 1982–1993.
Pascoe, M. C., Thompson, D. R., & Ski, C. F. (2017). Yoga, mindfulness-based stress reduction and stress-related physiological measures: A meta-analysis. *Psychoneuroendocrinology, 86*, 152–168.
Singh, S., Kyizom, T., Singh, K. P., Tandon, O. P., & Madhu, S. V. (2008). Influence of pranayamas and yoga-asanas on serum insulin, blood glucose and lipid profile in type 2 diabetes. *Indian Journal of Clinical Biochemistry, 23*(4), 365–368.

51 Pullen, P. R., Seffens, W. S., & Thompson, W. R. (2018). Yoga for heart failure: A review and future research. *International Journal of Yoga, 11*(2), 91–98.

52 Gangavati, A., Hajjar, I., Quach, L., Jones, R. N., et al. (2011). Hypertension, orthostatic hypotension, and the risk of falls in a community-dwelling elderly population: The maintenance of balance, independent living, intellect, and zest in the elderly of Boston study. *Journal of the American Geriatrics Society, 59*(3), 383–389.

53 As cited in Ladage, D., Schwinger, R. H., & Brixius, K. (2013). Cardio-selective beta-blocker: Pharmacological evidence and their influence on exercise capacity. *Cardiovascular Therapeutics, 31*(2), 76–83.

54 Bloom, H. L., Vinik, A. I., & Colombo, J. (2014). Differential effects of adrenergic antagonists (carvedilol vs metoprolol) on parasympathetic and sympathetic activity: A comparison of clinical results. *Heart International, 9*(1), 15–21.

55 Amza, A. G., Deaconu, A. I., Iorgulescu, C., & Dorobantu, M. (2018). Neurohormonal response in heart

failure and effects of beta-blockers on blood-pressure, heart rate variability and NT-proBNP plasma levels in a patient with newly diagnosed heart failure. *Journal of Hypertension Research*, *4*(2), 66–71.

56 Ladage et al., Cardio-selective beta-blocker.

57 Margolis, K. L., Buchner, D. M., LaMonte, M. J., Zhang, Y., et al. (2019). Hypertension treatment and control and risk of falls in older women. *Journal of the American Geriatrics Society*, *67*(4), 726–733.

58 As cited in Ladage et al., Cardio-selective beta-blocker.

59 Turner, R. M., & Pirmohamed, M. (2020). Statin-related myotoxicity: A comprehensive review of pharmacokinetic, pharmacogenomic and muscle components. *Journal of Clinical Medicine*, *9*(1), 22.

60 Turner & Pirmohamed, Statin-related myotoxicity.

61 Edgell, H., Moore, L. E., Chung, C., Byers, B. W., & Stickland, M. K. (2016). Short-term cardiovascular and autonomic effects of inhaled salbutamol. *Respiratory Physiology & Neurobiology*, *231*, 14–20.
Moore, L. E., Kapoor, K., Byers, B. W., Brotto, A. R., et al. (2019). Acute effects of salbutamol on systemic vascular function in people with asthma. *Respiratory Medicine*, *155*, 133–140.

62 Edgell et al., Short-term cardiovascular and autonomic effects (p. 9).

63 De, A., & Mondal, S. (2019). Immediate effect of yogic postures on autonomic neural responses. *Research in Cardiovascular Medicine*, *8*(4), 106–113.

64 Smith, W. G. (2014). Beta2-agonists for exercise-induced asthma. *Paediatrics & Child Health*, *19*(7), 355–356.

65 Cramer, H., Langhorst, J., Dobos, G., & Lauche, R. (2016). Yoga for metabolic syndrome: A systematic review and meta-analysis. *European Journal of Preventive Cardiology*, *23*(18), 1982–1993.
Pascoe, M. C., Thompson, D. R., & Ski, C. F. (2017). Yoga, mindfulness-based stress reduction and stress-related physiological measures: A meta-analysis. *Psychoneuroendocrinology*, *86*, 152–168.
Singh, S., Kyizom, T., Singh, K. P., Tandon, O. P., & Madhu, S. V. (2008). Influence of pranayamas and yoga-asanas on serum insulin, blood glucose and lipid profile in type 2 diabetes. *Indian Journal of Clinical Biochemistry*, *23*(4), 365–368.

66 Gangji, A. S., Cukierman, T., Gerstein, H. C., Goldsmith, C. H., & Clase, C. M. (2007). A systematic review and meta-analysis of hypoglycemia and cardiovascular events: A comparison of glyburide with other secretagogues and with insulin. *Diabetes Care*, *30*(2), 389–394.

67 Singh et al., Influence of pranayamas and yoga-asanas.

8

Assessing Musculoskeletal Balance in Yoga Therapy

RACHEL KRENTZMAN AND MARLYSA SULLIVAN

Yoga therapy's skill set and scope of practice differentiate the modality from other fields, such as physical therapy and psychotherapy, while complementing the work of other healthcare providers. Assessment procedures, including in the realm of *annamaya kosha*, are key in distinguishing yoga therapy and set the stage for its unique therapeutic process.

Yoga therapists use their professional skills and knowledge combined with informed intuition to plan and deliver yoga therapy tools to fit each individual's condition and constitution. Their diverse methods have yet to be discussed across lineages and schools of yoga therapy. It is therefore important to determine the foundational aspects of assessment and intake that align with yoga therapy's scope of practice to both meet client needs and integrate into healthcare settings. In addition, as yoga therapy enters more medical institutions, the field requires a means to communicate with other health professionals that establishes the profession as unique and complementary, with clear outcome measurements that assess the benefit to each individual.

Because yoga therapists often work with individuals and groups with specific diagnoses and medical conditions, their knowledge of anatomy, kinesiology, and pathology must surpass that available in yoga teacher training programs. As yoga therapist and teacher Aadil Palkhivala, C-IAYT, said, "Yoga teachers learn the rules of yoga, while yoga therapists may have to break those very rules to allow for healing" (personal communication, April 24, 2020).

Without a solid foundation and practice, it is impossible to begin to know how to tailor practices to suit each client's needs. Beginning yoga therapists are well-served by adopting a clear lens that takes into account the *panchamaya kosha* model but is rooted in an understanding of current biomedical science. This chapter focuses on annamaya, specifically the musculoskeletal system and structural considerations. However, its concepts of assessment and documentation are relevant for all of the koshas.

The musculoskeletal approach in this chapter is based on foundational kinesiology principles and movement science,[1] presented within the framework and scope of practice of yoga therapy. Not all yoga therapy training programs include detailed instruction on physical or orthopedic assessment; yoga therapists who do not have additional licensure or specific training must take care to remain within the scope of practice of yoga therapy.[2] The basic passive range-of-motion and simple tests mentioned in this chapter are appropriate for yoga therapists who have received adequate education in their use. Additional specialized skills are needed to assess specific populations, such as people with sciatica, knee pain, or scoliosis, from the yoga therapy perspective.

The Yoga Therapy Perspective: Musculoskeletal Assessment

Yoga therapists aim to assess each client holistically. Similarly, musculoskeletal assessment begins with an investigation of the connected movement patterns of the body rather than isolated parts. Starting with observation of posture and movement provides a zoomed-out perspective to evaluate functional movement patterns. Areas of potential tightness and/or weakness can be identified along with their effect on overall function and movement.

Based on the authors' years of experience in physical therapy, kinesiology, and clinical yoga therapy practice, several themes are key to understanding bodies: where the client falls on a continuum of stability versus mobility; concepts of collapse, prop, yield;[3] structure versus function. Based on these observations decisions can be made about what to test in a more specific way. In other words, the first part of an assessment is more global, the next more narrow and focused.

Symmetry versus alignment

Alignment is often defined in terms of straight lines, which adds to mistaken beliefs that there is one proper position into which everyone should fit. In fact, healthy musculoskeletal alignment is more about the correct *relative* position for each client.

Being in alignment is not the same as being symmetrical. Alignment carries with it a sense of ease, non-forcing, and being in tune with the flow of life.

Alignment includes harmony in thoughts, feelings, and actions. Humans are rarely symmetrical, with exactly equal parts on either side, but they can still be in alignment.

With this in mind, it is important to understand the difference between normal structural or functional deviations and imbalances that cause pain or dysfunction. Structural asymmetry does not always cause a loss of function or diminish one's ability to meet needs or participate in activity. Clients can learn to move more efficiently and effectively in ways that minimize pain and suffering while releasing the need to appear symmetrical or perfectly aligned as they move through life (see Box 8.1).

BOX 8.1 SYMMETRY VERSUS ALIGNMENT: THERAPEUTIC APPLICATION

Consider a client with a severe lumbar scoliosis, upper and lower back pain, and chronic migraines and dizziness. An artist in her late 40s and a mother of three, she stated that she had been struggling with depression and low energy.

Yoga therapy sessions explored finding balance and ease in movement, increasing body awareness, modifying activities, and discovering a new relationship with herself as she entered a new phase in life. After working with her for a few months, her scoliosis was less prominent and her pain had diminished significantly. In addition, she experienced dizziness and headaches less frequently, and she had stopped smoking and begun regularly attending a group yoga therapy series.

This client was able to live an active, fulfilling life—with the scoliosis still present but without pain or limitation. She learned that certain yoga postures were not beneficial for her and found a way to be in alignment with herself, despite the asymmetry of her spine.

The yoga therapy perspective recognizes that the contributors to pain or patterns of weakness or tightness in the body might lie in other koshas. For example, thoughts, emotions, beliefs, and one's relationships to others and to life circumstances can relate to patterns of tension or disconnection, leading to altered movement, pain, and decreased function. Working with the client's beliefs, emotions, sense of self, and relationship to life circumstances can have a profound effect on the physical patterns that contribute to pain or dysfunction.

Stability versus mobility

A client's relative predominance of stability and mobility is another important determinant in assessment and in development of an appropriate plan of care. Physical stability is seen when the parts move in coordination with the whole, resulting in less compressive force and more evenly distributed forces throughout the body during movement.[4] Harmonious movement happens when there is appropriate stability in the system.

Instability refers to a decrease in integrity of joints that may lead to inefficient movement patterns that create stress on soft tissue and joint surfaces. Dys-synchrony and disorganization of movement of joints, muscles, and sections of the body can limit function or contribute to pain. This distortion in optimal movement can be due to altered muscle recruitment patterns, decreased soft tissue integrity, and decreased body awareness. People with pain syndromes such as low back pain or headaches often demonstrate altered muscle recruitment that leads to abnormal movement patterns and possibly pain or decreased function. A client with headaches, for example, might have increased engagement of the upper trapezius and scalenes to compensate for weakness of the deep cervical flexors that should stabilize the neck. This altered pattern of muscular control creates uneven force distribution and stress and strain of the soft tissue as well as joints, contributing to pain.

In addition to localized instability, widespread alterations in connective tissue structure are also possible. Ehlers-Danlos syndrome is one such example of a systemic hypermobility condition. Any form of hypermobility can lead to uneven and excessive movement in areas of the body. Focusing on stretching and mobility without stability can be at best unhelpful and at worst harmful, leading to injury.[5]

Often, those who experience hypermobility crave stretching because they have an altered sense of proprioception—of where their body begins and ends in space.[6] They therefore tend to push into extreme postures, going beyond healthy limitations until eventually injury or inflammation occurs in the form of a strain, muscle or ligament tear, or tendonitis. Working with individuals with hypermobility can be challenging because they need to learn to establish new boundaries by holding back and building strength.

On the other end of the spectrum is hypomobility. Restrictions in joints, soft tissue, and muscles can limit functional mobility and contribute to pain. For those who are hypomobile, safe stretching can be beneficial. (The definition of a safe stretch varies for each individual and could include a range of approaches from static to dynamic.[7]) It is important for the yoga therapist to help discern and educate the client on where they are on this continuum of mobility or stability in relation to *asana* practice.

Additionally, an individual may have areas that are more mobile or unstable and areas that are hypomobile. For example, a client may present with excess mobility through the lumbar spine but decreased mobility in the hip joints. This individual would need to learn how to stabilize the spine as they create ease in their hips. Understanding how to both strengthen that which needs to be stabilized and stretch that which needs to be lengthened represents the essence of yoga—awareness.

Yield versus prop versus collapse

Yielding can be seen as the client's relationship to the earth—their ability to surrender into the support of the ground, to root down and respond by lifting as in a state of rebound or recoil. In yogic terms, this quality represents a state of *sattva* (balance) and a relationship to gravity that expresses the trust, connection, and strength that come with a state of ease. Yielding is the physical representation of *sthira sukham asanam*—the balance of effort/steadiness and ease described in Yoga Sutra 2.46[8] and sought in each posture. When the client is able to yield with enough integrity of structure to create a sense of lift, the breath flows effortlessly and *prana* remains unimpeded.

Collapsing is a state in which the client sinks into the earth without the ability to respond by lifting—a sense of sitting or resting on the bones, ligaments, and joints rather than maintaining structural integrity and focus by using the appropriate muscle activation. Collapsing can create compression in the joints and overstretch ligaments. Breath may be shallow and lethargic when one is in a collapsed state, and the energy is often depressed, as if the person has given up. Many individuals come to yoga in this state. In terms of the *gunas*, collapse could be referred to as *tamas*, a state of heaviness, laziness, lethargy, and lack of mobility or moving forward in life (see Chapter 3).

Propping is a state in which a client holds themselves up with excess force against gravity. Propped postures show muscle and joint tension through locked knees, held breath, tightened gluteals, lifted shoulders, or a puffed-out chest. Lack of ability to trust and surrender into the earth can result in propping. Propped physical postures may be a response to self-reliance, with the underlying belief that no support exists in the world, that one "must stay strong at all costs."

Propping is a strategy of protection. It is the posture adopted from being in a state of fight or flight, and muscles that correspond with sympathetic nervous system activation (e.g., iliopsoas, scalenes, quadratus lumborum, and upper trapezius) become tight and overactive. Through the lens of the gunas, this would be termed a *rajasic* state. Excess rajas is overactivity, aggression, anxiety, or too much chaotic movement in both body and mind. Breath and prana cannot flow freely in this state.

During musculoskeletal assessment, it is useful to observe the client through the lens of quality of movement using the categories of yield, collapse, and prop. This map is one way of seeing beyond the physical and provides information on how to better encourage the client to engage with the plan of care. For individuals in a state of collapse, example cues are "engage," "lift," "energize," and "root to lift," with a focus on extending the inhalation. For those who tend to prop, the aim is to create a sense of relaxation and ease by using language such as "let go," "melt," or "release," with a focus on extending the exhalation. Ultimately, the goal of yoga therapy is to create a means for the client to achieve a state of sattva, or balance, in each posture.

Structural versus functional limitations

Moving from a bigger picture of observation of alignment and stability/mobility, the next step of client evaluation is to discern between functional and structural limitations. Functional limitations are those caused by musculoskeletal or soft tissue imbalances rather than joint or skeletal limitations. According to Vladimir Janda's theory, patterns of musculoskeletal facilitation or inhibition emerge from the nervous system that controls them.[9] "Facilitation" refers to the level of contraction, activation, or tension the muscle holds and its timely initiation of movement for stability and functional mobility. "Inhibition" refers to a muscle's lack of activation to initiate functional motion. Janda's approach can be useful for yoga therapists, as its organized model illustrates common imbalances that lead to altered movement (Table 8.1).

Table 8.1 Common muscular imbalances

Area of Dysfunction	Weak or Inhibited Muscles	Tight and/or Short Muscles
Low back, hip, knee	Transversus abdominis Gluteus medius/minimus Gluteus maximus Pelvic floor Quadriceps (vastus medialis)	Iliopsoas Hamstrings Adductors Pelvic floor Quadriceps (rectus femoris) Piriformis Quadratus lumborum

Shoulder, neck	Lower and middle trapezius Serratus anterior Deep cervical flexors	Upper trapezius Levator scapulae Pectoralis major and minor Latissimus dorsi Scalenes Sternocleidomastoids

Adapted from Table 9.1 in Sullivan, M., & Robertson, L. C. H. (2020). *Understanding yoga therapy: Applied philosophy and science for health and well-being* (p. 193). Routledge.

As a result of a heightened stress response certain areas of the body are held in a facilitated or tight state. Many of these tight muscles are the fight/flight muscles activated in a stress response. For example, neck muscles, such as the upper trapezius or scalenes, are used for faster, shallower breathing and to scan the environment to evaluate and respond to danger. Tension in these muscles may begin with an injury to structures of the cervical spine, or the tension may arise from living in states of prolonged stress, fear, or anxiety. Regardless of the cause (physical, emotional, or otherwise), these muscles tend to overengage and contribute to altered breathing patterns or maladaptive postures such as anterior head carriage (forward head), rounded shoulders, and a collapsed chest. People with these patterns may experience pain or even structural deformation to the cervical spine such as disc injury or osteoarthritis. Looking for these underlying patterns as described by Janda enables yoga therapists to promote greater synchrony and alignment at the physical layer.

The clarity provided from a thorough musculoskeletal assessment enables the yoga therapist to discern whether the suffering that the client is experiencing is fundamentally functional (e.g., a result of a dysfunctional muscle-firing pattern), structural (e.g., related to the shape of a bony structure, as mentioned below under "Passive range of motion"), or affected by involvement of the other koshas.

Following skillful attention to physical issues, yoga therapist and client may together explore the effect of the mind's function on the body's lived experience from *pranamaya* through *anandamaya kosha*.

Yoga therapy application

Clients with lower back pain may present any of these patterns of facilitation or inhibition of muscles, leading to various postural and movement dys-synchronies or to altered function. Although two individuals may experience similar symptoms, addressing the source of the problem may require two very different interventions. For example, two of the most common presentations that may result from these postural imbalances and lead to back pain are

- rounded shoulders, forward head posture, decreased lumbar lordosis, posterior pelvic tilt, tight or short hamstrings, and externally rotated hips; and
- overarched lumbar spine (hyperlordosis), decreased abdominal activation, anterior pelvic tilt, flattened thoracic spine, decreased cervical lordosis, splayed ribs, and weak adductors and hip/pelvic musculature

These two patterns may contribute to uneven stresses on the joints of the low back, hip, and knee as well as the disc and soft tissue structures, leading to pathology in any of these areas. Each pattern creates stresses for different reasons. In one case, decreased flexibility of muscles such as the hamstrings or psoas may compress the vertebral structures, leading to pain, inflammation, and possibly disc deformation. In another individual, instability and uncontrolled mobility may cause repetitive-stress injuries as well as compression of the vertebral structures. In both cases, the symptom is lower back pain, but the intervention for each individual would be very different.

The nervous system also provides a link between these musculoskeletal patterns and the other koshas. Emotional states can affect how the individual relates to and connects to the body as well as how they hold their posture. In essence, beliefs affect bodies. A rigid mental outlook or need for control can create a similar physical pattern in which muscles are held in constant tension, unable to let go. Another individual may have a fragile sense of self, not knowing their place in the world and feeling unstable or ungrounded. This might appear as weakness in the legs, core, and/or sacroiliac (SI) joint. Recognizing such intangible contributors to physical presentation takes skilled inquiry and work with the yoga therapist over time, as each individual is unique. Once all the koshas are assessed, a personal program can be tailored to take into account any physical limitation along with underlying beliefs.

The idea of similar physical results arising from different patterns can also be illustrated in the upper body. Clients with shoulder pain may present with various imbalances contributing to pain, for example,

- rounded shoulders, tight pectorals, weak upper back and shoulder musculature, forward head posture, increased kyphosis, decreased thoracic movement, and shallow breathing; or
- shoulder hypermobility, collapsing through the shoulders in postures such as downward dog, disorganized scapulohumeral rhythm, weak scapular and shoulder stabilizers, scapular winging, unstable cervical spine or a feeling of "not knowing where the head should sit," and decreased cervical lordosis

In both patterns, the shoulder structures, such as the rotator cuff or bursae, can become compressed, inflamed, and painful, although the causes are different. In addition to shoulder dysfunction, these imbalances can lead to pain or structural dysfunction of the cervical spine, elbow, or wrist. Whether the diagnosis is tennis elbow, carpal tunnel syndrome, cervical disc disease, or rotator cuff tendonitis, the yoga therapist can assess the underlying functional movement patterns contributing to uneven stresses. Once the source of the problem is established, targeted asana and pranayama tools can be offered for optimal pain relief.

The Assessment Process

The assessment process enables both the yoga therapist and client to move from the big picture to greater detail around contributors to movement dysfunction. This allows the yoga therapist to determine possible musculoskeletal imbalances of tightness, decreased range of motion (ROM), or weakness. Muscle tests can be used to help discern these imbalances so that the plan of care is targeted to these contributors.

Figure 8.1 provides a map for use when assessing a client. As each individual is unique, the tools for assessment will vary depending on how the client presents and what the yoga therapist observes. It is important to remain curious about what emerges in the co-creation of the client's plan of care.

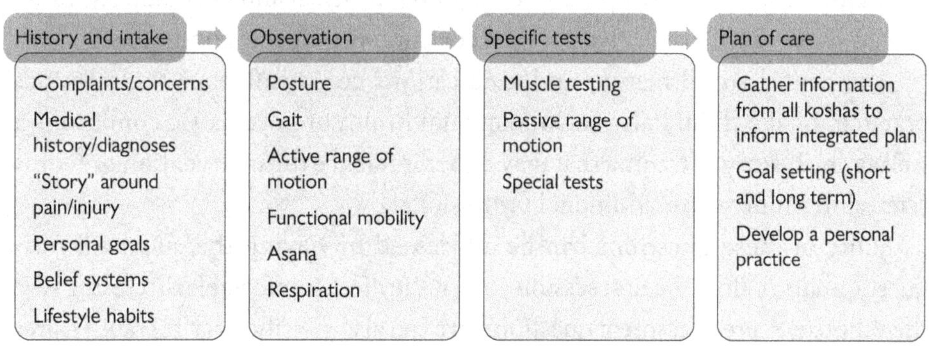

FIGURE 8.1 CLINICAL ASSESSMENT MAP

Yoga therapists investigate the physical, mental/emotional, and spiritual sources of any physical problem rather than simply pacifying the symptoms. Any hypothesis is based on observations that are followed up with more specific testing to determine accuracy or whether additional inquiry is required.

Consider a client who presents with an anteriorly tilted pelvis, pronounced lumbar lordosis, and collapse in the lower back in postures such as downward dog, warrior I, and warrior II. One could deduce that the psoas may be tight, causing an excessive lordosis, or that the abdominals may be weak and unable to provide adequate support in the posture. Perhaps there is hypermobility in the shoulder joint or weakness in the shoulder and upper back musculature. More specific muscle tests could help to differentiate among these possible sources of the client's presentation and identify appropriate tools for a plan of care focused on the specific area of dysfunction.[10] Additionally, cues that specifically address areas of dysfunction will help the client achieve both ease and integrity in asana practice.

The assessment map can be considered step by step.

History and intake

The story the client tells will point the yoga therapist in the right direction. Deliberate presence and deep listening skills then enable one to see beyond the story and focus on the storyteller's experience in addition to the details of the physical concern. Such assessment practices not only help the yoga therapist to gather information, but also to provide a safe space for the client to be seen and heard in the co-creation of the eventual plan (see Chapter 14).

Gathering as much pertinent information as possible helps the yoga therapist to decide what direction the assessment should take. Perhaps the problem is not physical at all but falls under one of the other koshas or in a more psychospiritual area. This chapter stays within the realm of the physical and energetic layers and how to proceed with tools that support common orthopedic conditions.

A client's medical history and medications could influence their physical practice. Intake should also include mental health or psychiatric conditions as well as any history of trauma that may either influence the intervention or require referral to a different or additional professional.

Some of these questions can be addressed by having the client fill out a questionnaire before the first session so that they feel comfortable disclosing what they choose. A preassessment questionnaire can also give the yoga therapist a great deal of information as to how to prepare for meeting the client for the first time. A flexible approach is important, as the intended direction may change as the yoga therapist interacts with the client in person. The map proposed in this chapter may help the practitioner to assess musculoskeletal imbalance, but it is in no way a complete yoga therapy assessment in and of itself.

Physically oriented questions (annamaya) usually begin the intake, offering the opportunity for the client to articulate the reasons they decided to participate in yoga therapy sessions. Here the yoga therapist also begins to establish a clear idea of the client's personal goals and expectations.

Was there an injury? Is there pain? What is the quality of the pain? How does the pain behave? What are some other symptoms? When did the pain begin? What was happening in their life at the time? What makes it better? What makes it worse?

During what activities is the pain present? Does it affect their daily life in a significant way? If so, how? Does it affect their sleep, their relationships? What is the source of their suffering?

Questions like these should offer an idea of the specific assessments that would be useful. Observation of posture and movement then provides more objective information.

BOX 8.2 RED FLAGS

Red-flag symptoms suggest a more serious problem that may require immediate medical care by a physician or other appropriate healthcare provider. The following red flags warrant referral out before beginning yoga therapy.

- **Pain all the time, regardless of activity or positioning**, may suggest something other than an orthopedic or mechanical reason for pain.
- **Progressive numbness or weakness in any limb** may indicate compression on spinal nerves or the spinal cord, which may require medical intervention.
- **Bowel or bladder dysfunction** may signal a spinal cord lesion.
- **Excessive swelling, redness, or heat in any joint** is a potential sign of infection.

Observation

Client observation begins even before the formal start of the session, when there is an opportunity to notice posture and overall movement patterns.

How does the client sit during the intake interview? Are the shoulders rounded? Is the head tilted to one side? Do they stand with one leg turned out?

These observations may turn out to be irrelevant, but careful noticing when the client is just being themselves is important.

Next comes consideration of overall standing posture from all angles—anterior (front), posterior (back), and sides. The following sections point yoga therapists toward the causes of physical complaints. Throughout the assessment process the dynamics between symmetry and alignment, stability and mobility, collapse/prop/yield, and structural versus functional limitations should always be considered.

Standing posture: Tadasana

- Feet: weight distribution (more on ball or heel of the foot, more on the left or right, collapsed arches/pronated feet or high arches/supinated feet).
- Knees: knee alignment (locked, hyperextended); relationship to pelvis and feet, knock-kneed (*genu valgum*) or bow-legged (*genu varum*), direction the patellae point, surrounding muscle tone, any evidence of quadriceps weakness/atrophy.
- Hips and pelvis: pelvic alignment (one side higher, one side rotated forward or back, overall excessive anterior or posterior tilt); hips internally or externally rotated (one or both feet turned in/out).
- Torso: decreased or increased lumbar, thoracic, and/or cervical curves; breath and movement of the ribs in concert with breath; balance and fluidity of movement of the torso in relation to the upper and lower body (i.e., integration).
- Shoulders: rounded, scapular winging, shoulder height (one side higher), muscle tone around the shoulders and neck.
- Neck: forward head posture, muscle tone around the neck and jaw, decreased cervical lordosis (flat neck).

Gait/walking pattern

After observing standing posture, it is a good idea to observe the gait pattern, especially if the reason for seeking yoga therapy involves back, hip, knee, or foot pain. While the client walks comfortably, specific observations can be made, as illustrated in Table 8.2.

Table 8.2 Points to observe during ambulation

Body Area	Points to Observe
Feet and legs	Quality of steps (evenness/rhythm, limping) Range of motion of hips and legs, including degree of hip extension at the end of stride Length of stride Heel-toe pattern Collapse or overpronation (roll toward the midline) and rigidity or supination (outward roll) of the feet or ankles Fluidity of movement Compensatory patterns (e.g., excess circumduction [circular movement] or hip hiking, knee hyperextension) Limping or uneven weight distribution
Trunk and pelvis	Integrated movements of pelvis and rib cage Amount of trunk rotation Mobility of spine and pelvis Breath during ambulation Spinal curves during ambulation
Upper body	Arm swing Position of shoulders (rounded or open) Lifted or collapsed chest Tension in neck and shoulders Accessory breathing
Overall integration of movement	Overall fluidity or rigidity during ambulation Ability to yield vs. collapse and/or prop

Active range of motion

Based on client complaints, history, and observation of posture and gait the yoga therapist can move on to ROM testing. Active ROM refers to movement that the client does on their own to help understand or explore muscular function and recruitment patterns. Passive mobility, discussed later, involves the yoga therapist assisting the movement to explore tissue tension and joint limitation.

It is important to understand the quality of motion with which the client presents before asking them to perform complex movement patterns like asana. For example, pain with active arm raising may lead the yoga therapist to limit postures that require weight-bearing on the arms.

Active ROM can demonstrate

- available range
- quality of movement, including the presence of compensatory patterns
- pain with motion

See Figure 8.2 for the basic planes through which the body moves. Example movements include

- neck flexion, extension, rotation, lateral flexion (sidebending)
- shoulder abduction, flexion, external rotation, internal rotation
- spinal rotation, lateral flexion, flexion, extension
- pelvic mobility: anterior and posterior tilt, rotational/circular movement; integration between pelvis and spine
- hip flexion, extension, abduction, adduction, internal and external rotation
- knee flexion and extension
- ankle dorsiflexion, plantarflexion, pronation, supination

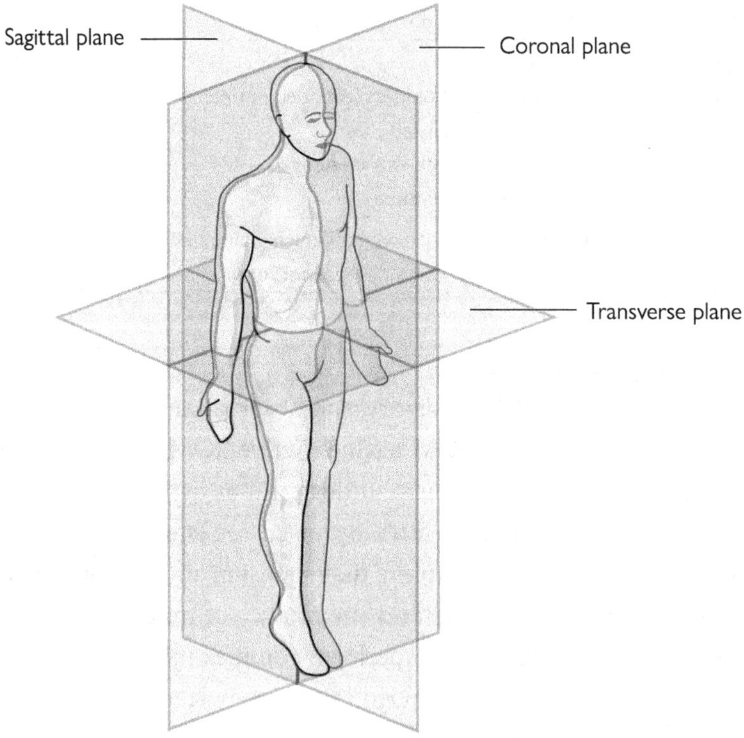

FIGURE 8.2 BASIC PLANES OF MOTION

Functional mobility

Before moving to the asana assessment, it is appropriate to assess the client's overall functional mobility. Transitions between positions provide information about joint mobility, pain, balance, ROM, endurance, coordination, and ability to perform physical asana. The yoga therapist can note whether modifications and props are needed.

Examples of functional mobility explorations include the following.

- Sit to stand: Can the client do this without using the hands? Is momentum required to stand?
- Balance:
  - Stepping forward or moving from sitting to standing (assess ability to transition from one position to another without assistance from a wall or chair).
  - Base of support (quality of balance when the feet are closer together vs. wider apart).
- Ability to transfer to and from the floor can help assess leg strength and balance. Does the client need assistance from a person, chair, or wall? (This can help to determine the need for a table or chair rather than working on the floor.)
- Ability to bear weight on hands and knees: Is there pain in the knees or wrists? Does this challenge the client's balance?

Asana

As a general rule, yoga therapists ask clients to perform foundational asana that can provide information about ROM, strength, flexibility, balance, coordination, proprioceptive awareness, tone, quality of movement, and ability to transition between positions. Included in observation are qualities of yield/collapse/prop as well as where the client falls on the continuum of mobility and stability.

Table 8.3 outlines recommended postures to assess. However, it is important to understand that the choice of asana varies depending on relevance to the client's primary concern and yoga practice experience.

Table 8.3 Recommended asana for assessment

Asana	Musculoskeletal Observations
Standing mountain pose (*tadasana*)	Shoulder position, respiratory pattern, spinal curves, collapse/prop/yield, pelvic tilt, abdominal tone and integrity, hip/knee/foot position
Tree pose (*vriksasana*) or one-leg balance, with or without external hip rotation	Overall balance, gluteus medius strength, leg strength, possibly external rotation in lifted leg
Chair pose (*utkatasana*) or shallow squat	Range of motion in ankles, knees, hips, pelvis, spine; strength of lower extremities; knee position (genu valgum/varum); abdominal tone
Triangle (*trikonasana*)	Length of hamstrings, adductors, quadratus lumborum, erector spinae; lateral spinal flexion and rotation; balance; external rotation of front leg; abdominal tone; shoulder abduction and external rotation; neck position and muscle tension
Warrior (*virabhadrasana*) I	Hip flexor (including iliopsoas) length, lower extremity strength, balance, shoulder range of motion, abdominal tone
Warrior II	Hip adductor length; hip abductor strength; abdominal tone; leg strength (quads, hamstrings, gluteals); hip range of motion (external rotation and abduction); lumbar spine control and stability; shoulder abduction (including scapular strength and compensatory tone of upper trapezius)
Standing forward fold (*uttanasana*)	Hamstring length, spinal and pelvic mobility, scoliosis/rib humps
Cat/cow (*marjaryasana/bitilasana*)	Ability to move from flexion to extension throughout spine, areas of limitation, ability to coordinate breath with movement, ability to articulate at each vertebral level
Child's pose (*balasana*)	Hip and knee mobility, shoulder flexion range, spinal flexibility
Plank (*phalakasana*)	Strength of serratus anterior, abdominals, triceps
Downward dog (*adho mukha svanasana*)	Hamstring and Achilles length, pelvic mobility and position, lumbar position and stability, abdominal tone, scapular stability and serratus anterior strength, neck tension, shoulder mobility/latissimus dorsi length, shoulder/elbow/wrist position
Cobra (*bhujangasana*)	Thoracic and lumbar mobility in extension, cervical position and stability, fluid and balanced spinal movement throughout vertebral segments, pectoralis length, erector spinae strength, scapular strength and balance between rhomboid/middle traps and lower traps
Seated staff pose (*dandasana*)	Hamstring length, spinal and pelvic mobility and stability
Easy seat (*sukhasana*; cross-legged)	Hip range of motion, spinal and pelvic mobility and position

Seated or supine spinal twist	Spinal rotation range, fluidity and balance of spinal movement throughout vertebral segments, limitations at different levels (e.g., decreased thoracic mobility, excessive lumbar mobility), tightness in pectorals and shoulders
Corpse pose (*savasana*)	Ability to relax, shoulder position (rounded, forward, lifted), head and neck position, jaw/facial tension, overall respiratory quality, position of hips and legs

During this portion of the assessment, active ROM as well as quality of movement and patterns of recruitment in different postures are observed. Areas of pain, restriction, and compensation are of interest here. A full yoga therapy assessment would also consider quality of breath, interoceptive awareness, energy levels and flow, emotions, and beliefs that may arise in the practice of an asana.

The clinical reasoning process carries the yoga therapist from observation to discerning possible contributors so that an appropriate intervention can be designed. For example, in downward dog a client may have a rounded upper back with most of the weight falling onto the upper extremities. Possible causes of this imbalance include decreased shoulder ROM, short/tight latissimus dorsi, short/tight hamstrings, and decreased thoracic mobility. To determine which issue is the culprit, the assessment continues.

In this example, the yoga therapist might next ask the client to bend their knees to release tension along the hamstring complex which, when shortened or tight, can pull on the pelvis and affect the position of the spine in downward dog. If the person can elongate the spine with bent knees, the yoga therapist can deduce that they likely have tight or short hamstrings. If flexing the knees did not change the thoracic hyperkyphosis, the client might next be asked to lie down and take their arms overhead; limited shoulder flexion in this position would indicate tight or short latissimus dorsi muscles. Confirmation that the latissimus rather than the shoulder joints are the problem could be obtained by performing a passive ROM to test whether limitation or pain occurs at the end of the range (see next stage of assessment). Finally, thoracic mobility could be assessed by having the client come into different postures, including spinal twists, to observe any movement limitations in the upper back.

The examples in Figure 8.3 illustrate the clinical reasoning process when looking at asana, moving from the posture to the imbalance and possible contributors. The next step in assessment is to determine which of these possible contributors may be the underlying issue.

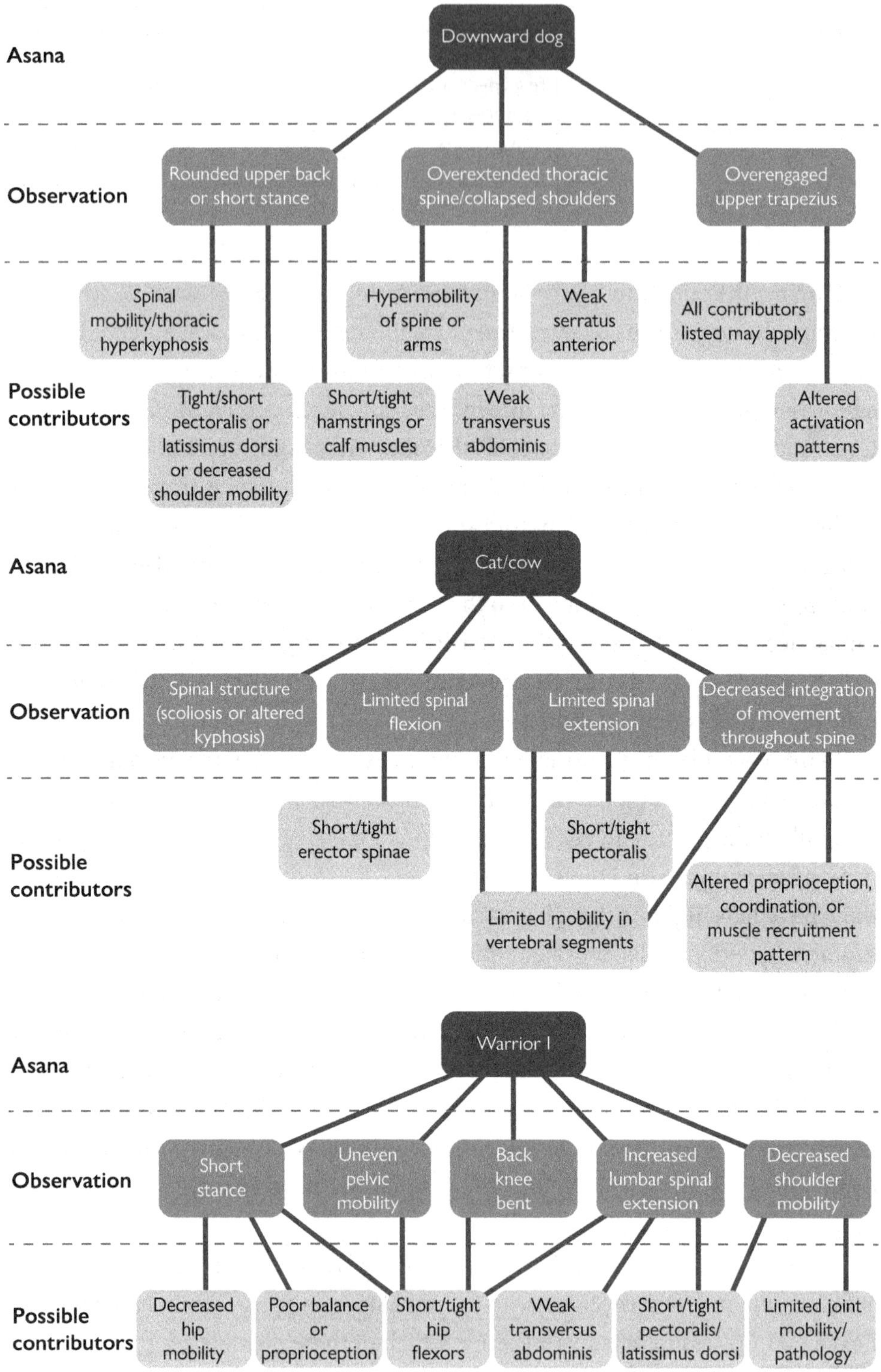

FIGURE 8.3 CLINICAL REASONING IN ASANA

Multiple additional contributors are possible for all of these observations.

Specific tests

The information gathered during observational assessment can prompt further testing to confirm suspicions. Is the limitation in downward dog from tight latissimus dorsi, shoulder joint limitations, and/or pain from tendonitis? Passive ROM testing, muscle testing for strength, and special tests can rule out or confirm the possible causes of dysfunction or pain. Once the cause is determined, the yoga therapist can decide what can be done within the scope of practice or whether a referral is needed.

Passive range of motion

In the example of the individual with shoulder limitation during downward dog, passive shoulder flexion would determine whether the joint has full range. The yoga therapist would gently assist the body part to move in its normal range (180 degrees) without any additional pressure or force. It is important to distinguish whether any limitation is from a joint limitation, muscle tightness, or pain from inflammation of a tendon, or bursae. Here again, the yoga therapist needs specific education, but a joint limitation generally would appear as a block to movement beyond a certain range (a bone contacting a bone); muscle tightness feels more like a stretch at the end of the range. Inflammation would be indicated by pain or a pinching sensation anywhere along the range of motion.

Muscle tests

The yoga therapist can choose specific muscle tests to look at length, strength, and recruitment patterns based on the information gathered through observation of asana and passive range. Again given appropriate training, the yoga therapist may employ manual muscle testing, in which the client holds the body part in a certain position while the yoga therapist applies manual pressure as resistance. Muscle testing provides information about the client's ability to use the muscle and its strength, as well as whether pain is present with resistance, which could signal an injury to the muscle. Muscle tests also help support the identification of which imbalances are present to provide a relevant and focused plan of care. For instance, this example client would likely need to build strength in the scapular stabilizers (serratus anterior and the lower/middle trapezius) and rotator cuff muscles.

Special tests

Several simple tests are appropriate for yoga therapists to use to help identify common imbalances or the need for a referral for a more extensive Western orthopedic evaluation (Table 8.4). In the above example, special tests could suggest the presence of impingement (painful-arc test) and rotator cuff dysfunction (empty-can test). Each yoga therapy training has its own focus and may teach students to perform these tests when assessing clients; staying within the scope of practice of yoga therapy requires working within the limits of one's professional training.

Table 8.4 Recommended special tests

Body Area	Test
Shoulder	Empty-can test (supraspinatus weakness/inflammation) Painful-arc test (shoulder impingement)
Knee	Ober test (iliotibial band tension)
Hip	Thomas test (iliopsoas tension) Trendelenberg sign (weak gluteus medius)
Lower back	Slump test (disc herniation or neural tension) Straight-leg raise (lumbar disc herniation, sciatica)
SI joint	March test (SI joint dysfunction)
Abdominals	ASLR (abdominal weakness, instability)

Depending on the yoga therapist's training, referral to another professional, such as a physical therapist or chiropractor, may be necessary for this type of assessment.
SI = sacroiliac; ASLR = asymmetric straight-leg raise.

Plan of care

Creating a plan of care follows observation of limitations and testing to confirm the possible cause of the dysfunction and rule out the need for immediate referral to another professional. Based on the findings, the yoga therapist can create short- and long-term goals that will inform the direction of each session and help to determine priorities. Once the problem areas have been identified and goals outlined, the following questions need to be answered:

- Which asana would best address the problematic area and underlying causes of dysfunction?
- What instructions and style of cueing will help the client meet their goals?
- How will physical assessment findings be integrated with the other koshas to create a meaningful, effective practice?

Summary

A clear, detailed musculoskeletal assessment is vital for the yoga therapist to understand a client's condition, learn about possible sources of discomfort, identify red flags, and determine short- and long-term goals for the plan of care. Without it, the intervention may lack focus and fail to address underlying factors, resulting in decreased effectiveness and delayed healing.

A defined assessment is also important as a means of communicating with other health professionals to ensure cohesive, integrated care. The path outlined in this chapter is a clear map for exploring potential causes for the client's concerns and an aid to developing practices suited to their physical needs. Yoga therapy can then proceed with an integration of all other koshas—pranamaya, manomaya, vijnanamaya, and anandamaya—into the plan of care.

Additional Resources

Cohen, B. B. (2014). *Sensing, feeling and action: The experiential anatomy of body-mind centering* (3rd ed.). Contact Editions.

Frank, C., Page, P., & Lardner, R. (2009). *Assessment and treatment of muscle imbalance: The Janda approach.* Human Kinetics.

Endnotes

1 See, e.g., Frank, C., Page, P., & Lardner, R. (2009). *Assessment and treatment of muscle imbalance: The Janda approach.* Human Kinetics; Houglum, P. A., & Bertoti, D. B. (2011). *Brunnstrom's clinical kinesiology* (6th ed.). F. A. Davis Company.

2 International Association of Yoga Therapists. (2020). Scope of practice for yoga therapy. https://cdn.ymaws.com/www.iayt.org/resource/resmgr/docs_certification_all/2020_updates_scope_ethics/2020-09_sop_v2.pdf
Compliance with local and other laws, which vary by jurisdiction, must also be ensured.

3 Cohen, B. B. (2014). *Sensing, feeling and action: The experiential anatomy of body-mind centering* (3rd ed.). Contact Editions.

4 See, e.g., Frank et al., *Assessment and treatment*; Houglum & Bertoti, *Brunnstrom's clinical kinesiology.*

5 See, e.g., Mueller, M. J., & Maluf, K. S. (2002). Tissue adaptation to physical stress: A proposed "physical stress theory" to guide physical therapist practice, education, and research. *Physical Therapy, 82*(4), 383–403.

6 See, e.g., Mueller & Maluf, Tissue adaptation.

7 Hakim, A. J., Keer, R. J., & Grahame, R. (Eds.). (2010). *Hypermobility, fibromyalgia and chronic pain.* Elsevier Health Sciences.

8 Desikachar, T. K. V. (1999). *The heart of yoga: Developing a personal practice* (p. 180). Inner Traditions.

9 Frank et al., *Assessment and treatment.*

10 For guidance that helps to distinguish the scope of practice of yoga therapy from that of physical therapy or other disciplines, please see International Association of Yoga Therapists, Scope of Practice for Yoga Therapy; Bhavanani, A. B., Sullivan, M., Taylor, M. J., & Wheeler, A. (2019). Shared foundations for practice: The language of yoga therapy. *Yoga Therapy Today*, Summer, 44–47.

9

Human Development and Sensory Integration: Pediatric Yoga Therapy

YANA KOFMAN

The human developmental sequence progresses through five hierarchical levels: gross motor skills, fine motor skills, speech and language development, cognitive, and socioemotional skills. This chapter focuses on the role of movement development and its connection to voluntary breath control in yoga therapy with pediatric populations. Speech and language development and cognitive development are not discussed here, although practices such as vocalized mantra and chanting could be considered to interact with these developmental levels.

For yoga therapists to apply appropriate therapeutic baselines, they must first have an understanding of clients' developmental stages in terms of gross and fine motor skills and emotional development. Broadly identifying gross motor and emotional skills provides a picture of the bottom and top of the human developmental sequence. An integrated approach enables yoga therapists to establish a framework for the whole client—and the family—to optimize outcomes.[1] Those who choose to work with pediatric populations require extensive background and training in understanding child psychology, neuromotor patterns, reflex integration, etc.; an overview of motor skills and socioemotional development is provided here.

Motor Skills

In pediatric yoga therapy, the ongoing relationship between postures and controlled breathing can teach a child about intrinsic balance and forces of gravity. Yoga therapists can introduce proper breathing techniques and encourage positions that enable clients to learn the qualities of diaphragmatic breath.

Counter to what often happens in adults, separating breath from movement aids in guiding the child away from their cognitive and analytical mind and toward their emotional engagement system. As the child becomes aware of inner sensations and connects them to feelings, inviting in the analytical self can etch the work into memory.[2]

Developmental structure and breath

Breath is deeply connected with human development. In typical trajectory, a child learns to clear their sinuses as young as age 2, breathing out using forced exhalation with their nostrils to cleanse the passages in a technique similar to *kapalabhati*. With an inverse breathing pattern, breath is forcibly inhaled, creating a hyperventilatory response and precluding forced exhalation.

An assessment of rib movement, diaphragmatic control, and their interrelationship may demonstrate a lack of rib cage expansion and areas where tension hinders mobility. Yoga therapy work in these cases might focus on diaphragmatic breathing and controlled forced exhalation, which helps with cleansing, waste elimination, and bilateral neurological control and integration.

Yogic breath practices may strengthen a child's lungs, promoting relaxation and a sense of well-being.[3] *Pranayama* also stimulates vital areas of the central nervous system, including the brain. Combining pranayama with *asana* enhances the benefits of each, although, as noted above, it may be necessary to de-link breath from movement initially.

Embryology

The embryonic musculoskeletal system begins to develop as early as 12 weeks of gestation. The formation of the "notochord"—a skeletal rod that supports the body and later becomes the spine, spinal cord, and brain—begins in the third week after conception. Arms and legs begin to develop in the fourth week. The limbs (first the arms, hands, and fingers, then the legs, feet, and toes) elongate between the fifth and eighth weeks; the lowest point of the backbone, the coccyx, also develops by the end of the fifth week. The process of osteoneogenesis (development of bone) does not complete until well after birth. Ossification (the process whereby tissue becomes bone) of most bony nuclei of the long bones and round bones begins about the third month of fetal life and is completed by late adolescence.

The four main types of human bones are

- long (the arm and leg bones)

- short (the small bones in the wrists and ankles)
- flat (the bones of the skull or the ribs)
- irregular (vertebrae)

Newborn bones have multiple ossification centers from which bone growth begins. Bones lengthen at the epiphyseal plate. Osteoblasts then move in and ossify the matrix to form bone. This process continues throughout adolescence until cartilage growth slows and eventually stops.[4]

Spinal curves

When viewed laterally (from the side), the spine's natural lordotic (inward) and kyphotic (outward) curves resemble an S (Figure 9.1). The thoracic and sacral areas of the spine form the normal kyphoses, otherwise known as the primary curves; the cervical and lumbar areas of the spine form the normal lordoses (secondary curves). Each spinal curve works to distribute mechanical loading the body experiences while static and in motion.

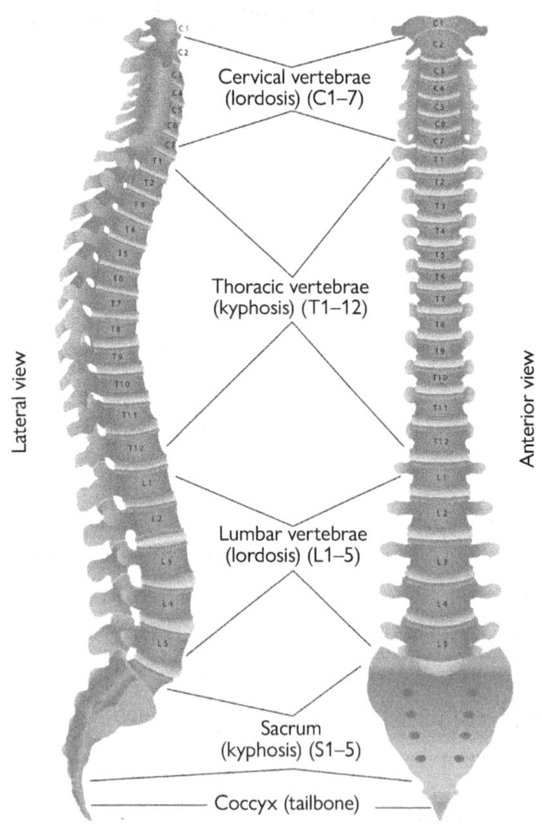

FIGURE 9.1 THE SPINAL COLUMN'S NATURAL CURVES

The primary curves (Figure 9.2) form during fetal development. These curves are protective in nature, safeguarding the fetus from trauma during pregnancy. The secondary curves (Figure 9.3) form after birth. The cervical spinal curve develops as a result of infants lifting their heads against gravity. Between the ages of 3 and 6 months, infants typically pick up their heads while prone (on their stomachs), eventually creating the forward neck curve (normal cervical lordosis). The lumbar spinal curve develops as a result of the infant crawling and later walking. At age 6–12 months, crawling aids in development of the forward low back curve (lumbar lordosis).

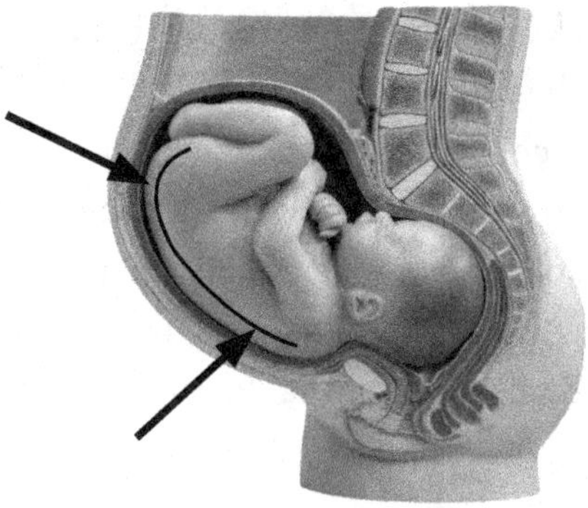

FIGURE 9.2 PRIMARY "NEWBORN" CURVES (THORACIC AND SACRAL SPINES)

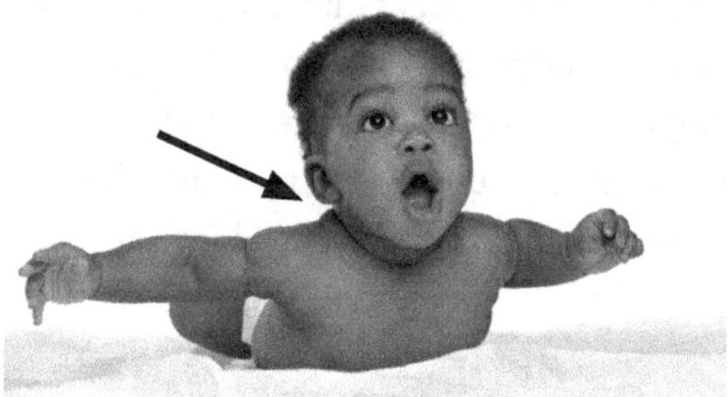

FIGURE 9.3A CERVICAL SPINE LORDOSIS (PART OF THE SECONDARY CURVES)

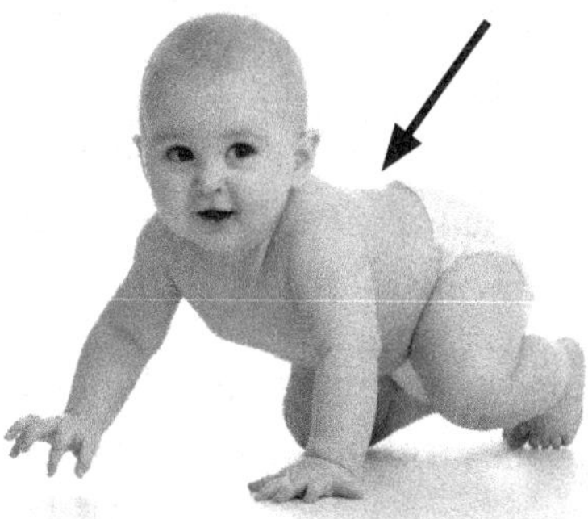

FIGURE 9.3B LUMBAR SPINE LORDOSIS (PART OF THE SECONDARY CURVES)

Infants' heads must be supported due to lack of cervical strength and antigravity control. Some do not develop strong neck muscles and struggle with holding their heads upright even after 6 months, when most babies have developed this ability. This weakness limits the development of the first secondary curve of the spine, the arch of the neck (Figure 9.3a). Pediatricians therefore advise new parents to encourage their babies to spend time prone. When on their tummies, infants tend to raise their arms and legs in the air and wiggle as if they are swimming; their head is arched up, eventually creating the cervical lordosis. These actions are necessary patterns in development as the body prepares the baby for each stage of spinal development. Spending time prone also lays the groundwork for the second secondary curve, the low back lordosis (Figure 9.3b). This second secondary curve continues to develop when the baby begins to crawl.

Parents may wrongly encourage early walking, causing children to miss critical practice with creeping and crawling to the detriment of their spinal curve development. Walkers and some carriers put babies in an upright posture before the spine is ready to support this weight. Encouraging a baby to stand before the low back arch has developed may lead to a flat lower back, or "lumbar kyphosis."

Gross and Fine Motor Skills

In neurotypical development, the infant undergoes a predicted sequencing as the body develops antigravity and postural control. As babies move their limbs, they develop stronger motor patterns. Head control gradually develops as caregivers continually support the infant's head. As the neck muscles strengthen, the baby is able to hold up their head without support, the dominant milestone in an infant's gross motor development.

Developmental posture sequencing

Yoga asana directly correlate to normal human development, inviting one to revisit the neurotypical sequences of movement experienced during the first year of life. Yogic practice enables the experience of all three planes of movement, promoting the development and maintenance of healthy spinal mobility. The developmental progression mirrors the following sequence of yoga postures.

- **Supine:** In the primary sequence in development, observed in newborns, infants lie on their backs with the spine and cranium weight bearing.
- **Prone:** The infant lies face-down with the head turned to one side. Prone

posture, the second sequence in infant development, is the antecedent to the critical cervical spinal curve development.

- **Seated:** In the third sequence in development, the infant bears weight on their sit bones (ischial tuberosities). The ring sit (*baddha konasana*, or cobbler pose)—with the knees flexed and the hips externally rotated, with soles of the feet touching—is the first upright position infants assume on their own.
- **Quadruped:** In the fourth sequence in infant development, weight is borne on the palms and knees with the ankles extended and plantar flexed (tabletop pose).
- **Tall kneeling:** The infant can kneel on the floor with the weight distributed below the knees (*vajrasana*, or thunderbolt). This posture helps to develop strength in the posterior (back) of the body, including the trunk, hips, and lower legs.
- **Half kneeling:** The infant is able to bring one foot forward with the knee bent while maintaining the other leg in the kneeling position (*anjaneyasana*, or low lunge).
- **Standing upright:** *Tadasana* (mountain pose).

BOX 9.1 THERAPEUTIC APPLICATION

Yoga therapy that employs these sequencing patterns might focus on gentle stretching, body alignment, assisted pose practice, and improvement of bilateral integration and coordination. Improving dynamic standing and seated balance and enhancing ability to transition between postures via controlled and purposeful fluidity may be therapeutic goals when working with motor skills development. Sessions would include positional changes in supine and seated; they could also focus on hand-to-foot spatial orientation by bringing the upper and lower limbs toward each other, as well as on bringing the left and right sides of the body to the midline.

Continuously challenging young clients to work on developmental postures and sequencing helps to build strength and attention, in turn improving developmental patterns. Using a yoga block under the seat for support in squatting, for example, may help to increase lower abdominal strength, hip flexibility, and muscular control.[5] Over time, gravity assists clients to develop increased tolerance to positional changes, in turn improving overall aerobic endurance.

Analyzing the motor components that infants use to attain each milestone can guide yoga therapists toward a developmentally sound care plan. Infants develop increased proficiency in motor skills by practicing and problem-solving when interacting with different environmental properties such as the type of surface they are on, the size and weight of their toys, and the physical distance and positioning of a caregiver relative to them. Babies also spend a prolonged amount of time playing with their fingers, hands, wrists, feet, and toes. These critical explorations, experienced while the spine is non-weight bearing (supported by the floor or other surface in a supine position), lay the groundwork for infant brain development.

A number of elements critical for body movement in space evolve within the first 6 months of life:

- symmetry between right and left sides
- extremity extension and flexion
- head alignment
- ability to hold head upright (against gravity)
- no head lag when pulling up to sit
- ability to lift head off the floor and assist when being pulled up to sitting (around 6 months)
- midline orientation (ability to evenly orient the right and left sides of the body around an imaginary central line)
- controlled, purposeful movements
- alternating coordinated movements (synchronous repetition of movements with opposite limbs, e.g., an infant alternating sucking on their big toes)
- lying prone (midline orientation is present in all positions, with visual fixing)

The following red flags indicate possible motor disturbances that could lead to poor postural stability. If a young client exhibits these issues, referral to an appropriate professional is warranted:

- absence of or limited flexor movements of the trunk
- strong asymmetries and inability to maintain a midline alignment
- absence of bilateral symmetrical flexor muscle control
- insufficient flexor muscle activity to balance the extensors
- delayed development of lateral spinal flexion
- poor visual control/downward visual gaze and visual convergence
- inability to achieve forearm weight bearing
- poor chin tuck
- excessive low tone ("frog" posturing)
- excessive muscular tone (arching and pushing into extension)
- lack of antigravity flexion (inability to bring feet to mouth, tight back muscles)
- overactive spinal extensors (poor trunk control, poor rib cage stability, arching)
- inability to roll to side-lying and/or rolling to prone via cervical hyperextension

These sequences develop as the body experiences gravity and explores movement. Supine and prone are the most critical positions in a child's motor development, as they are the cornerstones of the qualitative components of movements and govern postural control development. Supine and prone positions are also critical for developing correct breathing patterns in the rib cage and diaphragm. When the trunk is non-weight bearing, compensatory breathing patterns and breath control can be reeducated.

BOX 9.2 IDENTIFYING BEHAVIORAL VERSUS MOTOR CHALLENGES

Yoga therapy has been shown to enhance the acquisition of age-appropriate gross motor skills.[6] Developing the ability to mirror, repeat, and practice the actions of others is a milestone referred to as *imitation of body movement*. Babies as young as 8 months of age demonstrate the ability to clap hands together, wave, and play pat-a-cake and peek-a-boo.[7] These actions represent the beginnings of body-on-body imitation. Children begin to imitate multistep actions, such as putting one hand on their head and pointing with the other hand, around the age of 18 months.[8] More complex gestures and imitation tasks continue to evolve rapidly and include the ability to point an index finger, scratch a surface, open and close fists, drum hands on a surface, pull an earlobe, and pat a cheek.[9]

Young clients may not be developmentally ready or lack the cognitive attention to follow motor patterns. If the inability to follow motor patterns is instead behavioral in nature, a developmental approach of engaging and bonding with the yoga therapist would be used. Children with developmental challenges often have a history of delayed acquisition of motor skills, making it difficult to roll over, crawl, run smoothly, write, manage stairs, ride a bicycle, catch a ball, climb monkey bars, pump themselves on a swing, and so on. Clients may present with clumsy and awkward patterns of movement, exhibiting rigid gait, poor posture and postural control, and deficits in visual-perceptual and visual-motor coordination.

Sensory Integration

Healthy sensory development begins in infancy. Learning to lift the head and gaining postural and movement control—sitting, standing, rolling—are the first sensory-processing skills to develop. Babies often put objects in their mouths, exploring and learning by using the oral-motor system.

Additional relevant aspects of the sensory spectrum involve the body's eight sensory systems:

1. visual (sight)
2. auditory (hearing)
3. olfactory (smell)
4. gustatory (taste)
5. tactile (touch)
6. vestibular (balance and movement)
7. proprioceptive (muscles and joints, particularly involved with spatial awareness/orientation)
8. interoceptive (internal sensations; see Chapter 16)

This chapter focuses on the auditory, visual, tactile, vestibular, and proprioceptive systems, as they are instrumental in pediatric yoga therapy applications. Well-developed sensory processing positively influences cognitive development, communication, self-regulation, motor skills, and interactions with the environment.[10]

The tactile system

Everything felt in the environment using touch sensations, including vibrations, temperature, textures, and pain, is part of the tactile system. The skin organ is the largest receptor that sends signals to the brain. The skin's two most superficial layers are the epidermis, the outer layer, and the dermis, the deeper layer that contains various tactile receptors.

In a well-modulated nervous system, a child can perceive tactile stimuli accurately and respond appropriately based on their age to touch sensations.[11] Through natural developmental curiosity, children rapidly learn to interact with the environment safely and to protect themselves, without an excessive need for touch.

Problems may arise when the brain's neurological discrimination and perception pathways have difficulty deciphering sensory input. Possible observed behaviors stemming from tactile dysfunction are clumsiness, grasping a pencil too tightly or not tightly enough, inability to identify familiar objects by touch, poor fine motor skills, fear of the dark, messy appearance, point localization difficulty, and poor position sense (which occurs through the proprioceptive sensory system feedback via receptors in the joints).[12] Those with tactile dysfunction may also be unable to differentiate between light and hard touch, discriminate among sensations including textures, and have altered stereognosis (the mental perception of depth or three-dimensionality by the senses, usually in reference to the ability to perceive the form of solid objects by touch).

Examples of tactile defensiveness or avoidance (over-responsiveness) are a strong dislike of crowds, being extremely ticklish, walking on tiptoes, picky eating habits, or avoidance of being barefoot. Examples of tactile input-seeking (under-responsiveness) are engagement in biting, pinching, hitting, or headbanging; being unaffected by temperature; or enjoying strong flavors.

The auditory system

The auditory system is one's sense of hearing. The brain receives auditory messages from two separate pathways that work together: the peripheral auditory system, which includes the outer, middle, and inner ear, and the central auditory system, which only receives messages from the cochlear nucleus.

Examples of auditory defensiveness (over-responsiveness) are crying in response to loud noises or being distracted by minor background noises. Examples of auditory input-seeking (under-responsiveness) are enjoying background noises, not responding to important sounds like alarms, or speaking loudly.

An infant's auditory system fully develops in utero. Premature birth can result in delays in auditory system development. Children who have speech and language delays receive audiology testing to rule out hearing loss.

The visual system

The visual pathway is the neural pathway through which optical input travels to the brain. This pathway consists of the eye, optic nerve, optic chiasm, optic tract, lateral geniculate nucleus (LGN), optic radiation, and visual cortex. The first cells in the visual pathway, photoreceptors, are located in the retina. A photoreceptor is a sensory cell that converts light energy into a neural impulse (signal for the brain). That impulse travels from the retina, through the optic nerve, and along the visual pathway until it reaches the visual cortex (located in the cerebellum). Each eye sees from a different perspective and transmits a different signal to the brain. The visual cortex converts this information into a single, stable image—what one "sees."

The visual system is a primary system for future balance development. It is refined with acuity and clarity daily as a baby's brain develops and strengthens neuronal connections.

Modulation difficulties in the visual system occur with over- or under-responsiveness to optical input. Examples of visual defensiveness or avoidance (over-responsiveness) are avoidance of group activities, inability to estimate distances, avoidance of bright light, or fear of moving objects. Examples of visual input-seeking (under-responsiveness) are looking at items close up, enjoying patterns and bright colors, or staring at moving objects.

The proprioceptive system

The sense of the body's position in space is called the proprioceptive system. Joints, muscles, connective tissue, and skin all have sensory receptors that work together to create the perception of the body in space. These receptors communicate within the peripheral nervous system to allow for a sense of body position without the use of sight.

Proprioception is a secondary system for future balance development. Initially, proprioception depends on the visual system to provide knowledge of location while the body is supported and held by a caregiver. The receptors in each joint develop as a baby starts to sit upright around 6 months of age.

As with the other systems, modulation difficulties in proprioception occur when there is over- or under-responsiveness. Examples of proprioceptive defensiveness or avoidance (over-responsiveness) are difficulty walking up and down stairs, inability to climb ladders, light handwriting, or poor posture and low energy. Examples of proprioception input-seeking (under-responsiveness) are walking heavily and bumping into things, enjoying deep-pressure massage, or being unable to sit still.

The vestibular system

The vestibular system, involved with the sense of movement, is controlled by the inner ear, vestibular nerve, and semicircular canals. Difficulties become apparent when the brain's neurological discrimination and perception pathways cannot decipher sensory input. Possible observed behaviors of vestibular dysfunction are poor balance, odd posture, disorientation, and clumsiness.

The vestibular system is the tertiary and most advanced system for future balance development. Its function depends heavily on the visual system's development. The vestibular system activates when the eyes track horizontally off of midline and/or the head rolls.

Examples of vestibular defensiveness or avoidance (over-responsiveness) include fears about falling, stairs and uneven surfaces, or unexpected movement. Vestibular input-seeking (under-responsiveness) might include enjoyment of spinning and intense movement.

BOX 9.3 THERAPEUTIC APPLICATIONS

Tactile over-responsiveness

Age-appropriate oral-motor input can be encouraged during and before a yoga therapy session. Activities such as breastfeeding, using pacifiers, and bringing a child's favorite chewing toy or chewable snack to the yoga session encourage oral-motor input and organization, which will increase parasympathetic dominance. The chewing process uses bilateral temporomandibular joints (TMJ), providing inputs that activate the connection of both brain hemispheres. This activation in turn provides a calming influence and sends messages to the gastrointestinal system to initiate rest-and-digest responses.

Auditory over-responsiveness

Peaceful, serene environments, including waiting areas that minimize stressful stimuli, may soothe auditory over-responsiveness. Use of soft voices and adding background noises such as water fountains and noise-canceling machines might be helpful. Advance warnings about loud sounds, heavy curtains to block out sound, and closed doors for toilet flushing are useful.

Visual over-responsiveness

Blindfolds or eye masks reduce visual stimuli during a yoga therapy session. Use of soft lighting is highly recommended. Sensory integration can be developed by using postures that include rolling on the floor in linear directions. In addition, frequent breaks from visual input can be provided by encouraging a child to place their arm over their eyes or simply close them.

Proprioceptive over-responsiveness

Proprioceptive input is best provided with a child-directed strategy in mind at all times. Slow, steady, and calm inputs and activities—and avoiding active and rapid movements—are useful for working with proprioceptive over-responsiveness. Deep-pressure massage is an instrumental strategy in helping a child to organize their limbs toward the midline and in preparation for static prolonged weight-bearing postures, so referral to an appropriate provider may be necessary. These calming approaches encourage positive experiences during the yoga therapy session.

Vestibular over-responsiveness

Many of the same strategies for modulating the proprioceptive system apply to providing vestibular input. Linear forward and backward directions are easier for the brain to process and should be done before rotary directions (around one's own axis) are introduced. Working on one direction at a time, gentle postures with slow rocking, and, when appropriate, slowly and rhythmically bouncing on the lap, may be useful. Linear movement can be practiced until a child is fully comfortable and enjoys the input.

For more information on therapeutic applications in infants, see the work by Eeles and colleagues.[13]

Socioemotional Neurotypical Development

Erikson's psychosocial development theory considers human development through eight distinct stages (Table 9.1).[14] During each stage, the person must overcome a "psychosocial crisis." Triumph over each stage's crisis will result in a healthy personality and assimilation of a basic virtue. The first three stages are the most germane to pediatric yoga therapy. Identifying a client's psychosocial developmental stage is vital in developing a holistic yoga therapy approach.

Table 9.1 Erikson's psychosocial development theory

Stage	Age	Psychosocial Crisis	Basic Virtue
1	Birth to ~12 months	Trust vs. mistrust	Hope
2	12 months to ~3 years	Autonomy vs. shame	Will
3	3 to ~6 years	Initiative vs. guilt	Purpose
4	6 to ~12 years	Industry vs. inferiority	Competence
5	12 to 18 years	Identity vs. role confusion	Fidelity
6	18 to 40 years	Intimacy vs. isolation	Love
7	40 to 65 years	Generativity vs. stagnation	Care
8	65+ years	Ego integrity vs. despair	Wisdom

These stages do not always correlate to chronological age and may overlap. For example, an 11-year-old client attending a fifth-grade regular educational program may be demonstrating difficulties with ambition and responsibility, issues that usually occur during stage 3, while at the same time experiencing typical stage 4 issues. The child is therefore moving between two stages.

Early patterns of trust or mistrust in stage 1 play an influential role in individuals' emotional interactions for the remainder of their lives. A healthy relationship with a caregiver will help an infant to develop a sense of trust and security. Much yoga therapy work is rooted in issues that stem from the trust versus mistrust stage of socioemotional development.

The second stage of Erikson's theory, autonomy versus shame and doubt, occurs between the ages of 12 months and approximately 3 years because it is often correlated to the child's ability to walk independently. Children at this stage develop a sense of independence and physical control as they explore their environments. Stage 2 is also known as the "by myself" stage, when the toddler begins to show clear preferences for toys, food, and clothing and to act autonomously. At this stage, children begin to learn that controlled actions merit specific results. They also test boundaries to establish independence, resolving doubt into autonomy. Without a chance to explore the environment, toddlers may develop low self-esteem and shame.

Children begin to assert themselves more often as they deal with the issue of initiative versus guilt in the third stage of socioemotional development. This stage often occurs between the ages of approximately 3 and 6 years. A sense of ambition and responsibility develops as caregivers allow exploration within limits. During stage 3, it is important for children to investigate interpersonal skills through interactions and playing with their peers. Proper exploration helps to develop a sense of initiative to make decisions along with feelings of security. As interest in the world grows, the child will begin to ask many questions; this inquisitive stage is normal to emotional development, and not treating a child's questions as trivial helps to avoid embarrassment.

Effects of caregiver relationships and external environment on emotional regulation

The depth of the relationship between a child and their caregiver(s) is intrinsic to the success of pediatric yoga therapy. The emotional connection between a parent and infant is based on an intuitive responsiveness to meet the child's needs. Infants experience caregivers' physical contact, voices, and facial expressions before being able to completely comprehend them. These building blocks of healthy socioemotional development translate into normal emotional regulation.[15] Erikson's stage 1 emphasizes the trust toward caregivers in infancy as an essential milestone to forming trusting relationships with others. The cultivation of such a relationship is also critical to a healthy bond between yoga therapist and client.

Environmental stimuli deeply affect the understanding and expression of emotion. A supportive, accepting, and warm social environment during childhood supports optimal nervous system regulation and creates the trust necessary for successful yoga therapy outcomes. Lack of the appropriate environmental surroundings mentioned above will delay a child's emotional development.

Summary

This chapter is split into two main sections: motor skills and socioemotional development. In the former section, yoga is discussed as an integrated relationship between asana and pranayama; in the second, socioemotional development is related to yoga practice.

Respiratory development is discussed, followed by the developmental sequences of postures (supine, prone, seated quadruped, tall kneeling, half kneeling, standing upright). The sensory systems most instrumental in pediatric yoga therapy applications are the auditory, visual, tactile, vestibular, and proprioceptive systems. Well-developed sensory processing positively influences cognitive development, communication, self-regulation, motor skills, and interactions with the environment.

Humans progress from birth to adulthood in developmental stages. Learned motor skills are expanded with motor sequencing, coordinated patterns, and anatomically favored breathing patterns. The basic embryonic development of the spinal column is also useful for yoga therapists to understand. Yoga postures can be progressed to correlate with gross motor development.

Finally, yoga therapists should also understand the body's eight sensory systems and their relevance to the sensory integration of stimuli. Socioemotional development, described here using Erikson's psychosocial stages, may also provide useful support for yoga therapy applications. The effects of caregiver relationships and external environments on emotional regulation are critical for favorable outcomes.

Endnotes

1 Jagannathan, A., Nagarathna, R., Ramakrsihna, J., & Villacres, M. D. (2014). Decoding the integrated approach to yoga therapy: Qualitative evidence based conceptual framework. *International Journal of Yoga*, *7*(1), 22–31.

2 Bazzano, A. N., Anderson, C. E., Hylton, C., & Gustat, J. (2018). Effect of mindfulness and yoga on quality of life for elementary school students and teachers: Results of a randomized controlled school-based study. *Psychology Research and Behavior Management*, *11*, 81–89.

3 Telles, S., Gupta, R. K., Gandharva, K., Vishwakarma, B., Kala, N., & Balkrishna, A. (2019). Immediate effect of a yoga breathing practice on attention and anxiety in pre-teen children. *Children*, *6*(7), 84.

4 Netter, F. (2011). *Atlas of human anatomy*. Saunders/Elsevier.

5 Bly, L. (1994). *Motor skills acquisition in the first year: An illustrated guide to normal development.* Psychological Corp.

6 Radhakrishna, S. (2010). Application of integrated yoga therapy to increase imitation skills in children with autism spectrum disorder. *International Journal of Yoga*, *3*(1), 26–30.

7 Coplan, J. (1993). *Early language milestone scale*. Pro-Ed.

8 Bayley, N. (2006). *Bayley scales of infant and toddler development* (3rd ed.). Harcourt Assessment, Inc. Parks, S. (2004). *Inside HELP: Hawaii Early Learning Profile administration and reference manual.* VORT Corp.

9 The Motor Imitation Scale assesses these physical skills in young children. See Dadgar, H., Alaghband Rad, J., Soleymani, Z., Khorammi, A., McCleery, J., & Maroufizadeh, S. (2017). The relationship between motor, imitation, and early social communication skills in children with autism. *Iranian Journal of Psychiatry*, *12*(4), 236–240.

10 Cherland, E. (2012). The polyvagal theory: Neurophysiological foundations of emotions, attachment, communication, self-regulation. *Journal of the Canadian Academy of Child and Adolescent Psychiatry*, *21*(4), 313–314.

11 Dunn, W. (2001). The sensations of everyday life: Empirical, theoretical, and pragmatic considerations. *American Journal of Occupational Therapy*, *55*, 608–620.

12 Eeles, A. L., Spittle, A. J., Anderson, P. J., Brown, N., et al. (2013). Assessments of sensory processing in infants: A systematic review. *Developmental Medicine & Child Neurology*, 55, 314–326.

13 See, e.g., Eeles et al., Assessments of sensory processing.

14 Orenstein, G. A., & Lewis, L. (2020). Erikson's stages of psychosocial development. StatPearls Publishing. www.ncbi.nlm.nih.gov/books/NBK556096

15 Bronson, M. (2000). Recognizing and supporting the development of self-regulation in young children. *Young Children*, 55(2), 32–37.
Lagattuta, K. H., & Thompson, R. A. (2007). The development of self-conscious emotions: Cognitive processes and social influences. In J. L. Tracy, R. W. Robins, & J. P. Tangney (Eds.), *The self-conscious emotions: Theory and research* (pp. 91–113). Guilford Press.

10

Neurological Foundations: An Integrative Approach

KELLI BETHEL

According to the US Centers for Disease Control and Prevention, "Chronic diseases are defined broadly as conditions that last 1 year or more and require ongoing medical attention or limit activities of daily living or both."[1] It has been estimated that nearly 100 million Americans are affected by at least one of the thousands of chronic neurological diseases that exist, with these numbers expected to rise as the population ages.[2] The World Health Organization estimates that 6 million people die of stroke across the world each year.[3] Neurological disorders ranked as the leading cause of years lost to ill health (disability-adjusted life years) globally in 2015 and were the second leading cause of death.[4]

Between 1990 and 2015, the number of people affected by these disorders has increased, leading to more deaths and poor health across the lifespan.[5] Clients with neurological conditions require lifelong management and an integrative team approach to assist them in living well. The yoga therapist can play an integral role on such a team. Yoga therapists must learn to work collaboratively with clients, their families, and other healthcare professionals. Communication is an essential part of working as a member of a patient's integrative team. Evaluations, plans, and session notes must be written in a way that both clients and other providers can understand.

Neurological diseases and illnesses are complex, and for many are a chronic and/or progressive illness. Individuals with the same diagnosis, with the same area of the brain involved, may present and recover differently. Multiple factors impact clients, including neurological damage, trauma, and aging, along with social, emotional, spiritual, psychological, economic, cultural, environmental, and political factors. Each interacts and affects the health and well-being of the client and their families and friends.

For yoga therapists, individual evaluation of each client is essential, and all areas must be assessed. Only when the client is considered in their entire context of being can the yoga therapist support them on the journey to health and well-being with a chronic illness.

Evidence-Informed Yoga Therapy Practice with Clients with Neurological Conditions

Evidence-informed yoga therapy practice incorporates in equal parts current scientific evidence, clinical expertise, and client values and needs.[6] In working with clients with a neurological injury or disease, no single protocol can be applied to a specific diagnosis. Instead, the yoga therapist must follow the model of evidence-informed practice.

Current evidence has shown that the brain can grow new neurons and build new pathways around damaged circuits. The term *neuroplasticity* is used to describe this capacity in both healthy and injured brain tissue. Research in neuroscience, neurorehabilitation, motor learning, social cognitive theories, and yoga therapy is all relevant in developing a care plan for the neurologically involved client.[7]

The field of neurologic rehabilitation, as well as studies specific to yoga therapy and neurologically involved clients, have significantly increased since 2010.[8] Integrating both evidence-informed strategies from neurorehabilitation and yoga therapy allows the therapist to direct their evaluations and care plans to provide optimal client support. Current literature in neurorehabilitation has led to the development of an evidence-informed care model that includes three equally important areas: capacity, neuroplasticity and motor skills learning, and motivation.[9]

Capacity

For a client with a neurological condition, *capacity* may include range of motion, strength, pain endurance, walking speed, breathing pattern, musculoskeletal alignment, and considerations such as anxiety or depression. To work with the client toward increasing their capacity in any areas identified by evaluation, the yoga therapist needs to have an understanding of the client's medical diagnosis and any relevant contraindications. For example

- Is the client cleared to drop their head below their heart?
- Have they had recent brain surgery that would prevent them from lying flat on the ground?

- Is the client affected by temperature?
- Does the client have loss of sensation in their feet, hands, etc.?
- Do they have loss of vision?

More broadly, is the client's prognosis one that is expected to improve, stay the same, or progress? What are the client's physical and cognitive capabilities?

The yoga therapist also needs to consider scientific evidence from both the conventional and yogic perspectives:

- Are there relevant exercise science and clinical guidelines in either yoga therapy or medical communities?
- What are the evidence-based yoga studies?
- What yogic practices are relevant?
- Are any postures, breath practices, meditations, or philosophical principles known to benefit the diagnosis or any other area of need identified in the client evaluation?
- What are the appropriate yogic precautions and contraindications based on the client's medical history and assessment results?

Neuroplasticity and motor learning

This area focuses on the principles of motor relearning and exercise physiology. "Motor learning is a set of processes associated with practice or experience leading to relatively permanent changes in the capability for skilled movement."[10] For motor learning to occur, repetition and integration must prompt changes in the brain.[11] *Exercise physiology* is the application of principles that guide physical fitness in individuals, including regularity, progression, overload, variety, recovery, reversability, and specificity.

In this area, care strategies should be goal-directed and meaningful for the client. *Asana* that address balance and mobility must be task-specific and challenging. A focus on optimal alignment for each client rather than on "perfect" alignment supports clients' motor learning.

Sleep is another essential factor in neuroplasticity and motor skills acquisition. The brain needs down time (offline learning) to integrate skills and strategies. Yoga therapists can work with clients to develop and implement optimal sleep hygiene strategies.[12]

Motivation

Motivation is the third component of the neurorehabilitation model. Here, social-cognitive theories, neuroscience, and yogic philosophy provide a crucial intersection for work with clients with neurological conditions. In this area, the yoga therapist needs to focus on interventions that encourage and improve client self-efficacy. Therapies should be directed toward intrinsic motivation and client-identified meaning and purpose (see Chapter 13).

The yoga therapist must continuously question their choices: Does each one support the client's goals? In this area, yogic philosophy is intertwined with care strategies. The philosophical principles provide a set of guidelines that helps clients navigate their journeys with chronic illness. Understanding this foundation and encouraging the client to develop and use support mechanisms, including spirituality and religion (see Chapter 17), are powerful tools for clients with neurological conditions.

Social relatedness is another vital concept in working with this population. Depression and social isolation are high in those with neurological conditions.[13] Small-group yoga therapy programs may help while allowing for the therapist to address individual client goals.[14]

Yoga Therapy Strategies

Although each neurological client requires a unique medical assessment and treatment plan, commonly seen issues include

- abnormal muscle tone
- aggressive behavior
- aphasia
- ataxia
- balance loss
- brace/sling use
- cognitive impairments
- coordination and proprioception issues
- emotional control deficits
- fatigue

- gait disturbance
- heightened or decreased/lost hearing
- impaired judgment
- impaired strength
- irritability
- loss of mobility
- loss of range of motion
- loss of sensation
- medication influences
- neglect
- orthopedic issues
- seizures
- vestibular problems
- visual disturbances

Furthermore, common comorbidities with neurological conditions include

- blood pressure issues
- brain surgery
- carotid stenosis
- depression and social isolation
- diabetes
- obesity
- senior age
- substance-use issues
- trauma

The above lists are far from complete and vary by diagnosis, but clients with these identified issues may benefit from similar strategies to help mitigate the deficit, improve their capabilities, and keep the yoga therapist and client safe. The following suggested strategies may support yoga therapists working with clients with many such issues. The topics of trauma, posttraumatic stress, and substance abuse are more extensive than this chapter will address; it is recommended that yoga therapists employ well-studied yogic strategies to address these areas, modifying as appropriate for neurological clients.

Abnormal muscle tone

Muscle tone, by definition, refers to a muscle having the optimal amount of tension at rest. The client can move, or not move, the muscle on command. Muscle tone, commonly confused with strength, is often affected by a neurological injury or disease. "Normal muscle tone" can range from low-tone normal to high-tone normal. Low-tone normal is most often seen in clients who are hyperflexible—the resting length of the muscle is greater than average and causes joint hyperextension. (Conditions such as myasthenia gravis and collagen-vascular disorders like Ehlers-Danlos syndrome can cause low muscle tone, so yoga therapists should be aware of clients' medical diagnoses and the associated contraindications.)

For clients with low-tone normal musculature, asana practice should focus on strength and staying out of end ranges of motion. If such clients over time continue to work in hyperextension, they may experience joint damage and injury.

In those with high-tone normal musculature, the resting muscle length is shorter than average, with more rigidity, and clients may require more time to allow for a muscle to stretch.

Abnormal muscle tone occurs outside the range of normal. (Some clients may have both abnormal low tone and high tone in different areas of the body.) On the low-tone abnormal side, a client may exhibit flaccidity (no movement) or low tone, where the extremity appears floppy but some movement is possible. These impairments can lead to dislocation, balance issues, swelling in the extremity, pain, gait disturbances, difficulty with activities of daily living, and increased fall risk.

Modifications and supports need to be put in place to allow for safe alignment of a low-tone extremity. Props, walls, and chairs can be used to promote optimal alignment. Prone postures are challenging for clients with abnormally low muscle tone and are often contraindicated for those who have flaccid extremities, especially the arms. Clients may hyperextend a joint to create stability and require verbal and, at times, physical cues to enable them to work in a safe range of motion.[15]

Clients may also have abnormal high muscle tone and even rigidity. Abnormal high tone, often referred to as spasticity, manifests as extreme muscular rigidity.

As in those with low tone, high tone can impair activities of daily living, balance, and gait, potentially causing pain and putting such clients at risk for falls.

For some clients, spasticity in the lower extremities allows them to stand and ambulate, as they use their spasticity in place of functional voluntary muscle movement. Careful evaluation by a physical therapist or other appropriate healthcare provider is often warranted to determine the cost/benefit of using the high tone for mobility. Over time, clients may be trading mobility for the destruction of a joint; those with spasticity may also develop joint contractures.

When helping these clients work through range of motion, care must be taken to avoid going beyond the client's available range. Slow, static stretch at one joint may help relax the spasticity throughout the entire body; weight-bearing through the joint, in an appropriate range of motion, may also help to decrease spasticity.[16]

Conventional treatment for spasticity can include medication, Botox, and, in more severe cases, insertion of a Baclofen pump or surgical release.[17] If a client is placed on a medication to decrease their spasticity, the therapist needs to be aware that the medication may impact the entire body, not just the affected extremity. Botox injections, which are accompanied by a period of rehabilitation, may provide a short-term decrease in spasticity, but the client may then exhibit an underlying weakness. It is recommended that the yoga therapist consults with the client's treating physician and rehabilitation therapist to develop an understanding of the surgery itself and any contraindications.

Aphasia

Aphasia, an impairment of the language area of the brain, affects the production or comprehension of speech and/or the ability to write, do math, or tell time. Rather than a cognitive impairment, aphasia is a language impairment. Age increases the risk of aphasia.

There are three types of aphasia: Broca's, Wernicke's, and global. Broca's, or "expressive," aphasia occurs when there is damage to the brain's speech center that allows the formulation and expression of words, fluent speech, naming, and counting. Clients with expressive aphasia understand everything but cannot form words themselves or use incorrect words. Wernicke's, or "receptive," aphasia is due to brain damage that causes the person not to understand speech. Those with receptive aphasia can form words, but their speech emerges incongruent. They often lose the ability to read, tell time, perform math calculations, and discern the right and left sides of the body. Global aphasia is the combination of expressive and receptive aphasia.

Yoga therapists can use several empowering modifications when working with clients with aphasia. Evaluations need to be scheduled to allow for extra time for communication and discussion. Intake forms can use picture symbols instead of words. When speaking with these clients, it is important to not interrupt or attempt to finish sentences for them. Speak slowly and provide adequate time to answer questions.

In yoga therapy sessions, a multisensory approach is needed. Such an approach involves more than one sense and may include demonstration, auditory cues, and physical cues to help the client learn. Rooms should be free of noise and distractions. Maintain clients' attention, use simple speech and single-step directions, and avoid cues that incorporate right and left direction or counting. Presenting material in the client's primary language is extremely helpful, as those with aphasia have greater challenges with non-native language. They may benefit from having movements demonstrated and may, in some cases, need hand-over-hand assistance to understand the movement.

Give clients permission not to talk; they may feel as if they have "used up" their words for the day. Speaking is often exhausting for those with aphasia, and permission to be silent can be restorative. As noted, when working with someone with aphasia it is recommended that speech be kept simple and direct. This enables the client to follow the conversation and allows time to pause and reflect. Instructions need to be broken down into small, simple steps. Lengthy or wordy meditations will likely be frustrating for this group.

Journaling, or personal writing practices, are often difficult for clients with aphasia. It can be helpful to encourage clients to tap into areas of the brain that are not damaged; for example, music and smell are often useful tools in a yoga therapy session. Offering reminders that yoga therapy is not about perfection while creating practices that are challenging and work within clients' capabilities will help to foster self-efficacy.

Ataxia and proprioception

Clients with ataxia will have difficulty coordinating movement. Those with proprioception issues will have trouble sensing the body's position, motion, or equilibrium. Clients without proprioception issues can discern whether their arm is above their head or hanging by their side when blindfolded; those with proprioception issues cannot orient themselves in space or tell whether their arm is elevated or hanging by their side.

Working with clients with ataxia and proprioception deficits can be challenging and requires a multisensory approach. Assuming that they are able to stand, clients need to work on both sitting and standing balance. Asana should be modified to allow balance to be addressed while providing support to keep both client and yoga therapist safe. Seated asana may be better done in a chair versus seated on the floor.

The use of assistive devices such as a cane or walker may be challenging for this population. Using a wall for standing poses is supportive and provides proprioceptive input to help clients orient themselves in space. Additional input through supported touch or possibly light weights, such a 1-pound wrist weight, may help clients with ataxia to orient themselves. Guided meditations and breath practices that help clients to reconnect with their bodies may be beneficial.

Balance deficits

A balance problem exists when an individual has difficulty maintaining a stable and upright position either seated or standing. One or more factors can cause balance problems, including

- muscle weakness
- joint stiffness
- inner-ear (vestibular) problems
- somatosensory system issues
- vision alterations
- sensation alterations
- proprioception deficits
- altered postural reflexes
- medications (e.g., those prescribed for depression and high blood pressure)
- lack of activity or a sedentary lifestyle
- simple aging, as the vestibular system, somatosensory system, strength, flexibility, and nervous system cause slowed information relay

Balance is a multifaceted issue, and improving it requires more than having clients simply work on standing balance poses.[18] The range of motion of the joints, strength, and balance all need to be addressed. Yoga therapy work should be progressive and continue to challenge clients' balance as appropriate.

Cognitive impairments

Cognitive impairments not only affect how the yoga therapist works with clients but may impact the safety of the client, the yoga therapist, and those around them. Clients with cognitive impairments may have difficulty moving as directed. They may be easily distracted and unable to follow multi-step instructions. Certain types of brain damage may result in impulsivity and decreased safety awareness. These clients will need a multisensory approach and clear boundaries. If safety awareness is an issue, any asana offered should be challenging but also safe for the client, the therapist, and others who may be in a group.

Emotional impact

Emotions can be affected by neurological injury or disease. The grieving process that often accompanies a neurological diagnosis may significantly impact the client. Additionally, emotional reactivity and lability can be seen when there is damage to the area of the brain responsible for a particular type of emotional processing. Common emotional changes may include

- pseudobulbar affect[19]
- depression
- frustration
- anger
- lack of motivation

Modifications for these clients may include small-group sessions that allow for an informal support group. Remind clients of their progress and encourage positive self-talk, as this may be beneficial as well.[20] Sleep hygiene is crucial for these clients because lack of sleep can cause emotional changes.[21] Encourage rest and restoration as appropriate. Clients may need a referral to a mental health practitioner.

Fatigue

Fatigue is a significant issue for clients with a neurological injury or disease, who may describe feeling like they have "hit a wall" physically, mentally, or emotionally. This type of fatigue differs from being tired, and rest does not always alleviate it. Depression, lack of sleep, specific medication, pain, and decreased mobility all influence fatigue.

There are several techniques a yoga therapist can use to support a client who is experiencing fatigue. Clients should be encouraged to discuss their fatigue. They need to understand the importance of rest and be encouraged to do so. Yoga therapy sessions can incorporate energy-conservation techniques such as pacing and attention to posture; check in to make sure that sessions are not so exhausting that clients cannot complete their daily activities. Sleep hygiene techniques can also be taught and implemented into clients' daily schedules. Many clients with neurological conditions do better with mid- to late-morning appointments, especially if they have mobility impairments.

Loss of sensation

It is essential to know whether clients with neurological impairments have lost sensation. The sensation loss may include complete loss of sensation or numbness (anesthesia), a sense of "heaviness," tingling (paresthesia), hypersensitivity (hyperesthesia), pain (allodynia), difficulty perceiving temperature, or not being able to tell where the limbs are in space (proprioception deficit). Effects vary: For example, some clients may feel light touch but have no pain, whereas others may not be able to feel light touch but can tell hot from cold.

Sensation loss may occur because of damage anywhere between the affected tissue (which could be anywhere in the body) and the somatosensory cortex in the parietal lobe. When the cortex is damaged, the area of the body impacted will vary based on the location of the cortical damage.

Yoga therapists should always err on the side of caution with clients with sensory loss, who are at risk of injury. They may not be able to interpret pain sensations and cannot always tell if they have gone too deeply into an asana. Clients with sensory loss should use a yoga mat for all poses, and those with sensation loss in their feet may need to wear shoes for standing postures.

Neglect

Neglect is a lack of awareness on a client's involved side. Neglect usually involves damage to the right hemisphere of the brain and will therefore involve the left side of the body. This deficit is not a visual problem but rather one of perception. Clients with neglect may, for example, brush only half their hair or eat half a plate of food. They may not know when someone is standing next to them on their involved side. Age seems to increase the severity of neglect symptoms. Recovery is complicated and affects every area of a client's life.

Yoga therapists should take every opportunity to bring the client's awareness to the neglected side. This can include sitting and talking on their involved side. Clients may need hand-over-hand assistance, and care should be taken to make sure that all limbs on the neglected side are protected from injurious alignment.

Vestibular problems

The vestibular system includes the parts of the inner ear and brain that process the sensory information involved with controlling balance and eye movements. When the system is damaged, the client may present with

- imbalance or unsteadiness
- vertigo (a spinning or whirling sensation; an illusion of the self or the surrounding world moving)
- dizziness (a lightheaded, floating, or rocking sensation)
- blurred or bouncing vision
- nausea
- hearing changes
- problems with coordination, thinking, and memory

When working with clients with vestibular impairments, it is useful to understand what may trigger the vestibular response as well as what may help. These clients have a higher risk of falls. Limiting visual information can be helpful, perhaps by employing *drishti* (deliberately focused gaze), keeping lighting consistent, and eliminating distracting décor (keep walls neutral and flooring free of patterns). Props are especially helpful for clients with vestibular disorders.

Common Neurological Diagnoses

Following is an overview of the most frequently encountered neurological conditions. For more detailed information, refer to the sources suggested in the Additional Resources.

Brain injury

Brain injury is described as either traumatic or acquired based on the cause. An acquired brain injury is not hereditary, congenital, degenerative, or induced by birth trauma.

Traumatic brain injury (TBI), one type of acquired brain injury, is defined as an alteration in brain function or other evidence of brain pathology caused by an external force. Clients may report having "seen stars" and may not remember the injury. The symptoms can range from reporting feeling dazed and confused to loss of consciousness, coma, and death. TBIs can range from a mild concussion to severe subdural hematomas. Recovery may take weeks or months, even for those with a mild concussion. In some cases, the damage may be permanent. Falls account for 48 percent of all TBIs, with children and older adults most often affected.[22]

Stroke also falls into the acquired brain injury category. A stroke, also known as a cerebrovascular accident (CVA), occurs when there is interrupted blood flow to the brain, resulting in brain cell death. CVA is commonly caused by a thrombosis (stationary clot), embolism (floating clot), or hemorrhage (bleeding) in the brain. According to the American Stroke Association 795,000 people suffer a new or recurrent stroke each year in the United States, and nearly one in four people has had a stroke.[23]

The length of recovery and degree of lasting impairment differ for each brain injury survivor. Sensorimotor function and aerobic capacity can continue to improve for many months after a stroke.[24] Despite continued recovery postrehabilitation, brain injury survivors risk complications from inactivity because of decreased motor skills, depression, social isolation, and the need to reduce the risk factors that may have led to their brain injury.[25]

Multiple sclerosis

Multiple sclerosis (MS) is the most common chronic neurological disease in young adults, with women diagnosed two to three times more often than men.[26] This unpredictable disease process causes a disconnect between the brain and body and within the brain itself.[27] It is characterized by axonal injury, inflammation, and nerve demyelination. The exact cause of MS is still unknown, but it is believed to result from a combination of environmental and genetic factors. Clients with MS are often classified into one of four categories.[28]

- **Clinically isolated syndrome** is the first episode of neurological symptoms that last at least 24 hours; it may or may not develop into MS.
- **Relapsing-remitting MS** is the most common type; it is characterized by attacks or exacerbations followed by partial or complete recovery.
- **Secondary progressive MS** is characterized by progressive worsening of symptoms over time.
- **Primary progressive MS** is progressive loss of neurological function from the onset of symptoms with no remission.

The demyelination of the nerve sheath that occurs in MS impairs autonomic function and makes systemic temperature regulation less efficient. Heat exposure can increase symptoms for the client living with MS. This means the appearance of or heightening of fatigue, numbness, blurry vision, tremor, confusion, imbalance, and weakness. For this reason, yoga therapy sessions should not cause clients to become overheated; room temperatures should also not be too warm (and definitely not hot). Fatigue is a frequent complaint of clients with MS, so energy-conservation techniques need to be taught and reinforced both in and outside sessions.

Parkinson's disorder

Parkinson's disorder (PD) is a progressive neurological condition characterized by shuffling gait, tremor, and masked facial expression. As the disease progresses, *motor freezing*, in which the client is unable to initiate or continue ambulation mid-gait, is seen. The disease also has several non-motor symptoms, including psychiatric issues, autonomic dysregulation, sleep disorders, and sensory impairments.[29] The exact cause of PD is unknown, but it is believed to result from multiple factors, including genetics, diet, and toxic exposures.

Movement is recommended for all clients with PD and should begin as soon as the diagnosis is confirmed. Exercise guidelines for people with PD are for a well-rounded weekly program that includes 2.5 hours of moderate-intensity exercise, 2 to 3 days of strength training, 2 to 3 days of flexibility training, and 2 to 3 days of balance training.[30] Some clients may benefit from daily stretching to help with stiffness.

Clients with PD may also demonstrate fatigue and depression that affect their daily lives. Practice variations discussed earlier in this chapter are appropriate for these clients. Additionally, it is critical that yoga therapists remember to work toward the client's intrinsic motivators.

Because PD is a progressive disease, frequent reevaluation and goal-setting are needed. Yoga practices that maintain or increase the range of motion of the limbs, trunk, and chest expansion are beneficial. Poses that promote balance and movement may help to modify the disease progression.[31] Relaxation techniques may ease the rigidity typically seen in clients with this diagnosis. As the disease progresses, gait changes are often seen and clients may experience "freezing" or short steps with walking. Visual and auditory cues such as a metronome, synthesized music, or lines on a floor may help clients to overcome these hindrances to movement.

Summary

Yoga therapists working with clients with neurological disorders must have a thorough understanding of their medical and yogic presentations. Each is equally important in co-development of a plan of care.

Yoga practices can be easily modified and adapted, regardless of the diagnosis or capabilities of the client. Yoga can improve strength, range of motion, respiration, activities of daily living, balance, body awareness, and fear of falling in those with neurological disorders. The practices can help with anxiety, depression, and social isolation and may also help with stress and disease management. Yet yoga is even more powerful, for it allows the therapist to support clients in unifying mind, body, and spirit and enabling them to find meaning, purpose, and joy in their lives.

Additional Resources

American Parkinson Disease Foundation: www.apdaparkinson.org

American Stroke Association: www.stroke.org/en

Brain Injury Association: www.biausa.org

BrainLine. (n.d.). Glossary of brain injury terms. www.brainline.org/article/glossary-brain-injury-terms

Brent, M. (n.d.). 7 principles of physical training. www.livestrong.com/article/528271-7-principles-of-physical-training

Gaal, M. (2012). 7 principles of exercise and sport training. www.teamusa.org/USA-Triathlon/News/Blogs/Multisport-Lab/2012/August/28/7-Principles-of-Exercise-and-Sport-Training

Multiple Sclerosis Society: www.nationalmssociety.org

Parkinson's Foundation: www.parkinson.org

Vestibular Disorders Association. (n.d.). Vision challenges with vestibular disorders. https://vestibular.org/educational-resources/vision-hearing/vision-challenges-vestibular-disorders

Endnotes

1 National Center for Chronic Disease Prevention and Health Promotion, US Centers for Disease Control and Prevention. (2021). About chronic diseases. www.cdc.gov/chronicdisease/about/index.htm

2 Gooch, C. L., Pracht, E., & Borenstein, A. R. (2017). The burden of neurological disease in the United States: A summary report and call to action. *Annals of Neurology, 81*(4), 479–484.

3 GBD 2015 Neurological Disorders Collaborator Group. (2017). Global, regional, and national burden of neurological disorders during 1990–2015: A systematic analysis for the Global Burden of Disease Study 2015. *Lancet Neurology, 16*(11), 877–897.
World Health Organization. (n.d.). Global action plan for the prevention and control of NCDs 2013–2020. www.who.int/nmh/events/ncd_action_plan/en

4 GBD 2015 Neurological Disorders Collaborator Group, Global, regional, and national burden.
World Health Organization, Global Action Plan.

5 GBD 2015 Neurological Disorders Collaborator Group, Global, regional, and national burden.
World Health Organization, Global Action Plan.

6 Fetters, L., & Tilson, J. (2012). *Evidence based physical therapy* (pp. 3–7). F. A. Davis.

7 Winstein, C. J., & Kay, D. B. (2015). Translating the science into practice: Shaping rehabilitation practice to enhance recovery after brain damage. *Progress in Brain Research, 218*, 331–360.

8 Green, E., Huynh, A., Broussard, L., Zunker, B., et al. (2019). Systematic review of yoga and balance: Effect on adults with neuromuscular impairment. *American Journal of Occupational Therapy, 73*(1), 7301205150.
Mooventhan, A., & Nivethitha, L. (2017). Evidence based effects of yoga in neurological disorders. *Journal of Clinical Neuroscience, 43*, 61–67.
Oken, B. S., Kishiyama, S., Zajdel, D., Bourdette, D., et al. (2004). Randomized controlled trial of yoga and exercise in multiple sclerosis. *Neurology, 62*(11), 2058–2064.
Wahbeh, H., Elsas, S. M., & Oken, B. S. (2008). Mind-body interventions: Applications in neurology. *Neurology, 70*(24), 2321–2328.

9 Winstein & Kay, Translating the science into practice.
Winstein et al., Infusing motor learning research.

10 Schmidt, R. A., & Lee, T. D. (2017). *Motor control and learning: A behavioral emphasis* (6th ed., p. 283). Human Kinetics.

11 Hayhurst, C. (2018). Using motor learning to help patients. *PT in Motion*, February.
Kenyon, L. K., & Blackinton, M. T. (2011). Applying motor-control theory to physical therapy practice: A case report. *Physiotherapy Canada, 63*(3), 345–354.
Winstein, C., Lewthwaite, R., Blanton, S. R., Wolf, L. B., & Wishart, L. (2014). Infusing motor learning research into neurorehabilitation practice: A historical perspective with case exemplar from the accelerated skill acquisition program. *Journal of Neurologic Physical Therapy, 38*(3), 190–200.

12 Ong, J. C., Manber, R., Segal, Z., Xia, Y., Shapiro, S., & Wyatt, J. K. (2014). A randomized controlled trial of mindfulness meditation for chronic insomnia. *Sleep, 37*(9), 1553–1563.
Wang, X., Li, P., Pan, C., Dai, L., Wu, Y., & Deng, Y. (2019). The effect of mind-body therapies on insomnia: A systematic review and meta-analysis. *Evidence-Based Complementary and Alternative Medicine, 2019*, 9359807.

13 Shi, Y., Yang, D., Zeng, Y., & Wu, W. (2017). Risk factors for post-stroke depression: A meta-analysis. *Frontiers in Aging Neuroscience, 9*, 218.

14 Christensen, E. R., Golden, S. L., & Gesell, S. B. (2019). Perceived benefits of peer support groups for stroke survivors and caregivers in rural North Carolina. *North Carolina Medical Journal, 80*(3), 143–148.
Fiske, A., Wetherell, J. L., & Gatz, M. (2009). Depression in older adults. *Annual Review of Clinical Psychology, 5*, 363–389.

15 In situations where the yoga therapist cannot touch the client (e.g., when state or territory law prohibits touch by unlicensed professionals, the yoga therapist lacks sufficient training to offer supportive touch appropriately, or the session is being conducted virtually), it may be possible to use walls and other props to provide feedback. Note that, depending on the client's symptoms, extra caution should be exercised when working with these populations online; it may not be possible to offer asana safely via an online platform.

16 Cleveland Clinic. (n.d.). Spasticity: Management and treatment. https://my.clevelandclinic.org/health/diseases/14346-spasticity/management-and-treatment
Page, P. (2012). Current concepts in muscle stretching for exercise and rehabilitation. *International Journal of Sports Physical Therapy, 7*(1), 109–119.

17 Chang, E., Ghosh, N., Yanni, D., Lee, S., Alexandru, D., & Mozaffar, T. (2013). A review of spasticity treatments: Pharmacological and interventional approaches. *Critical Reviews in Physical and Rehabilitation Medicine, 25*(1–2), 11–22.
Thompson, A. J., Jarrett, L., Lockley, L., Marsden, J., & Stevenson, V. L. (2005). Clinical management of spasticity. *Journal of Neurology, Neurosurgery, and Psychiatry, 76*(4), 459–463.

18 Youkhana, S., Dean, C. M., Wolff, M., Sherrington, C., & Tiedemann, A. (2016). Yoga-based exercise improves balance and mobility in people aged 60 and over: A systematic review and meta-analysis. *Age and Ageing, 45*(1), 21–29.

19 Clients with pseudobulbar affect may experience reflexive crying and labile (rapidly changing) mood, sometimes for no reason at all. They may cry, laugh, or become angry at inappropriate times or in ways not fitting to their mood.

20 Winstein et al., Infusing motor learning research.
Wulf, G., Chiviacowsky, S., & Lewthwaite, R. (2012). Altering mindset can enhance motor learning in older adults. *Psychology and Aging, 27*(1), 14–21.

21 Ong et al., Randomized controlled trial.
Wang et al., Effect of mind-body therapies.

22 US Centers for Disease Control and Prevention. (2019). TBI: Get the facts. www.cdc.gov/traumaticbraininjury/get_the_facts.html

23 Benjamin, E. J., Blaha, M. J., Chiuve, S. E., Cushman, M., et al. (2017). Heart disease and stroke statistics—2017 update: A report from the American Heart Association. *Circulation, 135*(10), e146–e603. [Erratum in *Circulation, 135*(10), e646.]

24 Billinger, S. A., Arena, R., Bernhardt, J., Eng, J. J., et al. (2014). Physical activity and exercise recommendations for stroke survivors: A statement for healthcare professionals from the American Heart Association/American Stroke Association. *Stroke, 45*(8), 2532–2553.

25 Billinger et al., Physical activity and exercise recommendations.

26 National Multiple Sclerosis Society. (n.d.). What is MS? www.nationalmssociety.org/What-is-MS
Rakel, D. (Ed.). (2018). *Integrative medicine* (4th ed.). Elsevier.

27 National Multiple Sclerosis Society, What Is MS?

28 Youkhana et al., Yoga-based exercise.

29 Rakel, *Integrative medicine.*

30 Ellis, T., DeAngelis, T. R., Dalton, D., & Venne, J. (2016). Be active and beyond: A guide to exercise and wellness for people with Parkinson's disease. American Parkinson Disease Association. www.apdaparkinson.org/wp-content/uploads/pdf_publications/Be-Active-Book_For-Web-90o.pdf

31 Umphred, D. A., Lazaro, R. T., Roller, M. L., & Burton, G. U. ([2012] 2019). *Umphred's neurological rehabilitation* (6th ed., pp. 607–619). Mosby.

11

Foundations of Mental Health

DORCIA J. TUCKER

How Is Mental Health Determined?

A surface consideration of the meaning of "psychological health" might assume that the idea simply indicates the absence of psychological illness. However, as defined by the American Psychological Association, mental health is "a state of mind characterized by emotional well-being, good behavioral adjustment, relative freedom from anxiety and disabling symptoms, and a capacity to establish constructive relationships and cope with the ordinary demands and stresses of life."[1] Mental health is not a fixed point, but a dynamic consideration of the individual within the context of time, circumstance, psychical environment, and culture. This chapter provides an overview of select perspectives on mental health from sources ranging from modern psychology to ancient philosophical texts.

Western perspectives on mental health

Within the field of behavioral health, four related perspectives stand out as being illustrative of a holistic framework for understanding individual psychological well-being and health: person-centered therapy, existential psychology, Maslow's hierarchy of needs, and positive psychology.

Person-centered therapy

Developed by Carl R. Rogers, person-centered therapy (now also called client-centered therapy) is an example of humanistic-experiential therapy (i.e., concerned with the phenomenology, or lived experience, of the individual). Person-centered therapy has at its core the idea that each individual has an innate tendency to actualize, or fulfill, their potential. Rogers saw this tendency as a "movement toward greater order, complexity, and interrelatedness"[2] that was mirrored in the natural world on a spectrum from the smallest organisms to the formation of galaxies.

Rogers assumed that human nature is essentially positive and that it strives to be creative, autonomous, and self-actualizing (striving to reach one's positive potential). This inherently healthy way of functioning requires a flexible, ever-evolving integration between one's experience of the world and one's sense of self. According to the person-centered perspective, dysfunction is either (1) the result of a lack of integration between an individual's experiential reality and their self-concept, or (2) the product of adverse conditions against which an individual must struggle to meet their own needs. In the former case, the individual has either denied the reality of certain needs or experiences or adopted needs that are not their own. In the latter case, the severity or duration of the adverse conditions may have warped the ingrained tendency toward growth, but the individual will continue to adjust, in their own fashion, to their perception of reality.

To understand fully any individual, one must take into account the subjective whole of that person's experiences. According to Rogers, the individual's experiential world is an integration of perceptions, those about the self, the self in relation to others, and the self in relation to the external environment.[3] Not only is each person influenced by their environment, but each person also makes choices that affect that environment. With these choices comes responsibility. The way that a person experiences their environment, makes choices (or chooses not to make choices), and deals with the repercussions of those choices in their environment are all part of that person's subjective experience of reality.

In experiential terms, change occurs when individuals remove the obstacles to growth and are able to experience the self from which they have been blocked. Congruence, self-acceptance, and self-understanding are the hallmarks of change on a continuum from subjective rigidity and stagnation to flexibility and openness to new experiences. The individual goes from habitually objectifying experiences to accepting and taking responsibility for the subjective quality of experiences. The locus of evaluation shifts from external (what one should do) to internal (what is best for oneself) and facilitates the subjective experience of autonomy. Progress toward congruence and increasing mental health is marked by the ability to "perceive the objects in his phenomenal field...with increased differentiation."[4]

From the perspective of person-centered therapy, the ultimate goal is the individual's full experience of the world and of the self.

Existential psychology

Existential psychology's focus is on what it means to exist as a human being. This perspective is concerned with the person as a unique individual, but also with their ever-changing relationship with the reality of being (e.g., death, freedom). The dynamic characteristics of this relationship ensure that tension is always present to varying degrees and at different levels of the individual's awareness. The primary source of tension, which within an existential framework manifests as anxiety, is the ever-evolving "conflict that flows from the individual's confrontation with the givens of existence."[5] Existential anxiety may be likened to the background noise or radiation of the universe: normative, ever present, and potentially informative if one can tune into it. In contrast, a diagnosable anxiety disorder involves objectively excessive fear and anticipation of a future personal threat (see Chapter 12).[6]

That any individual would feel anxiety about death is not surprising; everyone who lives must also die. Likewise, it is understandable that one would dread facing the knowledge that life is ultimately devoid of objective structure, that there is no grand design, and people are free to make of life what they will. The part of the psyche that craves objective structure would also like to believe that "no man is an island, entire of itself," but this does not reflect the reality of life.[7] The world an individual inhabits is a product of their actions, thoughts, perceptions, and choices, all compounded by the ways the individual uses them to navigate the objective realities of their existence. No human being can truly know how another experiences the world, and thus can never completely know another or even the world that they inhabit. This basic isolation is yet another source of anxiety.

Out of these three sources of angst comes meaninglessness. Meaning—or one's core beliefs about themselves and the world—guides one's thoughts and in turn one's behaviors. Raised to an existential level this equates with Nietzsche's assertion that "He who has a *why* to live for can bear with almost any *how*."[8]

According to van Deurzen, "Existential anxiety or *angst* is that basic unease or malaise which people experience as soon as they are aware of themselves. It is the sensation that accompanies self-consciousness and awareness of one's vulnerability when confronted" with the lack of underlying structure in the universe.[9] This angst accompanies the nagging realization that one is the final arbiter of one's own life. It is awareness and, more importantly, acceptance of this personal life-power that allows one to live with and be energized by the anxiety of being human. The end result of working through this angst is "not to suppress, disguise or deny anxiety, but to understand its meaning and gain the strength to live with it constructively."[10]

Existential psychology maintains an optimistic focus on the present and the potential for change and growth in the future. The essential attitudes are a belief in the worth of the individual and a willingness to acknowledge the objective realities of the human condition (i.e., the givens of human existence as well as the demands and constraints of living in the world). One of the paths through existential angst is to develop a way to harness one's anxiety for constructive, authentic living. This includes confronting responsibility avoidance, identifying wishes and feelings, removing obstacles to decision-making, addressing existential isolation, and moving obstacles to meaningful engagement in the world. Rather than being driven by one's anxieties, an individual can choose to become aware of and harness the realities of existence to create a personally meaningful life.

Maslow's hierarchy of needs

Abraham Maslow's hierarchy of needs[11] is one of the most well-known theories of human motivation. It hypothesizes that a human being's most basic need is for physiological survival via food, shelter, etc. Until this need can be reliably satisfied, the individual will be preoccupied with pursuing this goal above all others. If the individual attains the means of maintaining physical survival, their goal becomes the attainment of other ("higher") needs, such as safety, belonging and love, and then esteem. The most common model of Maslow's hierarchy, often depicted as a pyramid, places the need for self-actualization as the highest level of motivation. Indeed, Maslow did discuss "peak experiences" in the context of people who are acting according to the highest level of personal motivation.

Although he originally considered self-actualization (the fulfillment of one's individual potential) to be the highest level of need and to include the behavior of those who sought to be part of something greater than the singular self, Maslow later added an additional tier to the top of the motivational hierarchy.[12] Maslow's highest level of human motivation is "transpersonal," meaning that an individual at this stage has gone beyond the need for self-fulfillment and self-aggrandizement and seeks to transcend considerations of the self. Individuals who are fortunate enough to be able to meet the needs of previous stages seek meaning in pursuits or causes that involve a greater connection to community, service, spirituality, and similar ideals that extend beyond the boundaries of the individual ego.[13]

Because of the scope of this hierarchy of needs from survival to transpersonal, Maslow creates a bridge between each of the perspectives considered in this section: humanistic (focused on the phenomenology of the individual), existential (concerned with the greater meaning[s] in life), and positive psychology (giving prominence to the positive aspects of each individual's character, including the transpersonal).

Positive psychology

Positive psychology focuses on the recognition and facilitation of human flourishing at the level of subjective experiences (e.g., satisfaction, happiness, and optimism); the individual (e.g., a capacity to love others, creativity, and wisdom); and the collective (e.g., civic virtues and the institutions that support them).[14] Research in the field of positive psychology acknowledges both the strengths and weaknesses of the individual, pursues methods to resolve personal distress, and seeks to cultivate the best aspects of individuals and institutions for the collective good.[15] Researchers focused on prevention have uncovered "human strengths that act as buffers against mental illness: courage, future mindedness, optimism, interpersonal skill, faith, work ethic, hope, honesty, perseverance, and the capacity for flow and insight, to name a few."[16]

Two aspects of positive psychology mark it as a product of the final decades of the 20th century: the attention given to self-transcendence (e.g., flow states) and the acknowledgment of the reciprocal effects of the mind-body-spirit complex. Ideas about flourishing and the impact of character strengths and virtues on quality of life, although not new (e.g., Aristotle's concept of eudaimonia), have coalesced in the theories of positive mental health and have found receptive audiences in most areas of modern healthcare. Kang et al. suggest that cultivating a mindset that focuses on the well-being of others (i.e., one that is self-transcendent) can lower defensiveness to threatening health-related information, provoke transient changes in prefrontal cortex activation, and produce objectively measured increases in health-promoting behavior change, such as decreased sedentary behavior and increased physical activity.[17] The insights of positive psychology are gaining traction as more individuals and health professionals pursue the goal of "making normal people stronger and making high human potential actual."[18] Likewise, the triad of self-transcendence, mind-body-spirit, and flourishing illuminates the relevance of positive psychology to the field of yoga therapy.

Yogic perspectives on mental health

Samkhya philosophy

The *Samkhya Karika* sets the foundation for many of the concepts of mental phenomena found in yoga and ayurveda. The highest conceptualization of the Self (*purusha*) is viewed as the intangible yet pervasive spirit woven throughout reality. This Self lies within all things but is not identical to all things. (Similar to the idea of the Tao, if one can describe the phenomenon, then it is not the true phenomenon.) Purusha defies the containment of explicit (manifest) language; it is the elemental ineffability that lies within everything. The individual self—what Western psychology might term the "ego"—is a pale echo conditioned by the existential realities of living in a material world.[19]

The *gunas* (*rajas*, *tamas*, and *sattva*; see Chapter 3) are manifestations of material energy that interact and inspire action according to their energy. And imbalance in the gunas (too much rajas or tamas) blinds one to pure wisdom and leads to desire, anger, and greed.

Within Samkhya philosophy, mind is a function of *prakriti*, the material manifestation of purusha. By explaining the activation of purusha through the differentiation of prakriti, Samkhya provides a foundation of describing and assessing the aspects of the natural world, the individual, and their interplay. The juxtaposition of aspects, elements, properties, faculties, etc., allows for the description of individual qualities and their potential imbalances. The Samkhya conceptualization of the mind includes *buddhi* (equanimous witness, discriminative knowledge, wisdom, ability to discriminate between real and not real), *ahamkara* (that which receives information from manas, judging it as threat or neutral; limbic system and ego), and *manas* (the sensory-motor mind). Yoga therapy helps to cultivate buddhi through attention to differential sensation in *asana*, expansive states in *pranayama*, and insight in meditation (see Chapter 23).

Ahamkara, the manifested differentiation of self (as opposed to the absolute Self/purusha), is the aspect of prakriti that creates the impression of individuality and self-identity.[20] Another aspect of prakriti, manas, is related to/derived from ahamkara and may be considered a mediator between ahamkara and the sense organs (*indriya*) that are responsible for perceptions.[21]

The nature of the true Self/*Atman* is connection, whereas the nature of ahamkara/ego is separation and individuation.[22] Both self/ahamkara and Self/purusha are necessary for the creation of a healthy self-identity. From an amorphous state of Self as undifferentiated from the world/environment, a child gradually develops boundaries between self and other—the ego/ahamkara develops over time. One must first establish a mature sense of self as agent (and explore its boundaries and trials) before embarking on the path to shed the falsely individuated self and reconnect to the true Self. To prematurely seek and cling to spiritual attainment (e.g., Atman or *kundalini*) has been described by Welwood as "spiritual bypassing."[23] The relative state of equilibrium between Atman and the maturity of ahamkara determine the characteristics of one's self-identity.

Ayurveda

Ayurveda picks up the thread of the knowledge expounded within the *Samkhya Karika* and applies it to everyday life. Within this system, an aspect of prakriti is the holistic constitution with which one is born. It is the tabula rasa of one's way of being in the world, one's nature/tendencies without the influence of the environment or nurturance. *Vikruti*, by contrast, includes the cumulative effects of one's upbringing, environmental influences, and life circumstances. Vikruti can be understood as the effect of life/living on one's prakriti.

Prana serves as the foundational essence that underlies all functions of the mind-body (see Chapter 20). It can be considered the wellspring from which the other two vital essences (*ojas* and *tejas*) originate. Similarly, ojas may be considered the cornerstone from which prana and tejas derive their balances and stability. Tejas assists by integrating the vitality and stability of prana and ojas, respectively. Each vital essence adds the energy of vitality/mobility/coordination (prana), clarity/discernment/integration (tejas), and solidity/endurance/nourishment (ojas) that supports mental and emotional well-being.[24]

The three gunas exist along a continuum from the most stable/stagnant aspects of tamas, through the motion/chaos of rajas, to the most refined/balanced aspects of sattva.[25] From an ayurvedic perspective, mental healing also exists along a continuum.[26] The first stage is moving from stuckness/mental inertia (tamas) to self-determined action (rajas). The second stage involves pacifying the energy of rajas (in the form of actions motivated by self-interest) and beginning to develop more sattvic/selfless motivations. The third stage is a refinement of sattva—moving from a drive for action directed toward the external world to spiritual/internal development via meditation.

It is important to understand that as elemental energies, each of the gunas has positive aspects and can include the mind in health-promoting ways. Sattva can contribute to equanimity, calm, mindfulness, mental "flow," and clear perception. Rajas can motivate creativity, inspiration, and excitement, but it can also produce anxiety and delusion. Finally, tamas can instill stability, stoicism, nurturance, and rest, but it can also engender sadness and ignorance.

Patanjali's *Yoga Sutras*

Many consider that the text of the *Yoga Sutras* was written from a dualistic cosmological understanding of Samkhya philosophy (see Chapter 1). From this perspective, reality is believed to exist in the polarity of purusha (the subtle ground or observer) and prakriti (the mundane matter that is observed).[27] The *Yoga Sutras* provide a path for a purifying journey from the gross (how one interacts in the world and physical practices) to the most subtle (inner work toward a merging of the observed and observer). This effort of self-purification may be thought of as removing the defilements of prakriti to realize purusha.

Patanjali viewed the body (and by extension, the mundane elements of daily life) as something to be burned away in the heat of ascetic and devoted practice. The ultimate awareness and goal of practice (purusha) is placed outside the body/individual, to the point of being giving an avatar within the context of the *niyama* of *ishvara pranidhana* (recognition of the source). The self must be transcended to contact the Self. This idea is in contrast with some non-dual philosophies that see the Self (or the Absolute Reality) as an intrinsic aspect of the self that, while also being all-pervasive (as is purusha), is not defiled in its interbeing with the world (see Chapter 2).

On its path toward transcendence of the physical/manifest, each of the eight limbs of Patanjali's yoga facilitates greater progress with the next. Postural practice (*asana*) follows the restraints (*yamas*, such as non-violence) and observances (*niyamas*, such as cleanliness), and is in turn followed by the more subtle breath practices (*pranayama*). Continuing the movement from a focus on the external to the internal, withdrawal of the senses (*pratyahara*) marks the shift from physical to mental practices in Patanjali's formulation. Cultivation of the behavioral/physical practices directly supports one's ability to attain/sustain the mental practices. The final three practices are *dharana* (focus), *dhyana* (meditation), and *samadhi* (absorption, transcendence).[28]

The panchamaya kosha model

Subsequent to the yamas and niyamas, the eight limbs of Patanjali's yoga are arranged rather linearly from external/observable to internal/subjective.[29] The five *koshas* of the *panchamaya* model, however, are interrelated and interdependent.[30] Each layer of the individual, from the gross to the subtle, is interwoven with and affects all other layers. For the purposes of this discussion, the five sheaths can be thought of as the physical body (*annamaya kosha*), breath/life force (*pranamaya kosha*), somatosensory mind (*manomaya kosha*), wisdom/higher mind (*vijnanamaya kosha*), and bliss/connection/spirituality (*anandamaya kosha*).[31] The sheaths are each affected by practices designed to cultivate health (e.g., each limb of Patanjali's yoga). Conversely, each then has an effect on one's experience of the yogic practices (e.g., increasing interoception within annamaya or pranamaya may deepen asana or pranayama practice).

Summary

In general, each of the modalities discussed asserts that the multilayered subjective experience of the individual (e.g., from gross to subtle and physical to spiritual/transpersonal) must always be taken into account and that the creativity and generativity of the individual is as important as genetics and the environment (i.e., "nature and nurture").[32]

Each of the models presented views health as a progression toward increasing wisdom, discernment, and internal coherence of the mental landscape of the individual. For person-centered therapy, this comes in the form of congruence between one's holistic understanding of self and the experience of living in the world.[33] Within the realm of existential psychology, this progression presents as the capacity and search for meaning, actualization, and transcendence. Positive psychology characterizes mental health as the capacity for optimal functioning, which is supported by character strengths and virtues, psychological well-being, supportive communities, and a potential for transcendence. In yoga and ayurveda, mental health is attained via the mind-body-spirit as one reconnects with and integrates inherent wisdom. The intersections of these various orientations are fertile ground for enriching the practice of yoga therapy for individuals and groups.

BOX 11.1 SELF-CARE

Cultivating balance

Improving the quality of each of the vital essences improves one's ability to maintain a healthy mind-body-spirit and thus fosters psychological health. Directing awareness to sense objects that are nourishing rather than depleting will tend to increase mental and emotional well-being. If one associates with materials, behaviors, thoughts, people, institutions, practices, etc., that predominantly embody the qualities one is trying to cultivate (e.g., rajas, tamas, sattva), one is likely to move in the direction of greater health.[34] In other words, associating with the nourishment, sensory inputs, and individuals appropriate to one's needs will cultivate an internal reflection of the qualities characteristic of those same foods, inputs, and people.

"Right associations" can be cultivated in line with the ayurvedic method of cultivating the opposite of the observed imbalance. If the principal imbalance reflects an overstimulation of pitta, the right association will be with practices, substances, and circumstances that pacify excessive pitta (see Chapter 20).[35] Similarly, if there is a lack of strength/stamina or another quality that suggests deficiency in ojas, then the right association may include appropriate food/

herbs, increased rest, or the cultivation of nourishing activities.[36] Even when there is no clear imbalance or deficiency, significant association with inputs that have a strong energetic charge will tend to increase the expression of that particular energetic in oneself.

Responsive and proactive self-regulation

From a biomedical perspective, the human body has multiple mechanisms for maintaining functional balance. Homeostasis is maintained by returning function to a set parameter after every disruption (e.g., body temperature). This form of balance is a reactive response to stressors. The existential reality of life includes innumerable stressors, including changing environments and progression through different life stages. What is optimal in one stage of life (e.g., childhood) may be less desirable at a later stage (e.g., late adulthood). The optimal stress response will also vary over time. The ability to calibrate to a "new normal" is allostasis: a dynamic, adaptive response to a past, present, or even future stressor.[37] As a future-oriented response, allostatic adaptation can also mean attending to self-care proactively, to mitigate the effects of an anticipated stressor.

Self-reflection and interoception are important precursors to self-care. Before adaptive adjustments can be made, one must have some awareness of how their system reacts in the presence of stressors and an understanding that the stress response may differ according to the stressor, duration, intensity, stage of life, etc. Developing interoception and self-reflection into a habit of introspection has the potential to create space for growth. As many in the field of yoga therapy have discovered, individual development can be the foundation for professional development, as the yoga student becomes a yoga teacher and perhaps later a yoga therapist. It is the experience of knowing oneself that allows an individual to transcend self-knowledge and begin to deeply engage with others.

Endnotes

1 American Psychological Association. (2015). *APA dictionary of psychology*. American Psychological Association (p. 568).

2 Raskin, N. J., & Rogers, C. R. (2005). Person-centered therapy. In R. J. Corsini & D. Wedding (Eds.), *Current psychotherapies* (7th ed., pp. 130–165; p. 131). Brooks/Cole.

3 Rogers, C. R. ([1951] 2003). *Client-centered therapy: Its current practice, implications, and theory*. Houghton Mifflin.

4 Rogers, *Client-centered therapy* (p. 142).

5 Yalom, I. D. (1980). *Existential psychotherapy* (p. 8). Basic Books.

6 American Psychiatric Association. (2013). *Diagnostic and statistical manual of mental disorders* (5th ed.). American Psychiatric Association.

7 Donne, J. (1624). *Devotions upon emergent occasions: Meditation XVII*. In the public domain.

8 Nietzsche, F. (1889). "Maxims and arrows," *Twilight of the idols*. Quoted in Frankl, V. E. (1984). *Man's search for meaning* (revised ed., p. 97). Washington Square Press.

9 Van Deurzen, E. (2002). *Existential counselling & psychotherapy in practice* (2nd ed., p. 34). Sage Publications.

10 Van Deurzen, *Existential counselling & psychotherapy* (p. 35).

11 Maslow, A. H. (1943). A theory of human motivation. *Psychological Review, 50*, 370–396.
Maslow, A. H. (1954). *Motivation and personality*. Harper & Row Publishers.

12 Koltko-Rivera, M. E. (2006). Rediscovering the later version of Maslow's hierarchy of needs: Self-transcendence and opportunities for theory, research, and unification. *Review of General Psychology, 10*(4), 302–317.

13 Koltko-Rivera, Rediscovering the later version.
Maslow, A. H. (1969). The farther reaches of human nature. *The Journal of Transpersonal Psychology, 1*(1), 1–9.

Note that in this context, ego does not differ significantly from the yogic concept of *ahamkara*, described later in the chapter; both are self-differentiation, with likely ego-centricity, and both are to be held lightly and transcended.

14 Seligman, M. E., & Csikszentmihalyi, M. (2000). Positive psychology: An introduction. *The American Psychologist, 55*(1), 5–14.

15 Linley, P. A., & Joseph, S. (2004). Applied positive psychology: A new perspective for professional practice. In P. A. Linley & S. Joseph (Eds.), *Positive psychology in practice* (pp. 3–12). John Wiley & Sons, Inc.

16 Seligman & Csikszentmihalyi, Positive psychology (p. 7).

17 Kang, Y., Cooper, N., Pandey, P., Scholz, C., et al. (2018). Effects of self-transcendence on neural responses to persuasive messages and health behavior change. *Proceedings of the National Academy of Sciences of the United States of America, 115*(40), 9974–9979.

18 Seligman & Csikszentmihalyi, Positive psychology (p. 8).

19 Miller, R. C. (2012). *The Sankhya Karika: A new translation with embedded commentary*. Integrative Restoration Institute.

20 Bachman, N. (2010). *The yoga sutras: Workbook*. Sounds True.

21 Miller, *Sankhya Karika*.

22 Miller, *Sankhya Karika*.

23 Welwood, J. (1984). Principles of inner work: Psychological and spiritual. *The Journal of Transpersonal Psychology, 16*(1), 63–73.

24 Frawley, D. (1996). *Ayurveda and the mind: The healing of consciousness*. Lotus Press.

25 Frawley, D., & Kshirsagar, S. (2016). *The art and science of Vedic counseling*. Lotus Press.

26 Frawley, *Ayurveda and the mind*.

27 Bachman, N. (2011). *The path of the yoga sutras: A practical guide to the core of yoga*. Sounds True.

28 Bachman, *Path of the yoga sutras*.

29 Bachman, *Path of the yoga sutras*.

30 Desikachar, K., Bragdon, L., & Bossart, C. (2005). The yoga of healing: Exploring yoga's holistic model for health and well-being. *International Journal of Yoga Therapy, 15*, 17–39.
Lad, V. (2002). *Textbook of ayurveda. Vol. 1: Fundamental principles* (pp. 194–196). Ayurvedic Press.

31 Bachman, *Yoga sutras* (p. 285).

32 Raskin & Rogers, Person-centered therapy (p. 133).

33 Raskin & Rogers, Person-centered therapy (p. 131).

34 Frawley, *Ayurveda and the mind*.

35 Lad, V. (2012). *Textbook of ayurveda. Vol. 3: General principles of management and treatment*. Ayurvedic Press.

36 Frawley & Kshirsagar, *Art and science* (p. 178).

37 Tonhajzerova, I., & Mestanik, M. (2017). New perspectives in the model of stress response. *Physiological Research, 66*(Suppl. 2), S173–S185.

12

Mental Disorders and the Yoga Approach

MICHAEL J. DE MANINCOR

Mental health concerns are recognized worldwide as leading causes of disability, and their prevalence appears to be increasing.[1] Their impact can be significant in the lives of individuals, relationships, families, communities, and the workplace.

Mental health is defined by the World Health Organization (WHO) as "a state of well-being in which every individual realizes his or her own potential, can cope with the normal stresses of life, can work productively and fruitfully, and is able to make a contribution to her or his community."[2]

This positive dimension of mental health is also reflected in WHO's broader definition of health, contained in its constitution: "Health is a state of complete physical, mental and social well-being and not merely the absence of disease or infirmity."[3] WHO also emphasizes that "mental health is recognized as more than the absence of mental disorders, and is an integral part of health. Indeed, there is no health without mental health."[4]

These definitions are generally consistent with concepts, teachings, and practices of the yoga *darshana*, which embraces and works with people in a holistic manner and recognizes the central role of the mind in health, mental health, and well-being. These definitions also provide a useful context for working in yoga therapy with people who have mental health concerns.

In most countries today, mental health concerns are approached via a diagnostic-treatment model in which the difficulty is classified as a mental illness or disorder. Mental health conditions are generally characterized by some combination of dysfunctional thoughts, emotions, behavior, social engagement, and relationships with others and often associated with a neurological dysfunction or neurochemical imbalance. These conditions comprise a broad range of problems with different symptoms and in most countries categorized using an extensive range of medical or clinical diagnoses.

The most commonly used approaches for classification or diagnosis of mental disorders are the American Psychiatric Association's (APA) *Diagnostic and Statistical Manual* (DSM; currently in version 5)[5] and WHO's *International Classification of Diseases* (ICD; currently in version 10).[6] The most common forms of diagnosed mental disorders include depression, anxiety, addictions, posttraumatic stress disorder (PTSD), and eating disorders. The most prevalent of these are depression and anxiety, which are the most likely to be encountered in the work of a yoga therapist and form the focus of discussion in this chapter. Less common mental disorders include schizophrenia and bipolar disorder.

Therapeutic yoga, particularly in the area of mental health, is not necessarily based on this modern medicalized approach of treatment of an individual's diagnosed condition. Rather, the approach in yoga and yoga therapy relates to a recognition of, and working with, the whole person. This perspective includes the multidimensional nature of the human being (*panchamaya kosha*; see Chapter 3) and their situation, circumstances, and environment, and then fostering self-agency to bring about change and healing for themselves through an appropriate regular yoga practice. A yoga therapy approach may include reduction of symptom severity, supporting the person to improve quality of life, and, ideally, changing the underlying patterns that cause or contribute to the state of suffering (including *vasana* [experiences or feelings persisting after an event] and *samskara* [deeply ingrained patterns], as described in Chapter 3) into a greater sense of wholeness, freedom, connection, and well-being.

From a yogic perspective, mental health concerns are a reflection or manifestation of underlying imbalances in the *gunas* or patterns of mind, thoughts, and behaviors. These obstacles include the *kleshas* and *antarayas* as well as *svabhava* (an individual's predispositions), vasana, and samskara, and are related to the operational qualities of the mind.[7]

Understanding these yogic concepts is important and useful for working with people with mental health concerns in yoga therapy. An understanding of Western medical conceptualizations of these conditions is also helpful. Again, although the yogic approach to understanding mental health concerns can in many cases be related to the modern diagnostic approach of mental illness, yoga therapy assists and supports people to facilitate desired change rather than treating an illness or condition.

Current Treatments for Mental Disorders

Current treatments for mental disorders include medical, psychological, complementary, mind-body, and lifestyle interventions (including yoga), and combinations of these. In most industrialized countries, medical and psychological treatments are the most common. Medical treatments mostly focus on pharmaceuticals and interventions such as electroconvulsive therapy (ECT) and deep brain stimulation (DBS) for depression. Commonly used psychological treatments include cognitive behavioral therapy (CBT); interpersonal therapy; a "third wave" of mindfulness-based therapies including mindfulness-based cognitive therapy (MBCT) and acceptance-commitment therapy (ACT); and a range of other psychotherapeutic approaches.

Although extensive research provides an evidence base for the effectiveness of these interventions,[8] questions remain about their efficacy; unwanted, harmful, or adverse effects (often referred to as side-effects); placebo effects; cost-benefit; individual choice; barriers and access to services; compliance; ethics; and long-term benefits.[9] In particular, psychopharmaceuticals are known to have a number of limitations, including adverse or harmful effects.[10] Several reviews of the research found only small differences between antidepressant medications and active placebos, especially for mild/moderate depression.[11] Some people choose not to be medicated, and others do not improve despite medications (often described as "treatment resistant").[12]

Psychological treatments are generally free from side-effects. However, some people choose not to seek psychotherapy because of perceived stigma, cultural issues, financial cost, or service availability. Also, a number of barriers to the implementation of these interventions have been identified[13] at the level of the individual, practitioner, health system, society, and more.[14] Despite the availability of treatments, 40 percent of people with depression or anxiety do not seek treatment; of those who do, fewer than half receive beneficial or evidence-based treatments.[15] Problems associated with psychopharmaceuticals and conventional psychological interventions are well-recognized as reasons for seeking complementary and integrative therapies.[16]

Yoga is recognized as having a potential role as an evidence-based intervention for mental health concerns, especially for depression, anxiety, and PTSD.[17] Numerous systematic reviews and meta-analyses suggest benefits of yoga in reducing depression and anxiety.[18] However, variety in diagnoses, severity of symptoms, and types of interventions, as well as limitations of clinical trial methodology, reporting, and risk of bias, suggest that the findings must be interpreted with caution.[19] A common concern in the research reviews is studies' considerable heterogeneity and lack of detail, rationale, and consistency of approach in the types of yoga interventions.[20]

Understanding Depression and Anxiety

The following discussion of depression and anxiety is intended to assist the yoga therapist in understanding the current medical conceptualization of these conditions, not to enable the provision of a diagnosis or to offer a medicalized framework for yoga-based interventions.

Depression

The term *depression* is often used to describe various and sometimes overlapping experiences. For many people, being depressed means feeling sad, blue, tearful, downhearted, detached, or having a lowered mood. However, experiencing these feelings does not necessarily mean someone has depression. Such feelings are common, generally brief, and do not usually have significant or lasting effects on normal functioning. Although such individuals may be in need of support or assistance, they do not generally require a medical, psychological, or clinical intervention. Clinical depression is also common, but it is considered more serious and requires intervention. Without professional assistance, clinical depression can result in chronic disability and even death by suicide.

Depression can be conceptualized as a diagnosed mental disorder or illness in several ways. According to the ICD-10, a "depressive episode" is when the person suffers from lowering of mood, reduction of energy, and decrease in activity. Capacity for enjoyment, interest, and concentration are reduced, and marked tiredness after even minimal effort is common. Sleep is usually disturbed and appetite diminished. Self-esteem and self-confidence are usually reduced and, even in mild forms of depression, some ideas of guilt or worthlessness are often present. The lowered mood varies little from day to day, is unresponsive to circumstances, and may be accompanied by somatic symptoms such as loss of interest and pleasurable feelings, marked psychomotor retardation, agitation, weight loss or gain, and loss of libido; symptoms are generally worse in the morning.

A depressive episode may be mild, moderate, or severe depending on the number and severity of symptoms experienced. A "mild" depressive episode is characterized by two or three of the above symptoms, and although the person is usually distressed by these, they will probably be able to continue with most activities. A "moderate" depressive episode is characterized by four or more of the above symptoms; the person is likely to have great difficulty in continuing with ordinary activities. In "severe" depression, several of the above symptoms are marked and distressing, typically with loss of self-esteem and ideas of worthlessness or guilt. Suicidal thoughts and acts are common, and a number of the somatic symptoms are usually present. A severe depressive episode may also be referred to as "major depression."

"Recurrent depressive disorder" is characterized by repeated depressive episodes with varying degrees of severity and without any history of independent episodes of mood elevation and increased energy (mania). The person may, however, experience brief episodes of mild mood elevation and overactivity immediately after a depressive episode, sometimes precipitated by antidepressant treatment. The first episode may occur at any age from childhood to old age, onset may be acute or insidious (gradual), and duration varies from a few weeks to many months. The risk that a person with recurrent depressive disorder will have an episode of mania never disappears completely, regardless of the number of depressive episodes experienced. If such an episode does occur, the diagnosis is generally changed to bipolar affective disorder.

In many industrialized countries, the psychology and medical professions use the term *clinical depression*, rather than a depressive episode of varying severity as in the ICD-10, to refer to a diagnosable mental disorder. The term *major depressive disorder* (MDD), as defined by the DSM-5,[21] is also used. The APA describes MDD as a medical illness that affects how one feels, thinks, and behaves, causing persistent feelings of sadness and loss of interest in previously enjoyed activities. Similar to the ICD-10 definitions, episodes of MDD are also classified according to severity. The nature of symptoms (e.g., suicidal ideation and behavior) is also considered in assessing severity.[22]

Depression can lead to a variety of emotional and physical problems. It is seen as a chronic illness that usually requires long-term treatment, and many people with depression have concurrent physical and other mental health disorders ("comorbidities").[23]

It is important to distinguish depression from the sadness and grief experienced during bereavement.[24] Although the grief associated with such loss is often intense and long lasting, with many symptoms similar to depression, such emotions are considered a natural response to the loss.

Although symptom-based approaches to describing depression are well-established, debate continues regarding the adequacy and validity of such diagnostic descriptors.[25] In summary, depression may include a depressive episode of varying severity, or a medical or psychological diagnosis of MDD or clinical depression, or, in the absence of a diagnosis, a person may experience symptoms of depression with varying degrees of severity and duration.

Etiology, risk factors, and pathogenesis

Many factors predispose a person to or precipitate depression, including genetics, female gender, childhood experience, previous trauma, social and cultural factors, physical and physiological contributors (including substance abuse and physical health problems), and stress.[26] The etiology (cause) and pathophysiology of depression are complex. The role and interaction of genetics, stress, neurobiology and neurochemistry, perception and sense of self and self-worth, and other potential factors remain unclear. Factors that may initiate depression and those that maintain the condition are likely to be very different. Genetic and stress vulnerabilities interplay to initiate a cascade of neurobiological alterations that disrupt a dynamic and complex system. Structural and functional neurological abnormalities may potentiate progressive effects of recurrent and chronic depression.[27]

Because yoga therapy considers the individual where they are in the present moment, it may be neither necessary nor helpful for the yoga therapist to explore the underlying causes of the client's concerns. Often, these underlying causes remain unknown to the individual. In some cases, however, understanding contributing factors may be useful in the design of an appropriate yoga practice. The important consideration is that changes occur toward greater well-being. In many cases, especially with more severe depression, it is advisable (sometimes essential) for the yoga therapist to work in collaboration with a psychologist or psychiatrist.

Anxiety

Anxiety is generally described as feelings of fear, worry, or nervousness about something with an uncertain outcome. It reflects the thoughts and bodily reactions a person may have when presented with an event or situation they (believe they) cannot manage or undertake successfully.[28] The perceived threat may be in the present moment, triggered by a memory from a past experience, or imagined in the future. When a person is experiencing anxiety, their mind is actively assessing the situation, sometimes automatically and outside of conscious attention, and developing predictions of how well they will cope based on past experiences; such thought processes are sometimes seen as a normal part of everyday life. Although some anxiety is a natural response to a threatening situation, high anxiety levels may prevent a person from identifying an effective way of managing the threatening situation.[29]

Symptoms or feelings of anxiety include ongoing worry or thoughts that are distressing and interfere with daily living; confusion; trembling; sweating; faintness or dizziness; difficulty sleeping; increased heart rate; difficulty breathing; upset stomach or nausea; restlessness; avoidance behavior; and irritability.[30]

The Australian non-profit services organization Beyond Blue distinguishes between anxious feelings and anxiety, describing anxiety as:

> more than just feeling stressed or worried. While stress and anxious feelings are a common response to pressure, they usually pass once the stressful situation has passed, or [the] "stressor" is removed. Anxiety is when these anxious feelings are ongoing and exist without any particular reason or cause.[31]

Similarly, a distinction is often made between anxiety and anxiety disorders. Anxiety disorders are defined as a group of mental disorders characterized by various combinations of key features—excessive anxiety, fear, worry, avoidance, and compulsive rituals—associated with impaired functioning or significant distress.[32] According to this definition, and similar to the distinction between feelings of depression and a diagnostic disorder, the main distinctions between anxious feelings and a disorder are severity and duration.[33]

Specific types of anxiety disorders include generalized anxiety disorder (GAD), which is the most common, specific phobias including social phobia or social anxiety disorder, panic disorder, obsessive-compulsive disorder (OCD), and PTSD.[34]

GAD is the most common anxiety disorder presenting in primary care settings and the most substantive focus of research.[35] Other anxiety disorders, such as phobias and PTSD, have specific distinguishing features. The main differences between GAD and general symptoms of anxiety are severity and duration of the symptoms.

Etiology, risk factors, and pathogenesis

As mentioned previously, anxiety and depression are related and highly comorbid, and considerable overlap of symptoms and risk factors characterizes the disorders. It is important to note that there is ongoing controversy about whether anxiety and depression constitute a common underlying emotional disorder or distinct and separate disorders.[36]

It also remains unclear whether anxiety and depression share an underlying cause. Many of the factors related to etiology and pathogenesis certainly appear to be common to both conditions.[37] Similar to depression, many factors predispose a person to anxiety, including genes, childhood experience, previous or recent trauma, physical and physiological factors (including substance abuse and physical health problems), and stress.[38]

Putting it together

Although depression and anxiety are identified as diagnostically independent categories of mental disorders,[39] comorbidity of symptoms and diagnoses is well-recognized and common.[40] The many longstanding questions of the theoretical and clinical significance of their comorbidity[41] remain an important issue for treatment choice and outcomes.[42] The primary distinguishing feature in symptom presentation between the disorder categories can be summarized as anhedonia (loss of ability to feel pleasure) in depression and excessive worry in anxiety.[43] Some suggest that the two disorders represent more of a spectrum or mixed anxiety-depression disorder, with "anxious depression" as subtype of depressive disorders.[44]

Evidence for Yoga as a Mind-Body-Lifestyle Approach for Mental Health

Several factors and types of evidence support the notion of yoga for mental healthcare. First are the theoretical and historical proposition of the teachings and practice of yoga as a mental healthcare system, mentioned earlier and in Chapter 11. Second, extensive indirect or related evidence suggests the efficacy of interventions with yogic components. Examples include exercise, relaxation, breathing exercises, mindfulness and other non-yogic forms of meditation, and cultivation of values and positive aspects of mental health.

Finally, a growing body of research suggests positive effects of yoga-based interventions for mental health, particularly for depression and anxiety. However, the results and interpretations must continue to be treated with caution, and further research is required. In addition to methodological limitations (see Chapter 6), lack of details and heterogeneity of the yoga interventions make it difficult to draw robust conclusions about the benefits of yoga as a mental health intervention. Also, studies vary considerably in length of intervention and the intensity and frequency of yoga and include different types of active and non-active control comparisons. What is classified as a yoga intervention, including multi-component yoga-based mindfulness programs such as mindfulness-based stress reduction (MBSR), is another concern.

It is also possible that benefit derives from doing *anything* to improve one's mental health. To ascertain the benefit of the yoga itself, inclusion of active controls, as well as comparisons with conventional treatments, is recommended.

These issues and concerns are largely related to the "strength of evidence" for yoga-based interventions in mental health. This is not to say that yoga-based interventions are not effective—lack of evidence does not equal lack of effectiveness. However, these issues highlight the lack of clarity concerning what kinds of practices might be effective for different individuals with various mental health concerns.

Plausible Mechanisms of Action

Yoga might affect mental health via many possible mechanisms. Research has primarily focused on mechanisms related to biological (including neurophysiological), psychological (including emotional and cognitive), and behavioral factors.[45] These mechanisms have also been described as an integration of "bottom-up" (biological) and "top-down" (psychological) influences (see Chapter 13).[46] This section highlights potential psychoneurophysiological mechanisms.

Stress is a known contributor to depression, anxiety, and other mental health concerns.[47] The stress response involves a two-way communication between the brain (including a person's appraisal and perceptual experience in relation to a stressor) and the cardiorespiratory, immune, metabolic, and other systems via the autonomic nervous system (ANS), endocrine system, and hypothalamic-pituitary-adrenal (HPA) axis.[48] As noted in Chapter 7, *homeostasis* refers to the mechanisms that keep the parameters of one's physiological functions within the ranges necessary for survival.[49]

Allostasis is the adaptive process of maintaining stability during conditions that are outside of the usual homeostatic range, and *allostatic load* is the cost to the body for maintaining this stability during deviations from the usual homeostatic range (see Chapter 11).[50] More specifically, allostatic load refers to the cumulative effect of neurophysiological responses to perceived stressors, which include the release of a cascade of hormones (serotonin, melatonin, cortisol) and neurotransmitters (including the catecholamines epinephrine, norepinephrine, and dopamine, and gamma-aminobutyric acid [GABA]) that activate the HPA axis and the sympathetic branch of the ANS (see Chapter 7).

Prolonged activation and increased allostatic load contribute to overactivity of the HPA axis and functions of the sympathetic nervous system (SNS), with associated underactivity of the parasympathetic nervous system (PNS); imbalances in the endocrine system, hormones, and neurotransmitters; and potentially adverse changes in brain anatomy and physiology and neurological and cognitive functions.[51] An organism's responsiveness to internal and external challenges is limited by the need to maintain stability. Reduced capacity for responsiveness increases allostatic load.[52] All these factors are known to contribute to a range of physical and psychological health concerns.[53]

Numerous authors have proposed that the primary mechanism by which yoga practices affect mental health concerns such as depression and anxiety is by reducing the effects of stress and allostatic load, with associated neurophysiological changes.[54] This mechanism occurs via a number of pathways, including downregulation of the HPA axis, balancing the functions of the ANS (reduction of activity in the SNS and activation of the PNS, also known as the "relaxation response"[55]), vagus nerve stimulation leading to greater heart rate variability and neurotransmitter levels, and regulating hormonal imbalances via decreases of cortisol and catecholamines and increases of serotonin, melatonin, and GABA.[56]

Other potential factors associated with yoga practice may contribute to these and potentially other mechanisms of action, including the sheer effort of doing something (anything) to care for oneself, the therapeutic benefit of connection with the yoga therapist, social engagement and connection from participation in group classes, and an increased sense of purpose and meaning sometimes described as spiritual. These factors are well-known among yoga practitioners, teachers, and therapists but have not been given much attention in research.

Clinical Implications for Yoga Therapists

Yoga therapy includes assessment of the individual's needs, initial design and delivery of a suitable plan of care, and, ideally, ongoing review, refinement, and development of the plan of care. Both yogic and Western medical conceptualizations of mental health and mental health concerns are important to help inform these processes.

Ongoing research demonstrates the potential effectiveness of yoga-based interventions for mental health concerns, including reducing symptoms of depression and anxiety and less common and more severe types of mental health concerns, and improving general mental health, well-being, and resilience. However, further research is required for yoga interventions to be recognized as evidence-based approaches. This would also provide much-needed clarity around types of practices and specific yogic tools for individuals with different needs and abilities, contraindications and potential adverse effects, and how much yoga (dosage) is required for sustainable benefit.

Yoga is generally considered safe for most people with mental health concerns. Although some adverse events and injuries have been associated with yoga practice, these are usually related to more extreme types of physical postures and breathing techniques (especially for people with anxiety), practices unsuited to the particular individual, and the presence of preexisting conditions. (See Chapter 23 for a brief discussion of meditative yoga practice in the presence of serious mental health issues.) Cramer and colleagues have suggested that yoga "can be recommended to patients with physical or mental ailments, as long as it is appropriately adapted to their needs and abilities and performed under the guidance of an experienced and medically trained yoga teacher."[57] The recommendation for "medically trained" yoga teachers is ambiguous, but appropriate training, knowledge, and skills of yoga therapists for delivery of interventions for people with mental health concerns are generally considered necessary[58] and require further consideration in the field.

A final consideration for developing yoga as an effective intervention for people with mental health concerns is the significance of the therapeutic relationship or alliance (see Chapter 13). Therapeutic relationship has been given extensive attention in the psychotherapeutic research literature[59] and is central to the teaching tradition and healing applications of yoga therapy.[60] There is more to the healing process than the particular practices and techniques used.

It is well-recognized that people do not recover from mental health concerns in a single proven way. However, a range of potentially effective interventions can help people recover, stay well, and live more fulfilling lives. Offering the right intervention, including yoga-based interventions, for the individual's needs is important for beneficial outcomes and risk minimization.

Summary

This chapter offers a basic understanding of the common mental health concerns of depression and anxiety, primarily from a contemporary Western medical perspective. These concepts have been related to basic yogic understandings of mental health, and the research to date has been summarized.

A prescriptive approach of which techniques to use for particular mental health conditions (the diagnostic-treatment model) has not been offered. The research suggests that many, perhaps most, yoga-based interventions are at least safe and seem to have some benefit for different people with mental health concerns. Efficacy is somewhat independent of diagnosis or condition and instead related to the individual. Details and recommendations of specific yoga-based interventions to consider for helping people with mental health concerns are addressed elsewhere throughout the literature.

BOX 12.1 PHARMACOTHERAPY CONSIDERATIONS FOR YOGA THERAPISTS

MAMTA PARIKH

A basic understanding of the side-effects of common medications will help yoga therapists to know which practices may be best for a specific client and which are contraindicated. Medications used in the treatment of psychiatric disorders also have important monitoring parameters and key client education points. Having multiple professionals involved in monitoring and emphasizing these education points can help with outcomes.

Selective serotonin reuptake inhibitors (SSRIs), serotonin norepinephrine reuptake inhibitors (SNRIs), tricyclic antidepressants (TCAs), bupropion, mirtazapine, and monoamine oxidase inhibitors (MAOIs) are antidepressants used for treatment of major depressive disorder and anxiety disorders. These medications can take up to 4 to 8 weeks to be fully effective. Patients may feel jittery at the beginning of treatment, which can be addressed by the prescribing provider lowering the dose and titrating slowly. Abruptly discontinuing these medications can result in withdrawal; therefore, they need to be tapered. Sexual dysfunction is commonly reported with these medications, except for bupropion, which can be used as an alternative.

SSRIs (e.g., sertraline, paroxetine, citalopram, escitalopram, fluoxetine) and SNRIs (e.g., venlafaxine, duloxetine) are common first-line treatments for depression and anxiety disorders. They can cause gastrointestinal side-effects like nausea, vomiting, abdominal pain, constipation, and diarrhea, which tend to resolve within 1 to 2 weeks. A client may have discontinued one of these medications because of such side-effects. SNRIs, bupropion, and fluoxetine are activating; therefore, it is best to take these in the morning to avoid insomnia. Paroxetine is a sedating SSRI best taken at bedtime. SNRIs can also raise blood pressure as the dose is increased, so clients should be monitored by their prescribing providers.

Bupropion and mirtazapine are two more first-line agents. Bupropion, also used for smoking cessation under a different brand name, is activating, like fluoxetine and SNRIs. It can lower seizure threshold, so it must be avoided in those with seizure disorders. Mirtazapine is a sedating antidepressant, and it stimulates appetite, potentially resulting in weight gain, hyperglycemia, elevated lipids, etc.

TCAs (e.g., amitriptyline, nortriptyline, doxepin) are not the preferred agents for first-line treatment because of their significant side-effect profile. TCAs are sedating and have anticholinergic side-effects, meaning they inhibit parasympathetic functions. They can also affect the heart rhythm (QT prolongation) and lower the seizure threshold. MAOIs (e.g., phenelzine, tranylcypromine) are not commonly used because they interact with other pharmaceuticals such as dextromethorphan. MAOIs also interact with tyramine-containing products such as aged cheese, aged wine, fava beans, sourdough, etc.

Mood stabilizers, like lithium, valproic acid, lamotrigine, and carbamazepine, are commonly used in the treatment of bipolar disorder, schizoaffective disorder, and so forth. Lithium requires regular bloodwork to check complete blood count (CBC), serum electrolytes, and lithium levels. Those who have been prescribed lithium must remember to stay hydrated and avoid non-steroidal anti-inflammatories (NSAIDs). Valproic acid, lamotrigine, and carbamazepine are anticonvulsants; therefore, abrupt withdrawal of these agents may result in seizures. They interact with many medications, so the prescribing provider must have a complete medication list, including prescription, over-the-counter (OTC), herbal, and supplement products, and clients should be made aware of the risks for interaction. These drugs also carry risk of a serious reaction, Stevens Johnson Syndrome, so if a client on one of these medications reports a rash after starting therapy, they must be referred back to their prescribing provider immediately. Valproic acid and carbamazepine also require routine bloodwork from the prescribing physician.

There are two groups of antipsychotics: first generation (FGAs) and second generation (SGAs). FGAs (e.g., haloperidol, fluphenazine) carry an increased risk of extrapyramidal symptoms (EPS),[61] hyperprolactinemia (elevated levels of the hormone prolactin), and neuroleptic malignant syndrome.[62] Because of these side-effects, FGAs are reserved for after a patient has failed SGA therapy(ies). Clozapine is an SGA that is recommended when a patient has failed two adequate antipsychotic trials and has a Risk Evaluation and Mitigation Strategy (REMS)[63] that requires reporting of their absolute neutrophil count (ANC). SGAs (e.g., clozapine, olanzapine, risperidone) have a lower risk of EPS; however, they can cause significant metabolic abnormalities like weight gain, elevated blood glucose, and abnormal lipids. Routine EKG monitoring is needed with antipsychotics due to risk of QT prolongation. Haloperidol, fluphenazine, olanzapine, aripiprazole, risperidone, and paliperidone are available as long-acting injectable antipsychotics that can be given periodically on a regular schedule (e.g., every 4 or 6 weeks), so they are often used for those who have a history of medication non-compliance.

Hydroxyzine and benzodiazepines (e.g., alprazolam, lorazepam, diazepam) are used for the acute treatment of anxiety. They tend to be prescribed as needed. Benzodiazepine use should be limited to 2 to 4 weeks due to its side-effects and abuse potential; especially when used with opioids, they can cause respiratory depression. Benzodiazepines can also be used for the treatment of seizures.

It is important to obtain a comprehensive list of a client's medications, including prescription, OTC, herbal, and supplement products. Taking into consideration the side-effects and major interactions of common medications will better enable yoga therapists to offer practices that keep clients safe. Clients may also seek yoga therapy specifically to address a medication side-effect, so knowledge of what can be practically addressed and what may need to be referred back to the prescribing provider is part of creating an appropriate practice environment.

Additional Resources

Emerson, D., & Hopper, E. (2011). *Overcoming trauma through yoga: Reclaiming your body.* North Atlantic Books.

Mason, H., & Birch, K. (Eds.). (2018). *Yoga for mental health.* Handspring Publishing.

Miller, R. C. (2015). *The iRest Program for healing PTSD: A proven-effective approach to using yoga nidra meditation and deep relaxation techniques to overcome trauma.* New Harbinger Publications.

Stearns, M. N., & Stearns, R. N. (2010). *Yoga for anxiety: Meditations and practices for calming the body and mind.* New Harbinger Publications.

Weintraub, A. (2003). *Yoga for depression: A compassionate guide to relieve suffering through yoga.* Harmony.

Endnotes

1 GBD 2017 Disease and Injury Incidence and Prevalence Collaborators. (2018). Global, regional, and national incidence, prevalence, and years lived with disability for 354 diseases and injuries for 195 countries and territories, 1990–2017: A systematic analysis for the Global Burden of Disease Study 2017. *Lancet, 392*(10159), 1789–1858.

World Health Organization. (2019). Mental disorders [fact sheet]. www.who.int/en/news-room/fact-sheets/detail/mental-disorders

2 World Health Organization. (2014). Mental health: Strengthening our response. Fact sheet No. 220. www.who.int/news-room/fact-sheets/detail/mental-health-strengthening-our-response

3 World Health Organization. (1946). Basic documents. In *Constitution of the World Health Organization*. United Nations.

4 World Health Organization, *Mental Health.*

5 American Psychiatric Association (APA). (2013). *Diagnostic and statistical manual of mental disorders* (5th ed.). APA.

6 World Health Organization. (2015). *International classification of diseases* (10th ed.). http://apps.who.int/classifications/icd10/browse/2015/en#/F30-F39

7 In addition to Chapters 2 and 3 of this book, see Desikachar, T. K. V. (1999). *The heart of yoga: Developing a personal practice* (pp. 121–123). Inner Traditions.

8 Canadian Psychiatric Association. (2006). Clinical practice guidelines: Management of anxiety disorders. *Canadian Journal of Psychiatry, 51*(8 Suppl. 2), 9S–91S.
Ellis, P., & Royal Australian and New Zealand College of Psychiatrists (RANZCP) Clinical Practice Guidelines Team for Depression. (2004). Australian and New Zealand clinical practice guidelines for the treatment of depression. *Australian and New Zealand Journal of Psychiatry, 38*(6), 389–407.

9 Ankarberg, P., & Falkenstrom, F. (2008). Treatment of depression with antidepressants is primarily a psychological treatment. *Psychotherapy: Theory, Research, Practice, Training, 45*(3), 329–339.
Biegler, P. (2010). Autonomy and ethical treatment in depression. *Bioethics, 24*(4), 179–189.
Blumenthal, R., & Endicott, J. (1996). Barriers to seeking treatment for major depression. *Depression & Anxiety, 4*(6), 273–278.
Wang, P. S., Aguilar-Gaxiola, S., Alonso, J., Angermeyer, M. C., et al. (2007). Use of mental health services for anxiety, mood, and substance disorders in 17 countries in the WHO world mental health surveys. *Lancet, 370*(9590), 841–850.

10 Gartlehner, G., Gaynes, B. N., Amick, H. R., Asher, G., et al. (2015). Nonpharmacological versus pharmacological treatments for adult patients with major depressive disorder. *Comparative Effectiveness Review*, No. 161. Agency for Healthcare Research and Quality publication No. 15(6)-EHC031-EF.
Hindmarch, I. (1998). Cognition and anxiety: The cognitive effects of anti-anxiety medication. *Acta Psychiatrica Scandinavica, 393*(Suppl.), 89–94.

11 Fournier, J. C., DeRubeis, R. J., Hollon, S. D., Dimidjian, S., et al. (2010). Antidepressant drug effects and depression severity: A patient-level meta-analysis. *JAMA, 303*(1), 47–53.
Hougaard, E. (2010). Placebo and antidepressant treatment for major depression: Is there a lesson to be learned for psychotherapy? *Nordic Psychology, 62*(2), 7–26.
Moncrieff, J., Wessely, S., & Hardy, R. (2004). Active placebo versus antidepressants for depression. *The Cochrane Database of Systematic Reviews*, CD003012.

12 Fava, M. (2003). Diagnosis and definition of treatment-resistant depression. *Biological Psychiatry, 53*(8), 649–659.
Nierenberg, A., Katz, J., & Fava, M. (2007). A critical overview of the pharmacologic management of treatment-resistant depression. *Psychiatry Clinics of North America, 30*, 13–29.

13 Killackey, E., Jorm, A., Alvarez-Jimenez, M., McCann, T. V., Hides, L., & Couineau, A. L. (2008). Do we do what we know works, and if not why not? *Australian and New Zealand Journal of Psychiatry, 42*(6), 439–444.

14 Australian Bureau of Statistics. (2008). *National survey of mental health and well-being: Summary of results.* ABS.

15 Biegler, Autonomy and ethical treatment.
Tiller, J. W. (2013). Depression and anxiety. *Medical Journal of Australia, 199*(S6), S28–S31.

16 Astin, J. A. (1998). Why patients use alternative medicine: Results of a national study. *JAMA, 279*(19), 1548–1553.
Biegler, Autonomy and ethical treatment.
Killackey et al., Do we do what we know works?

17 Jeter, P. E., Slutsky, J., Singh, N., & Khalsa, S. B. (2015). Yoga as a therapeutic intervention: A bibliometric analysis of published research studies from 1967 to 2013. *Journal of Alternative and Complementary Medicine, 21*(10), 586–592.

Morgan, A. J., Reavley, N. J., Jorm, A. F., Bassilios, B., et al. (2019). *A guide to what works for depression* (3rd ed.). Beyond Blue.

18 Cabral, P., Meyer, H. B., & Ames, D. (2011). Effectiveness of yoga therapy as a complementary treatment for major psychiatric disorders: A meta-analysis. *The Primary Care Companion for CNS Disorders, 13*(4), PCC.10r01068.

Cramer, H., Lauche, R., Langhorst, J., & Dobos, G. (2013). Yoga for depression: A systematic review and meta-analysis. *Depression & Anxiety, 30*(11), 1068–1083.

Kirkwood, G., Rampes, H., Tuffrey, V., Richardson, J., & Pilkington, K. (2005). Yoga for anxiety: A systematic review of the research evidence. *British Journal of Sports Medicine, 39*(12), 884–891.

Pilkington, K., Kirkwood, G., Rampes, H., & Richardson, J. (2005). Yoga for depression: The research evidence. *Journal of Affective Disorders, 89*(1–3), 13–24.

Uebelacker, L. A., Epstein-Lubow, G., Gaudiano, B. A., Tremont, G., Battle, C. L., & Miller, I. W. (2010). Hatha yoga for depression: Critical review of the evidence for efficacy, plausible mechanisms of action, and directions for future research. *Journal of Psychiatric Practice, 16*(1), 22–33.

19 Cramer, H., Langhorst, J., Dobos, G., & Lauche, R. (2015). Associated factors and consequences of risk of bias in randomized controlled trials of yoga: A systematic review. *PLoS ONE, 10*(12), e0144125.

Cramer et al., Yoga for depression.

Uebelacker et al., Hatha yoga for depression.

20 Cramer et al., Yoga for depression.

Kirkwood et al., Yoga for anxiety.

Uebelacker et al., Hatha yoga for depression.

21 APA, *Diagnostic and statistical manual of mental disorders.*

22 APA, *Diagnostic and statistical manual of mental disorders.*

23 APA, *Diagnostic and statistical manual of mental disorders.*

24 APA, *Diagnostic and statistical manual of mental disorders.*

25 Kendler, K. (2002). Hierarchy and heritability: The role of diagnosis and modeling in psychiatric genetics. *American Journal of Psychiatry, 159*(4), 515–518.

Luyten, P., Blatt, S. J., Van Houdenhove, B., & Corveleyn, J. (2006). Depression research and treatment: Are we skating to where the puck is going to be? *Clinical Psychology Review, 26*(8), 985–999.

26 Ellis & RANZCP Clinical Practice Guidelines Team for Depression, Australian and New Zealand clinical practice guidelines.

27 Maletic, V., Robinson, M., Oakes, T., Iyengar, S., Ball, S. G., & Russell, J. (2007). Neurobiology of depression: An integrated view of key findings. *International Journal of Clinical Practice, 61*(12), 2030–2040.

28 Australian Psychological Society (APS). (n.d.). Anxiety disorders. www.psychology.org.au/publications/tip_sheets/anxiety

29 APS, Anxiety Disorders.

30 APS, Anxiety Disorders.

31 Reavley, N., Morgan, A., Jorm, A., Wright, J., et al. (2019). A guide to what works for anxiety: An evidence-based review. https://dpvhealth.org.au/app/uploads/2018/02/BB_A-guide-toAnxiety.pdf (p. 6).

32 Canadian Psychiatric Association, Clinical practice guidelines.

33 Boyce, P., Harris, A., Drobny, J., Lampe, L., Starcevic, V., & Bryant, R. (Eds.). (2015). *The Sydney handbook of anxiety disorders: A guide to the symptoms, causes and treatments of anxiety disorders.* University of Sydney.

34 APS, Anxiety Disorders.

35 Baxter, A. J., Scott, K. M., Vos, T., & Whiteford, H. A. (2013). Global prevalence of anxiety disorders: A systematic review and meta-regression. *Psychological Medicine, 43*(5), 897–910.

Gwynn, R. C., McQuistion, H. L., McVeigh, K. H., Garg, R. K., Frieden, T. R., & Thorpe, L. E. (2008). Prevalence, diagnosis, and treatment of depression and generalized anxiety disorder in a diverse urban community. *Psychiatric Services, 59*(6), 641–647.

Newman, M. G., Llera, S. J., Erickson, T. M., Przeworski, A., & Castonguay, L. G. (2013). Worry and generalized anxiety disorder: A review and theoretical synthesis of evidence on nature, etiology, mechanisms, and treatment. *Annual Review of Clinical Psychology, 9*, 275–297.

36 APA, *Diagnostic and statistical manual of mental disorders.*

Barlow, D. H., Allen, L. B., & Choate, M. L. (2016). Toward a unified treatment for emotional disorders—republished article. *Behavior Therapy, 47*(6), 838–853.
Newby, J. M., McKinnon, A., Kuyken, W., Gilbody, S., & Dalgleish, T. (2015). Systematic review and meta-analysis of transdiagnostic psychological treatments for anxiety and depressive disorders in adulthood. *Clinical Psychology Review, 40*, 91–110.
Tiller, Depression and anxiety.
Watson, D. (2005). Rethinking the mood and anxiety disorders: A quantitative hierarchical model for DSM-V. *Journal of Abnormal Psychology, 114*(4), 522–536.

37 APA, *Diagnostic and statistical manual of mental disorders.*

38 Katzman, M. A., Bleau, P., Blier, P., Chokka, P., et al. (2014). Canadian clinical practice guidelines for the management of anxiety, posttraumatic stress and obsessive-compulsive disorders. *BMC Psychiatry, 14*(Suppl. 1).
Reavley et al., *A guide to what works.*

39 APA, *Diagnostic and statistical manual of mental disorders.*

40 APA, *Diagnostic and statistical manual of mental disorders.*
Australian Bureau of Statistics, *National survey of mental health and well-being.*
Craske, M. (2012). Transdiagnostic treatment for anxiety and depression. *Depression & Anxiety, 29*(9), 749–753.
Hunot, V., Churchill, R., Silva de Lima, M., & Teixeira, V. (2007). Psychological therapies for generalised anxiety disorder. *The Cochrane Database of Systematic Reviews, 2007*(1), CD001848.
Keller, M., & Hanks, D. (1995). Anxiety symptom relief in depression treatment outcomes. *Journal of Clinical Psychiatry, 56*(Suppl. 6), 22–29.
Kendall, P. C., Kortlander, E., Chansky, T. E., & Brady, E. U. (1992). Comorbidity of anxiety and depression in youth: Treatment implications. *Journal of Consulting and Clinical Psychology, 60*(6), 869–880.
Kessler, R. C., McGonagle, K. A., Zhao, S., Nelson, C. B., et al. (1994). Lifetime and 12-month prevalence of DSM-III-R psychiatric disorders in the United States: Results from the National Comorbidity Survey. *Archives of General Psychiatry, 51*(1), 8–19.
Kessler, R. C., Sampson, N. A., Berglund, P., Gruber, M. J., et al. (2015). Anxious and non-anxious major depressive disorder in the World Health Organization World Mental Health Surveys. *Epidemiology and Psychiatric Sciences, 24*(3), 210–226.
Schatzberg, A. (2015). The chicken and egg of anxiety and depression. *Epidemiology and Psychiatric Sciences, 24*, 227–229.
Tiller, Depression and anxiety.

41 APA, *Diagnostic and statistical manual of mental disorders.*
Blanco, C., Rubio, J. M., Wall, M., Secades-Villa, R., Beesdo-Baum, K., & Wang, S. (2014). The latent structure and comorbidity patterns of generalized anxiety disorder and major depressive disorder: A national study. *Depression & Anxiety, 31*(3), 214–222.
Kendall et al., Comorbidity of anxiety and depression.

42 APA, *Diagnostic and statistical manual of mental disorders.*
Astin, Why patients use alternative medicine.

43 Zbozinek, T. D., Rose, R. D., Wolitzky-Taylor, K. B., Sherbourne, C., et al. (2012). Diagnostic overlap of generalized anxiety disorder and major depressive disorder in a primary care sample. *Depression & Anxiety, 29*(12), 1065–1071.

44 APA, *Diagnostic and statistical manual of mental disorders.*
Barlow et al., Toward a unified treatment.
Fawcett, J., & Kravitz, H. M. (1983). Anxiety syndromes and their relationship to depressive illness. *Journal of Clinical Psychiatry, 44*(8, pt. 2), 8–11.
Kring, A. M., & Sloan, D. M. (Eds.). (2010). Introduction and overview. In *Emotion regulation and psychopathology: A transdiagnostic approach to etiology and treatment* (pp. 1–9). Guilford Press.

45 Kinser, P., & Lyon, D. (2014). A conceptual framework of stress vulnerability, depression, and health outcomes in women: Potential uses in research on complementary therapies for depression. *Brain and Behavior, 4*(5), 665–674.
Riley, K. E., & Park, C. L. (2015). How does yoga reduce stress? A systematic review of mechanisms of change and guide to future inquiry. *Health Psychology Review, 9*(3), 379–396.

Uebelacker, L., & Broughton, M. (2016). Yoga for depression and anxiety: A review of published research and implications for healthcare providers. *Rhode Island Medical Journal*, *99*(3), 20–22.
46 Gard, T., Noggle, J. J., Park, C. L., Vago, D. R., & Wilson, A. (2014). Potential self-regulatory mechanisms of yoga for psychological health. *Frontiers in Human Neuroscience*, *8*, 770.
Schmalzl, L., Powers, C., & Henje Blom, E. (2015). Neurophysiological and neurocognitive mechanisms underlying the effects of yoga-based practices: Towards a comprehensive theoretical framework. *Frontiers in Human Neuroscience*, *9*, 235.
47 APA, *Diagnostic and statistical manual of mental disorders.*
Cohen, S., Janicki-Deverts, D., & Miller, G. (2010). Psychological stress and disease. *JAMA*, *298*(14), 1685–1687.
Hammen, C. (2005). Stress and depression. *Annual Review of Clinical Psychology*, *2005*(1), 293–319.
Van Praag, H., de Kloet, E., & van Os, J. (2004). *Stress, the brain and depression.* Cambridge University Press.
48 McEwen, B. (2007). Physiology and neurobiology of stress and adaptation: Central role of the brain. *Physiological Reviews*, *87*(3), 873–904.
49 McEwen, B., & Wingfield, J. (2010). What is in a name? Integrating homeostasis, allostasis and stress. *Hormones and Behavior*, *57*(2), 105–111.
50 McEwen, Physiology and neurobiology.
51 Kiverstein, J., & Miller, M. (2015). The embodied brain: Towards a radical embodied cognitive neuroscience. *Frontiers in Human Neuroscience*, *9*, 237.
McEwen, B. (2009). The brain is the central organ of stress and adaptation. *NeuroImage*, *47*(3), 911–913.
Reppermund, S., Zihl, J., Lucae, S., Horstmann, S., et al. (2007). Persistent cognitive impairment in depression: The role of psychopathology and altered hypothalamic-pituitary-adrenocortical (HPA) system regulation. *Biological Psychiatry*, *62*(5), 400–406.
Stewart, J. (2006). The detrimental effects of allostasis: Allostatic load as a measure of cumulative stress. *Journal of Physiological Anthropology*, *25*(1), 133–145.
52 Streeter, C. C., Gerbarg, P. L., Saper, R. B., Ciraulo, D. A., & Brown, R. P. (2012). Effects of yoga on the autonomic nervous system, gamma-aminobutyric-acid, and allostasis in epilepsy, depression, and post-traumatic stress disorder. *Medical Hypotheses*, *78*(5), 571–579.
53 APA, *Diagnostic and statistical manual of mental disorders.*
Belmaker, R., & Agam, G. (2008). Mechanisms of disease—Major depressive disorder. *New England Journal of Medicine*, *358*, 55–68.
Bogdan, R., & Pizzagalli, D. A. (2006). Acute stress reduces reward responsiveness: Implications for depression. *Biological Psychiatry*, *60*(10), 1147–1154.
Cohen et al., Psychological stress and disease.
Hintsa, T., Elovainio, M., Jokela, M., Ahola, K., Virtanen, M., & Pirkola, S. (2016). Is there an independent association between burnout and increased allostatic load? Testing the contribution of psychological distress and depression. *Journal of Health Psychology*, *21*(8), 1576–1586.
Innes, K. E., Vincent, H. K., & Taylor, A. G. (2007). Chronic stress and insulin resistance-related indices of cardiovascular disease risk, Part 2: A potential role for mind-body therapies. *Alternative Therapies in Health and Medicine*, *13*(5), 44–51.
McEwen, B. S. (1998). Stress, adaptation, and disease: Allostasis and allostatic load. *Annals of the New York Academy of Sciences*, *840*, 33–44.
McEwen, B., & Wingfield, J. (2003). The concept of allostasis in biology and biomedicine. *Hormones and Behavior*, *43*(1), 2–15.
Stewart, The detrimental effects of allostasis.
van Praag et al., *Stress, the brain and depression.*
54 Kinser, P. A., Goehler, L. E., & Taylor, A. G. (2012). How might yoga help depression? A neurobiological perspective. *Explore*, *8*(2), 118–126.
Pascoe, M., & Bauer, I. (2015). A systematic review of randomised control trials on the effects of yoga on stress measures and mood. *Journal of Psychiatric Research*, *68*, 270–282.
Streeter et al., Effects of yoga.
Uebelacker et al., Hatha yoga for depression.
55 Benson, H., & Klipper, M. (1976). *The relaxation response.* Avon.
56 APA, *Diagnostic and statistical manual of mental disorders.*

Gard, T. (2015). *The neural and psychological mechanisms of yoga and mindfulness meditation.* Maastricht University.
Innes, K., Bourguignon, C., & Taylor, A. (2005). Risk indices associated with the insulin resistance syndrome, cardiovascular disease, and possible protection with yoga: A systematic review. *Journal of the American Board of Family Practice, 18*(6), 491–519.
Kinser & Lyon, Conceptual framework.
Kinser et al., How might yoga help depression?
McCall, M. C. (2013). How might yoga work? An overview of potential underlying mechanisms. *Journal of Yoga and Physical Therapy, 3*(1), 130.
Riley & Park, How does yoga reduce stress?
Ross, A., & Thomas, S. (2010). The health benefits of yoga and exercise: A review of comparison studies. *Journal of Alternative and Complementary Medicine, 16*(1), 3–12.
Salmon, P., Lush, E., Jablonski, M., & Sephton, S. E. (2009). Yoga and mindfulness: Clinical aspects of an ancient mind/body practice. *Cognitive and Behavioral Practice, 16*, 59–72.
Schmalzl et al., Neurophysiological and neurocognitive mechanisms.
Streeter et al., Effects of yoga.
Uebelacker et al., Hatha yoga for depression.

57 Cramer, H., Krucoff, C., & Dobos, G. (2013). Adverse events associated with yoga: A systematic review of published case reports and case series. *PLoS ONE, 8*(10), e75515.

58 de Manincor, M., Bensoussan, A., Smith, C., Fahey, P., & Bourchier, S. (2015). Establishing key components of yoga interventions for reducing depression and anxiety, and improving well-being: A Delphi method study. *BMC Complementary and Alternative Medicine, 15*, 85.

59 Ankarberg & Falkenstrom, Treatment of depression.
Castonguay, L. G., Goldfried, M. R., Wiser, S., Raue, P. J., & Hayes, A. M. (1996). Predicting the effect of cognitive therapy for depression: A study of unique and common factors. *Journal of Consulting and Clinical Psychology, 64*(3), 497–504.
Gelenberg, A. J., Freeman, M. P., Markowitz, J. C., Rosenbaum, J. F., et al. (2010). Practice guideline for the treatment of patients with major depressive disorder: Third edition. *American Journal of Psychiatry, 167*(10), 13–118.
Kanter, J. W., Rusch, L. C., Landes, S. J., Holman, G. I., Whiteside, U., & Sedivy, S. K. (2009). The use and nature of present-focused interventions in cognitive and behavioral therapies for depression. *Psychotherapy, 46*(2), 220–232.
Malhi, G. S., Bassett, D., Boyce, P., Bryant, R., et al. (2015). Royal Australian and New Zealand College of Psychiatrists clinical practice guidelines for mood disorders. *Australian and New Zealand Journal of Psychiatry, 49*(12), 1087–1206.
McQueen, D., Cohen, S., St. John-Smith, P., & Rampes, H. (2013). Rethinking placebo in psychiatry: How and why placebo effects occur. *Advances in Psychiatric Treatment, 19*(3), 171–180.

60 Desikachar, T. K. V., & Cravens, R. (2011). *Health, healing, and beyond: Yoga and the living tradition of T. Krishnamacharya.* North Point Press.

61 These involuntary movements, such as tremors, muscle contractions, or restlessness (e.g., foot-tapping), may appear after one or many doses of a medication and can be acute or chronic.

62 This rare but serious condition affects the nervous system, resulting in symptoms such as high fever and muscle stiffness.

63 REMS is a drug safety program that the US Food and Drug Administration (FDA) requires for certain pharmaceuticals.

Section III

YOGA THERAPY PRACTICE AND TOOLS

Section IIIA Therapeutic Skills

This section describes therapeutic skills that enable the yoga therapist to create a healing environment and therapeutic relationship that contribute to the client's ability to move toward healing or co-created goals. Each chapter explores different approaches for applying the skills necessary for the yoga therapist to be in partnership with the client.

These skills cultivate safety in yoga therapy, from the environment to the client's internal feelings. By applying yogic teachings and through inquiry, these competencies support behavior change and self-agency.

A common thread is that the yoga therapist uses yogic teachings to attune and cultivate their own experiences and understanding so that they can affect the healing space. These skills reinforce personal resilience and interoception through the development of inner awareness and intrapersonal qualities. The same techniques guide the interpersonal relationship between yoga therapist and client, helping the client move toward equilibrium.

Client traditions can differ from those of the yoga therapist. In these instances, therapeutic skills and knowledge of the parallels in yogic and other traditions can bridge gaps and emphasize the transcultural aspects of healing. When approached with this sensitivity, yoga therapy supports women's health and even expanding awareness for those transitioning at the end of life.

Yoga therapists apply their therapeutic skills to integrate yoga techniques into the discernment of when and how to assist clients who could be in any stage of life. These diverse techniques and theoretical and experiential approaches enable clients to build personal skills and resilience within a transformational healing environment.

Marilyn Peppers-Citizen

13

Relationships in Yoga Therapy: Developing Collaboration Within a Healing Presence

TRACEY MEYERS

In every healing profession, developing a therapeutic relationship is one of the most important factors in helping a client to grow. Extensive research in psychotherapy and other healing professions demonstrates that the alliance between the professional and the client is important to treatment results. In psychotherapy, the therapeutic relationship has been described as the "quintessential integrative variable."[1] Research studies have demonstrated that the quality of the client-therapist relationship can predict positive clinical outcomes independent of the specific psychotherapeutic technique.[2] In medicine, a systematic review of clinical outcomes based on the doctor-patient relationship revealed a small but statistically significant improvement in outcomes when the relationship between the provider and patient was positive.[3]

Yoga therapy requires a strong personal relationship between the yoga therapist and client that may include physical touch, emotional support, and facilitation of a safe environment in which clients can experience and process. The establishment of a therapeutic relationship is the backbone of the definition of yoga therapy developed by the International Association of Yoga Therapists (IAYT) and figures prominently in the organization's code of ethics: "Yoga therapy is the professional application of the principles and practices of yoga to promote health and well-being *within a therapeutic relationship* that includes personalized assessment, goal setting, lifestyle management, and yoga practices for individuals or small groups"[4] (emphasis added).

The preamble to the Code of Ethics and Professional Responsibilities continues:

> As yoga therapists, we acknowledge our responsibility to create a safe environment for learning and healing for our clients/students. We are committed to conducting ourselves in a manner that is consistent with the principles of yoga. We value the ethical principles of yoga outlined by Patanjali in the first two limbs of the eight-limbed path (*yama and niyama*) and strive to incorporate these principles into our professional practice. IAYT-certified yoga therapists must be committed to responsible and ethical practice, to their own professional and personal growth, and to contributing to the growth and development of the field of yoga therapy. In furtherance of these commitments, we agree to be bound by the following Code of Ethics and Professional Responsibility.[5]

For many beginning yoga therapists, establishing a therapeutic relationship can be challenging. Even given a strong desire to help others, they may not know the appropriate steps to create and maintain a healthy professional relationship with clients. IAYT and accredited yoga therapy training programs have identified the therapeutic relationship as an important clinical issue that should be addressed in mentoring and supervision.[6]

From the perspective of a yoga therapist and clinical psychologist, the material in this chapter explores the development of a therapeutic relationship within a framework that is unique to yoga therapy. In addition, challenges, red flags, and strategies to enhance the clinical relationship in yoga therapy are considered, with emphasis on the unique role of yoga therapists as change agents.

Scope of Practice

According to the IAYT scope of practice, yoga therapists "[g]uide clients in implementing the therapeutic plan, aimed at prevention and health promotion."[7] Underlying this guidance is the establishment of a positive therapeutic alliance. However, the scope of practice guidelines clearly indicate that yoga therapists do not "[u]ndertake individual or group psychological counselling, unless appropriately qualified to do so," nor do they "[r]ecommend specific lifestyle or nutrition changes outside of a yoga therapy framework, unless appropriately qualified to do so."[8]

These guidelines can be confusing to those who may not fully appreciate the difference between the frameworks of yoga therapy and psychotherapy. Table 13.1 lists several of the important distinctions between the two professions, including fundamental models, procedures in sessions, and the role of the healer.

Table 13.1 Key distinctions between yoga therapy and psychotherapy

Psychotherapy	Yoga Therapy
Biopsychosocial model for assessment	*Panchamaya kosha* or other yogic model for assessment (sometimes accompanied by other comprehensive assessments, e.g., biopsychosocial-spiritual model, stage of change framework)
Diagnosis and treatment of a specific psychological disorder	Focus on the whole person including breath, musculoskeletal system, nervous system, and connection to self and others
Use of past history to better understand present-day challenges	Present-moment focus using yoga, somatics, mindfulness, etc.
Psychotherapist uses specific therapy/counseling techniques to promote change	Yoga therapist supports client in investigation of their own system's messages
Psychotherapist has specific training in human behavior and developing and selecting appropriate therapeutic techniques	Client becomes expert in self-exploration and investigates what supports change for them

These lists offer a brief overview of the two professions' approaches; they are not intended to be in any way exhaustive, nor to imply that the differences are absolute. For example, psychotherapists increasingly assess patients through a biopsychosocial-spiritual lens, and yoga therapists may use this model as a companion to yogic assessment tools such as the *gunas*, *vayus*, *dosha*, and *kleshas*.

Creating a Therapeutic Relationship

To stay within the scope of practice and fulfill the mission of yoga therapy, it is important to establish three key elements to create a healing therapeutic relationship: *self-congruence*, *unconditional positive regard*, and *empathy*. Carl Rogers, one of the most influential psychologists in the 20th century for his humanistic approach, identified these elements of therapeutic alliance.[9]

Although these components of a healing relationship originally come from the psychotherapy tradition, they are part of many modalities, including mindfulness-based meditation teacher training programs, mentoring, supervision, and coaching. The three key elements are also well within the scope of practice for yoga therapists, as they are sufficiently broad to encompass general healing relationships and are not specific to any one modality (e.g., psychotherapy). These three elements can serve as a guide for yoga therapists to foster these qualities in themselves (intrapersonal qualities) and between themselves and the client (interpersonal qualities).

Self-congruence

The first key element of a therapeutic relationship, self-congruence refers to the yoga therapist's ability to be themselves in front of the client. Rather than hiding behind a role or pretending to be someone they are not, they are able to demonstrate strengths and vulnerabilities without oversharing personal or irrelevant information that would redirect the focus away from the client's own exploration. For example, a yoga therapist might share their own physical injury with a client when describing how they modify a yoga pose to prevent further injury. They are modeling both non-harming, one of the foundations of yoga philosophy, and self-compassion (see Chapter 24). The yoga therapy client, in turn, learns the importance of listening to the body and sees the yoga therapist as a real person to whom they can relate. Self-congruence can be felt by the client as openness and genuineness, which can facilitate trust in the therapist.

Unconditional positive regard

Unconditional positive regard is the yoga therapist's ability to communicate warmth and care for the client regardless of what the client says, does, or feels. The foundations of mindfulness meditation describe this aim as paying attention in a "non-judgmental" way. Yoga therapists may convey unconditional positive regard in a variety of ways, including gentle physical assists, practicing *pranayama* alongside a client, and sitting in silence holding space for what is unfolding with the client. Unconditional positive regard leads clients to a feeling of being accepted, which can become the foundation for making changes later in the course of yoga therapy.

Empathy

The final key element of a therapeutic relationship is empathy or empathic understanding. In terms of a healing relationship, empathy is the yoga therapist's ability to respond with sensitivity and understanding to the client's experiences moment to moment throughout the session.[10] The important concept of moment-to-moment tracking appears in mindfulness-based stress reduction mediation programs, psychotherapy, and other healing modalities as "present-moment awareness" and being "in the here and now." When a yoga therapist is able to consistently track and stay with a client, the client feels heard, seen, and valued. Present-centered empathy goes beyond simple listening or repeating back a client's words; it requires active listening and tuning in to the yoga therapist's own inner responses. Yoga therapists might track their inner responses using the *koshas* (e.g., noticing physical sensations through *annamaya*) or somatics (noticing where in the body a particular emotional response is occurring) as a framework for tuning in.

Cultivating Healing Presence

To develop the three key elements of a therapeutic relationship, the yoga therapist can begin by cultivating an open and curious attitude. The attitudes of mindfulness described by Jon Kabat-Zinn[11] can be helpful to beginning yoga therapists.[12] Kabat-Zinn outlined seven specific attitudes that form a foundation for active listening and tuning in with another:

- non-judging
- patience
- beginner's mind
- trust
- non-striving
- acceptance
- letting go

Buddhist teacher Bhante Gunaratana emphasized the importance of an open-minded, curious, and relaxed approach to moment-to-moment awareness through a set of attitudes that includes accepting what arises, dropping expectations, letting go and flowing with all changes, being gentle with oneself, and viewing problems as challenges.[13]

In addition to the mindful attitudes described by Kabat-Zinn and Gunaratana, other practices that have been established in Buddhism, yoga, Western philosophy, psychotherapy, and somatic (body-based) therapies can facilitate a strong healing presence in yoga therapists.

Active listening and tuning in are practices taught by Buddhist scholar and meditation teacher Gregory Kramer. He describes his practice of Insight Dialogue as a relational or "interpersonal meditation practice"[14] that can allow one to remain connected to one's own self while meeting someone else fully and non-judgmentally in their moment-to-moment experience.

Kramer describes six steps that help practitioners to "pay attention to [their] bodies, thoughts, emotions, and storylines."[15] Each step for inner and outer tracking is interconnected with the others and can provide yoga therapists with valuable practices to develop interpersonal and intrapersonal awareness:

1. pause
2. relax
3. open
4. trust emergence
5. listen deeply
6. speak the truth

These steps can be practiced as an individual, self-directed meditation practice to tune and strengthen the yoga therapist's ability to remain present, which is the foundation for the three key elements described above. In addition, they can be used directly in dialogue with another to facilitate empathy and compassion.

Bottom-up techniques

In 1979, the psychotherapist and philosopher Eugene Gendlin developed a form of deep listening he called Focusing.[16] Focusing requires clearing a space, developing a felt sense, handling, resonating, asking, and receiving. Touching into a "felt sense," arguably the key to Focusing, involves bringing awareness inside the body to discover one's previously undiscovered feelings, physical sensations, and imagery. It starts from a place of not knowing and simply being curious and interested in one's own internal experience.

Through Focusing, yoga therapists can recognize what they truly feel and use these feelings to support the client. For example, if a yoga therapist notices pressure in their chest while working with a client, they may want to investigate whether the client is undergoing anxiety or some other emotional or physical constriction in their chest. They can then use specific yoga therapy practices to see how best to support the client.

This type of interpersonal resonance with another person can also be seen through a biomedical lens, as a process of response via mirror neurons, which "discharge both when an individual executes a motor act and when he observes another individual performing the same or a similar motor act."[17] In addition to actions, many studies have shown that a mirror neuron system is involved in human emotions, including empathy.[18] For example, if a client is crying, the yoga therapist may discover that they, too, are moved to tears. This does not necessarily indicate a strong countertransference reaction[19] or poor boundaries, but instead, the activation of emotional circuits in the brain through the close observation of another person.

Supportive practices

Three supports may be particularly useful to help beginning yoga therapists develop skills for active listening, tuning in, and interpersonal mindfulness:

1. **Create or purposely sustain a personal meditation practice.** Using a simple practice log, yoga therapists can complete and track a daily meditation practice for at least 30 minutes a day for 30 days to develop enhanced inner-listening abilities. These practices might include body scanning, breath awareness, and loving-kindness meditations.
2. **Develop a regular peer-to-peer active-listening practice.** Having a peer or buddy system is an excellent way for new therapists to begin to practice the tuning-in and deep-listening skills suggested by Kramer.[20]
3. **Seek individual supervision with an experienced yoga therapist.** Formal supervision with a mentor can be invaluable to a new therapist. During supervision, yoga therapists can enhance what Egan calls "visibly tuning in" skills,[21] being able to empathically listen to the client. To develop these skills, supervisors may ask yoga therapists to video themselves when they start working with new clients and ask themselves the following questions when watching the recording.
   - Overall, how do you feel toward the client? (Include attitudes, judgments, physical reactions, or emotions evoked when interacting with the client.)
   - What did your verbal behavior convey to the client? (Include tone, pace, content of questions, and responses to client dialogue.)
   - What non-verbal behaviors did you notice in the interview? (Consider eye contact, posture, and gestures.) What did these non-verbal behaviors convey to the client?
   - How was the quality of your attention during the interview (consistent/inconsistent, sustained/limited/poor)?
   - Were there are any internal or external distractions that interfered with maintaining your attention?

- What might strengthen your connection with the client going forward?

Yoga therapists often report, as they develop their tuning-in skills, that they are more aware of the personal reactions occurring. The more aware a yoga therapist is of personal thoughts, feelings, and emotions, the better they become at regulating verbal and non-verbal behaviors in the service of the client. For example, a yoga therapist might notice irritation when a client has not done the home practices discussed the week before. Recognizing these emotions, the yoga therapist can explore further about what is coming up for them. Perhaps they have unrealistic expectations for the client, or they feel disappointed by their lack of progress. Self-exploration can support the yoga therapist to respond to the client in a more effective and attuned manner.

The Clinical Interview in Yoga Therapy

Once the yoga therapist has firmly established the underlying skills needed to develop a sound therapeutic relationship, the next level of skill acquisition involves the use of clinical interviewing. Clinical interviewing can be thought of as a set of complex skills that require the ability to

- ask structured questions to obtain detailed and specific information
- ask open-ended questions to allow a client to describe their unique experience
- observe non-verbal cues, including eye contact, body language, and gestures
- allow space for the client to share their story, in their own words, about why they have sought yoga therapy and what they would like to change
- convey to the client that they are being listened to and understood
- set the stage for behavioral change

It is important for yoga therapists to view the clinical interview as the first opportunity to establish the therapeutic relationship. The initial intake interview should not be focused on getting to the bottom of the problem, but rather on a dialogue in which a safe space is created and unconditional presence is established.[22] The yoga therapy intervention begins the moment the client walks into the space or first contacts the yoga therapist, so it is important that the therapist develop the necessary skills to initiate a therapeutic dialogue.

However, new yoga therapists are often faced with the challenge of completing paperwork, following a prescribed set of yoga therapy assessment tools, and navigating a busy clinic or hospital room, usually in an hour or less. They may feel overwhelmed, which can make it difficult to sufficiently tune in to their clients as they try to write everything down and ensure that they are doing a complete assessment. As a result, they miss a critical window for establishing the therapeutic relationship.

Yoga therapists can instead view the clinical interview as extending across several sessions to enable sufficient time to establish the three essential elements for the therapeutic relationship. Although some are comfortable taking notes and conducting an interview at the same time, many yoga therapists find that they miss critical non-verbal behaviors and opportunities to provide support to the client if they are looking down and writing. An abbreviated personal intake form can help to ensure that they have captured key information, building confidence in their interviewing skills while allowing ample time during the session to attune to the other important interpersonal interactions that are occurring.

A short yoga therapy intake interview might include questions like these:

1. What brings you to yoga therapy today?
2. What would you like to get from our time together?
3. How much time each day are you willing to commit to feeling better? To healing?
4. What do you know about yoga?
5. What do you know about yoga therapy?
6. Do you have any questions for me?

Such inquiry can help beginning yoga therapists to become more comfortable asking open-ended questions that allow clients to share. These types of questions also help yoga therapists to understand the client's expectations for yoga therapy, allow them to notice their own reactions (felt sense), and begin to assess the client's readiness for change.

Readiness for change

Determining clients' readiness for change should be an important component of the clinical intake in yoga therapy. Sometimes yoga therapy students assume that because the person voluntarily came in for a yoga therapy intake, they must be motivated and ready to make lifestyle changes. However, it is important for the student to develop an understanding of change behavior to effectively create care plans that accurately match the person's readiness.

Prochaska and DiClemente developed the transtheoretical model of change, or stages of change, as a comprehensive way of considering how behavioral change occurs.[23] Originally focusing on smoking cessation, Prochaska and DiClemente proposed a two-dimensional model to modify behavior. Now recognized for multiple uses, the first dimension includes the five stages of change enumerated in the transtheoretical model:

1. precontemplation
2. contemplation
3. preparation
4. action
5. maintenance

Termination is sometimes included as a sixth stage that reflects the complete cessation of a behavior such as smoking. The second dimension of the stages of change model focuses on the process of change, including the activities and events that support modification of a behavior such as smoking, alcohol use, or overeating.

As part of the intake process, yoga therapists can assess clients' readiness for change across a variety of behaviors by using the stages of change model. Regardless of the stage at which a client initially presents, it is important for yoga therapists to remember the following:

- Most clients come to yoga therapy because they want something to be different.
- Creating space for something different in life requires change.
- Being in a helping relationship is supportive of behavior change.

By listening for what Rollnick et al. call "change talk,"[24] yoga therapists can establish a sound understanding of a client's current readiness. Change talk is an important indicator that a person is beginning to consider making changes in their life. Such phrasing usually means that the client has moved into the second (contemplation) or even third stage of change (preparation). On the other hand, the absence of change talk or resistance to considering changes likely indicates that the client may be in a precontemplation stage of change.

Ambivalent language around change, or what Rollnick et al. call "conflicting motivations,"[25] can be an important turning point for some clients who may be reluctant to fully embrace yoga therapy. Clients might say that "I know yoga is good for me, but I hate exercising," or "I know I should meditate, but my mind is too jumpy." These clients are likely moving toward early contemplation, which can begin to set the stage for change behavior.

Some change talk already includes commitment language, which may be evident in the clinical interview. Speech such as "I am ready to start doing meditation" or "I am going to join a yoga class at my gym" suggests that the client may be moving toward an action stage. In subsequent sessions, the yoga therapist can continue to evaluate the client's stage of change by noting change language that the client provides around different behaviors. Once a client shares specific steps that they have completed (e.g., "I did my morning yoga plan"), their stage of change has again shifted, this time into action, which can lead eventually to maintenance.

Beginning with the clinical interview, the yoga therapist can carefully assess each behavior and develop a tracking system to record the presenting problem(s), change language (present/not present), and stage of change on an ongoing basis. It is important to do this for each of the client's presenting problems because they may be at different stages of change for each problem. For example, one student at Maryland University of Integrative Health shared how a client came in to get help with hip pain. Throughout the clinical interview, the student carefully identified the client's stage of change by listening for key phrases. The client said, "I have to start doing yoga because I can't go on like this any more" (contemplation stage), but he also acknowledged that he did not want to change his extremely stressful work schedule. "I can't even go there around my schedule. It is set in stone." Continuing to work with the client around the areas they are most ready to address will likely result in a more successful outcome than focusing on a behavior where there is resistance, or ambivalence at best.

The clinical interview can help direct the yoga therapist to more closely focus on the areas in which the client will consider making changes. In the beginning of a course of yoga therapy, it is recommended to select the low-hanging fruit, the area(s) that the client is most receptive to addressing. Facilitating an accurate match between the stage of change and the type of yoga therapy work offered is a critical factor in creating a strong therapeutic partnership between the therapist and client, both in the short term and for the duration of the yoga therapy.

When clients are in a precontemplation stage of change, beginning yoga therapists may give up prematurely or try to push them toward work that is not appropriate for their readiness, producing resistance, frustration, and sometimes premature termination. It is important to recognize that care can be offered with successful outcomes at any stage of change as long as it matches the client's readiness. The modalities offered will differ depending on the stage of change, and flexibility in offering stage-appropriate interventions is crucial.[26]

Miller and Rollnick describe the critical conditions necessary for people to change.[27] Their technique of "motivational interviewing" includes a current assessment of a person's motivation and readiness for change. Yoga therapists can ask clients to rate their confidence and motivation for yoga therapy, which can provide important information about the client's readiness for change, by using open-ended questions like those below as well as a readiness ruler (Figure 13.1) modeled after those suggested by Rollnick and others around behavioral change.

- How important is it to you to seek yoga therapy? On a scale of 0 to 10, with 0 being not important at all, 5 being somewhat important, and 10 being very important, where would you place yourself?
  - Why did you select this number _____, and not a lower number like [1 or 2]? (Answers to this question tell the yoga therapist what the benefits the client sees in seeking yoga therapy.)
  - What might help to move your number a little higher?
- How certain are you that yoga therapy will help you with your problem? On a scale of 0 to 10, with 0 being not certain at all, 5 being somewhat certain, and 10 being very certain, where would you place yourself?
  - Why did you select this number ____, and not a lower number like [1 or 2]? (If the client chooses 0 or 1, the yoga therapist can instead ask why they chose such a low number.)
  - What would it take to move your number a little higher?

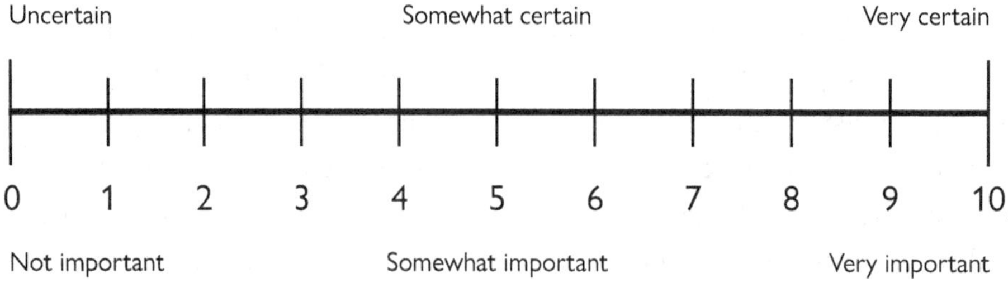

FIGURE 13.1 YOGA THERAPY READINESS RULER

If a client chooses consistently low numbers (0–2) during the initial interview, the yoga therapist should consider whether the client is ready to make changes before moving forward with the course of yoga therapy and be prepared to offer appropriate precontemplation or contemplation interventions. If they choose high numbers, they will be able to quickly move toward preparation and action interventions. Table 13.2 summarizes the stages of change and suggested appropriate yoga therapy interventions based on the model.[28]

Table 13.2 Stages of change in yoga therapy

Stage of Change	Hallmark Behaviors/ Statements	Stage-Appropriate Plan Goals	Stage-Appropriate Interventions
Precontemplation	Unaware of problem(s) Not ready or willing to make change(s) Not uncomfortable (enough) with current situation May feel coerced or pressured to seek help "I don't need to exercise."	Increasing information about one's self, problems, and feelings	Validation of lack of readiness Active listening Development of a therapeutic alliance around neutral/non-threatening areas If receptive, providing education
Contemplation	Aware problem exists and change needs to occur, but not committed yet to action Ambivalence to change "I know I should do yoga to help me relax, but I don't have the time."	Assessing and reflecting how one feels and thinks about oneself with respect to a problem Valuing clarification around what matters most	Continuing to validate client's perspective Paying attention to any change language Developing pros and cons of changing Visualizing consequences to changing/not changing behavior
Preparation	Intention and small behavioral changes are beginning to occur Increased motivation to take action in the near future "I bought a yoga mat last week, and I might try watching a video online."	Guiding future change steps and commitment Managing fears and anxieties around change	Commitment-enhancement techniques (e.g., motivational interviewing) Setting small, achievable goals Teaching basic skills to develop healthy behaviors Identifying healthy support system, including people and environment

Stage of Change	Hallmark Behaviors/ Statements	Stage-Appropriate Plan Goals	Stage-Appropriate Interventions
Action	Taking actual steps for change Practicing new behaviors Modifying behaviors, environment, or experiences to change old behaviors "I began a morning meditation practice and turned off my cell phone so I would not be disturbed."	Substituting adaptive or alternative behaviors for problem behaviors Encouraging positive self-talk	Teaching more advanced tools to learn new and effective skills (relaxation, meditation, yoga) Developing healthy routines and habits Assertiveness training and mindful communication Other treatments (e.g., psychotherapy, support groups)
Maintenance	New behavior(s) sustained for at least 6 months Shows active perseverance in maintaining these changes "I have a daily yoga practice and am thrilled about how much better I feel."	Positive reinforcement for gains made Relapse prevention Noticing early warning signs of slippage	Continuing skill building Developing a relapse-prevention plan Increasing alternatives for healthy living Focusing on self-efficacy and self-empowerment
Termination (optional stage)	Permanent cessation of behavior or full ongoing commitment to new behavior "I will never go back to feeling like I have no control over stressful situations."	Continued positive reinforcement	Fully engaged with healthy lifestyle

BOX 13.1 RED FLAGS

During the clinical interview and subsequent sessions, yoga therapists may occasionally identify a client who has serious mental health issues. These red flags warrant careful assessment and consideration for appropriateness for yoga therapy. Red flags, which extend beyond simple resistance or precontemplation behavior as described earlier, generally fall into the categories of active substance use, self-harm/suicidal behavior, violence/aggression, and active psychosis.

Many yoga therapists avoid asking questions around these sensitive areas because they feel it is out of their scope of practice. However, it is important to identify red flags as soon as possible when establishing the therapeutic relationship to ensure well-being and safety for both the client and the yoga therapist. Being caught off guard when a problem area arises can be anxiety-producing and overwhelming to a new yoga therapist. Therefore, it is wise to include some basic questions around substance use, mental health, and behaviors including aggression and self-harm in every intake. If these problem areas rise to the level of immediate concern, the yoga therapist can already have a plan on how to address them. This may include supervision with a mentor or trusted colleague, collaboration with a mental health professional, referral to a more appropriate professional, and emergency services/crisis planning. The plan will depend on the risk level and immediacy of concern of the behavior.

For yoga therapists working in an agency, clinic, or hospital, that particular facility will likely be required to complete forms for informed consent and release of information for medical and mental health professionals, as well as specific procedures around confidentiality, client rights, and risk issues. Yoga therapists in private practice are strongly advised to consider seeking consultation with other professionals and legal advisors to develop procedures for informed consent and risk issues.

Several good resources are available regarding questions/inquiry areas to include in a clinical interview if red-flag issues are identified.[29] If no red flags are identified, the yoga therapist may elect to omit these additional questions. Potential questions to ask in a clinical interview or follow-up session include the following.

Violence/aggression considerations:

- Diagnosis that includes violent or impulsive behavior
- Previous history of violent behavior
- Brain injury or other neurological conditions that affect thinking, judgment, or insight (see Chapter 10)
- History of abuse in family of origin or domestic violence
- Psychosis/autism spectrum disorders

Active psychosis considerations:

- Past history of major mental health issues
- Physical appearance (unusual body language, hygiene issues, talking to oneself [responding to internal stimuli])
- Evidence of active substance use (bloodshot eyes, odor of substance use)
- Thought content (paranoid, disorganized, delusional, fixated)

Suicidal ideation considerations:

- When did they last have a thought about killing themselves?
- How often do they think about killing themselves?
- Have they made a previous suicide attempt?
- Do they now have a plan to kill themselves?
- Can they carry out the plan?

Active substance use considerations:

- Current use (including self-report and evidence of active use [bloodshot eyes, odor of substance use])
- Type of substance
- Frequency, duration, and reason for use
- Interference with daily life
- Past use and treatment

Based on the additional information gathered during the clinical interview, the yoga therapist can feel more adequately prepared to determine the best care plan. The most appropriate next steps are evaluated depending on the red flags identified (see Box 13.1), the severity of the present issues, and potential immediate risk. It might be necessary to develop a collaborative plan with the client and mental health professionals or to advise the client to postpone yoga therapy until the more immediate risk issues are addressed. Yoga therapists should always seek support from a supervisor, agency director, or mentor for additional guidance.

Summary

Gathering important information during the clinical interview can help yoga therapists to build strong therapeutic alliances with clients. By creating a healing presence through the use of self-congruence, unconditional positive regard, and empathy, yoga therapists can develop a safe and trusting environment in which clients can explore their intentions for yoga therapy.

Developing the skills to ask questions that will elicit important information is key to clinical interviewing. By understanding the basic principles of stages of change and motivational interviewing, yoga therapists can obtain valuable information to help formulate goals for therapy that will maximize clients' potential for growth. Furthermore, by developing a strong set of interviewing skills, beginning yoga therapists will feel confident that they are working within their scope of practice and providing quality care to the clients they serve.

Additional Resources

Hanh, T. N. (2014). *The art of communicating*. HarperOne.

Levounis, P., Arnaout, B., & Marienfeld, C. (2017). *Motivational interviewing for clinical practice*. American Psychiatric Association Publishing.

Miller, W. R. (2018). *Listening well: The art of empathic understanding*. Wipf & Stock.

Prochaska, J. O., Norcross, J., & DiClemente, C. (1994). *Changing for good: A revolutionary six-stage program for overcoming bad habits and moving your life forward positively*. Quill.

Richardson, H., & Tomlin, K. M. (2005). *Motivational interviewing and stages of change: Integrating best practices for substance abuse professionals*. Hazelden Publishing.

Tull, D. E. (2018). *Relational mindfulness: A handbook for deepening our connections with ourselves, each other, and the planet*. Wisdom Publications.

Endnotes

1 Wolfe, B. E., & Goldfried, M. R. (1988). Research on psychotherapy integration: Recommendations and conclusions from an NIMH workshop. *Journal of Consulting and Clinical Psychology*, *56*, 448–451.

2 Ardito, R. B., & Rabellino, D. (2011). Therapeutic alliance and outcome of psychotherapy: Historical excursus, measurements, and prospects for research. *Frontiers in Psychology*, *2*, 270.
Horvath, A. O., & Bedi, R. P. (2002). The alliance. In J. C. Norcross (Ed.), *Psychotherapy relationships that work: Therapist contributions and responsiveness to patients* (pp. 37–69). Oxford University Press.
Norcross, J. C. (2002). *Psychotherapy relationships that work: Therapist contributions and responsiveness to patients*. Oxford University Press.

3 Kelley, J. M., Kraft-Todd, G., Schapira, L., Kossowsky, J., & Riess, H. (2014). The influence of the patient-clinician relationship on healthcare outcomes: A systematic review and meta-analysis of randomized controlled trials. *PLoS ONE*, *9*(4), e94207.

4 International Association of Yoga Therapists (IAYT). (2020). IAYT code of ethics and professional responsibilities. https://cdn.ymaws.com/www.iayt.org/resource/resmgr/docs_certification_all/2020_updates_scope_ethics/2020-09_code_of_ethics_v2.pdf

5 IAYT, *IAYT code of ethics*.

6 Forbes, B., Horii, C., Earls, B., Mashek, S., & Akshar, F. (2012). Clinical group supervision in yoga therapy: Model, effects, and lessons learned. *International Journal of Yoga Therapy*, *22*, 61–78.

7 International Association of Yoga Therapists (IAYT). (2020). Scope of practice for yoga therapy. https://cdn.ymaws.com/www.iayt.org/resource/resmgr/docs_certification_all/2020_updates_scope_ethics/2020-09_sop_v2.pdf

8 IAYT, *Scope of practice*.

9 Rogers, C. R. (1957). The necessary and sufficient conditions of therapeutic personality change. *Journal of Consulting Psychology*, *21*, 95–103.
Rogers, C. R. (1967). *The therapeutic relationship and its impact: A study of psychotherapy with schizophrenics*. University of Wisconsin Press.

10 Rogers, *The therapeutic relationship*.

11 Kabat-Zinn developed mindfulness-based stress reduction (MBSR), which recontextualizes Buddhist mindfulness meditation techniques in a Western scientific framework.

12 Kabat-Zinn, J. (2013). *Full catastrophe living: Using the wisdom of your body and mind to face stress, pain, and illness*. Bantam Books.

13 Gunaratana, H. (2011). *Mindfulness in plain English*. Wisdom Publications.

14 Kramer, G. (2007). *Insight dialogue*. Shambhala Publications.

15 Kramer's website (www.insightdialogue.org) describes specific ways in which interpersonal mindfulness practices can be done in a group format.

16 Gendlin, E. T. (1981). *Focusing*. Bantam Books. See also Chapter 16 of this book.

17 Acharya, S., & Shukla, S. (2012). Mirror neurons: Enigma of the metaphysical modular brain. *Journal of Natural Science, Biology, and Medicine*, *3*(2), 118–124 (p. 118).

18 Preston, S. D., & de Waal, F. B. (2002). Empathy: Its ultimate and proximate bases. *Behavioral and Brain Sciences*, *25*(1), 1–71.

19 The term *countertransference* originated with Sigmund Freud in the early 20th century and referred to the unconscious and unresolved conflicts of the therapist that are triggered by the patient and can interfere with treatment. Hayes et al. describe a countertransference reaction as "internal and external reactions in which unresolved conflicts of the therapist, usually but not always unconscious, are implicated" (p. 497): Hayes, J. A., Gelso, C. J., Goldberg, S., & Kivlighan, D. M. (2018). Countertransference management and effective psychotherapy: Meta-analytic findings. *Psychotherapy*, *55*(4), 496–507.

20 Kramer, G. (n.d.). Guidelines. https://insightdialogue.org/relational-practices/insight-dialogue/guidelines

21 Egan, G., & Reese, R. (2018). *The skilled helper: A problem management and opportunity development approach to helping* (11th ed.). Cengage Learning.

22 Egan & Reese, *The skilled helper*.

23 Lacey, S. J., & Street, T. D. (2017). Measuring healthy behaviours using the stages of change model: An investigation into the physical activity and nutrition behaviours of Australian miners. *BioPsychoSocial Medicine*, *11*(30), 1–8.
Miller, W. R., & Rollnick, S. (2002). *Motivational interviewing: Preparing people for change* (2nd ed.). Guilford Press.
Norcross, J. C., Krebs, P. M., & Prochaska, J. O. (2011). Stages of change. *Journal of Clinical Psychology*, *42*, 476–478.
Prochaska, J. O., & DiClemente, C. C. (1984). *The transtheoretical approach: Crossing traditional boundaries of therapy*. Dow Jones Irwin.
Prochaska, J. O., & DiClemente, C. C. (1985). Common processes of change in smoking, weight control and psychological distress. In S. Shiffiman & T. A. Wills (Eds.), *Coping and substance abuse* (pp. 345–363). Academic Press.
Prochaska, J. O., & DiClemente, C. C. (1986). The transtheoretical approach: Toward a systematic eclectic framework. In J. C. Norcross (Ed.), *Handbook of eclectic psychotherapy* (pp. 163–210). Brunner/Mazel.
Prochaska, J. O., DiClemente, C. C., & Norcross, J. C. (1992). In search of how people change: Applications to addictive behaviors. *American Psychologist*, *47*(9), 1102–1114.

24 Rollnick, S., Miller, W. R., & Butler, C. C. (2008). *Motivational interviewing in health care: Helping patients change behavior*. Guilford Press.

25 Rollnick et al., *Motivational interviewing*.

26 Prochaska et al., In search.
27 Miller & Rollnick, *Motivational interviewing.*
28 Lacey & Street, Measuring healthy behaviours.
Norcross et al., Stages of change.
Prochaska & DiClemente, *Transtheoretical approach.*
Prochaska & DiClemente, Common processes.
Prochaska & DiClemente, Transtheoretical approach.
Prochaska et al., In search.
29 Lukas, S. (1993). *Where to start and what to ask: An assessment handbook.* W. W. Norton & Co.
Sommers-Flannagan, J., & Sommers-Flannagan, R. (2016). *Clinical interviewing* (6th ed.). John Wiley & Sons.
Wiger, D. E., & Huntley, D. K. (2002). *Essentials of interviewing.* John Wiley & Sons.

14

Cultivating Resilience and Safety in Yoga Therapy Practice

NYA PATRINOS

Your trials did not come to punish you,
but to awaken you—
to make you realize that you are a part of Spirit
and that just behind the sparks of your life is the Flame of Infinity.

Paramahansa Yogananda

Yoga's ability to increase physical, mental/emotional, and energetic resilience is cited as one of its main therapeutic benefits.[1] Paramahansa Yogananda declared that life's trials are what enables humans to know that they are part of the Divine. An ancient metaphor for the yoga practitioner is that of the lotus flower, a symbol of resilience. The lotus grows out of the mud, rising up from adverse circumstance toward the sky; although the lotus resides in water, its petals do not get wet. Similarly, Buddhist monk Thich Nhat Hanh asserted that the secret to happiness is to be resilient by acknowledging and transforming suffering, not by running from it.[2]

Key components of resilience are optimism, altruism, a strong moral compass, faith/spirituality, humor, social support, influential role models, an ability to face fears, and connection to meaning and life purpose. Resilience can be defined as the ability to bounce back from adversity. Resilient people remain calm during crises and emerge from stressful situations without perceived long-term negative consequences:

> High resilience is correlated with quicker cardiovascular recovery following subjective emotional experiences, less perceived stress, greater recovery from illness or trauma and better management of dementia and chronic pain. Compromised

resilience is linked to dysregulation of the autonomic nervous system through measures of vagal regulation.[3]

Yoga therapists can cultivate client relationships that foster resilience by seeing clients' lotus potential while establishing a safe container of compassionate interaction, empathetic verbal and non-verbal communication, mutual respect, and deep listening.[4] The creation of a safe container requires care, patience, and interest as the yoga therapist assigns themselves the task of creating an optimal healing environment. Yoga therapists can develop this skill through education and practice. This chapter draws on yogic concepts as well as scientific literature to explore the cultivation of resilience and safety, an underpinning that facilitates resilience, in work with yoga therapy clients.

Building Resilience

Research on resilience has focused on how to explain why some people adapt more favorably in the face of adverse conditions. The findings suggest that supportive families, quality schools, engaged communities, and social policies encourage resilience.[5] In addition, resilience is "fostered by both downregulating defensive states and supporting more flexibility and adaptability in relationship to various phenomena of the BME (Body Mind Environment) to promote physiological restoration as well as positive psychological and social states."[6]

The term *resilience* is close to *samatvam* or *upeksha*, usually defined in yoga as equanimity. In the *Bhagavad Gita*, equanimity and yoga are considered the same: "Having abandoned attachment [and] become indifferent to success or failure. It is said that evenness of mind is yoga" (2.48).[7]

A blueprint for a yoga therapist who wants to foster equanimity or resilience within a safe container of practice is given in a popular version of the *Yoga Sutras*:

> To preserve openness of heart and calmness of mind, nurture these attitudes: Kindness to those who are happy. Compassion for those who are less fortunate. Honor for those who embody noble qualities. Equanimity to those whose actions oppose your values. (1.33)[8]

A *sankalpa* (sometimes translated as "intention") for yoga therapists could be to remain unattached to outcomes and embody the qualities of kindness, compassion, honor, and equanimity when working with a client. Practices like *trataka* (concentration),[9] *yoga nidra*,[10] *ujjayi pranayama* (victorious breath),[11] and *sama vritti* ("equal" breathing)[12] may help to develop and maintain samatvam/upeksha for both client and therapist.

A key difference between samatvam/upeksha and resilience is that when people are overly resilient they can become tolerant of unpleasant, counterproductive, harmful, and abusive circumstances. In addition, they may develop unachievable goals and false hopes. In such cases less resilience might result in people being called to action to make change, refusing to accept harmful conditions, and having a more realistic worldview.[13] The negative side of resilience is not found in samatvam and upeksha, "being able to keep the mind steady and balanced in all conditions of life."[14] States of samatvam and upeksha do not require a catalyst of adversity or something from which to bounce back to enable personal development and thriving, although they encompass those ideas.

Yogic resilience in practice

Yoga is a life skill that increases resilience by improving feelings of clear-mindedness, composure, elation, energy, life purpose, satisfaction, and self-confidence during stressful situations. One becomes resilient by remembering that the true Self is Divine:

> [W]e naturally identify less and less with external desires or wants. This perspective reveals that we are merely the temporary caretakers of whatever we possess. With this attitude, nothing binds us. As life bestows gifts upon us, we are delighted. With their revocation, we may feel momentarily upset, but with the grace of remembering our Divine Self, our emotional equilibrium is quickly restored.[15]

Even a short program of yoga is effective for enhancing emotional well-being and resilience to stress.[16] Yoga achieves these results through regulation of vagal function, reduction of allostatic load, facilitation of self-regulatory and coping skills, increased cardiopulmonary and central nervous system function, and induction of balance in the autonomic nervous system.[17] After 2 to 5 years of yoga practice, practitioners report reduced stress and increased feelings of well-being.[18] The more consistent the practice, the better the outcomes.[19]

Panchamaya kosha

One of the ways in which yogic tools foster resilience is through integration and unification of the five sheaths/bodies in the *panchamaya kosha* system (body, breath, emotions, wisdom, and spirit; see Chapter 3). Aligning the main sheaths of existence enables "one's own prana [to] heal, connect and unite the disintegrated individual thereby creating a chance for the bounce-back to happen."[20] *Asana* works on the levels of *annamaya* with physical practice of asana and *pranamaya* with concentration on and coordination with the breath while practicing asana. Asana also addresses *manomaya*, regulating and promoting resilience by altering the state of the autonomic nervous system during the physical practice of yoga. As people develop in their asana practice, they overcome self-defeating tendencies and re-form themselves mentally, emotionally, and physically.

Yogic techniques to become aware of the breath and shift unhealthy response patterns are the tools of self-regulation and resilience. On the level of pranamaya, breathwork affects vagal tone and facilitates shifts in the autonomic state with benefits to psychological health. Similar to asana, pranayama offers opportunities to mimic stressors and practice resilience by remaining calm when heightened mental or physical states are activated. A forceful breath such as *bhramari* (bee breath), for example, might ultimately enable the conscious release of built-up tension. The potential challenge of creating space where it did not previously exist, through a lengthened exhalation or a retention, might foster the expansion of awareness. Working with a client with both heating and cooling pranayama, with the opportunity to self-regulate for increased equanimity after the specific practice, may also facilitate resilience.[21]

Yoga asks one to move beyond limiting beliefs and toward upeksha/samatvam. Modalities that address *vijnanamaya* offer self-regulation techniques and mind training. These techniques include *pratyahara* (withdrawal from the senses through body scanning, progressive relaxation, yoga nidra, etc.), *dharana* (concentration practices including *mudra* and *mantra*), and *dhyana* (meditation/mindfulness) (see Chapter 23). "Meditations can help with maintaining relative calm in the body-mind *during* an activating practice"[22] (emphasis in original). When one relaxes and slows down through these practices with *savasana* (corpse pose), yoga nidra, or meditation, it is possible to rebuild and replenish resilience and achieve equanimity and a state of joy or bliss, *anandamaya*.

The gunas and polyvagal theory

Through the lens of the *gunas*, resilience is the process of moving from activation to calm,[23] or adversity back to equilibrium, which can be defined as the flow from *tamas* or *rajas* to *sattva* (see Chapter 3). Yoga provides "neural exercise, and a methodology of working with the gunas, for the regulation and resilience of the system."[24]

People have an individual range of sensitivity to sensation, stress, and arousal—a "window of tolerance" based on their personal history and lifestyle. When one is outside their window of tolerance, the nervous system becomes dysregulated. Sleep deprivation, trauma history, chronic stress, and adverse childhood experiences (ACEs)[25] are correlated with greater dysregulation (i.e., a smaller window of tolerance). Each person's dysregulation will push them away from sattva guna and move them toward rajas or tamas. The development of sattva strengthens resilience through discriminative wisdom, mental clarity, adaptability, and self-regulation. Developing sattvic qualities enlarges the window of tolerance and facilitates resilience.

The parasympathetic nervous system is the calming part of the autonomic nervous system, also known as the tend-and-mend or rest-and-digest system. The vagus nerve interfaces with the parasympathetic nervous system to regulate the heart, lungs, and digestive tract and works in opposition to the sympathetic nervous system, which is involved in fight, flight, and freeze behaviors. Polyvagal theory "posits that the neural platforms supporting social behavior are involved in maintaining health, growth and restoration."[26]

When considering yoga therapy alongside polyvagal theory, "resilience is represented by the capacity to recognize and shift states"; also indicative of resilience is an ability to change one's relationship to the fluctuations of the gunas and the neural platforms of the sympathetic nervous system, dorsal vagal complex, and ventral vagal complex.[27] Sattva can be increased by doing yoga practices that safely challenge the practitioner; meeting these challenges promotes resilience. No one will be in a sattvic state all the time; resilience is developed by continually moving back to sattva from tamas or rajas. Some evidence-based practices for developing sattva are *nadi shodhana*[28] (alternate-nostril breathing) and maintaining a varied asana practice that includes rajasic modalities like *vinyasa*[29] and more *tamasic* approaches (e.g., *yin*[30] and restorative[31] techniques) over a single session or a longer period.

The yamas and niyamas

Yoga also optimizes "autonomic control, providing greater physiological and psychological adaptability and resilience through reducing emotional reactivity and lowering the physiological set point of reactivity."[32] An integrated practice of the eight limbs of yoga is one strategy for resilience-building. Working with the *yamas* and *niyamas* promotes positive physiological states, prosocial behavioral responses, and a guide for reaction in response to phenomena.[33] Asana practice reinforces the niyamas of *tapas*, *svadhaya*, and *ishvara pranidhana*. (See Chapter 24 for a full discussion of the use of yamas and niyamas in yoga therapy.) Cultivating these characteristics may enable clients to stay present through activation and learn to return to a state of calm.[34]

With the permission and interest of the client, one can begin a yoga therapy session by setting an intention to examine the individual's responses to challenges, frustration, and uncertainty that surface during the practice. The skills of resilience are developed by keeping the mind and body safe, calm, and connected while in asana: The challenge of holding the postures with equanimity, even when charged feelings arise, offers the opportunity to practice controlling the body, develop willpower, manage and explore emotions, and develop concentration.[35] Dynamic practices, too, can provide a laboratory for flowing with rather than forcing through.

The discipline and steadiness learned in yoga will also be a support when clients work with difficult memories or emotional issues within or outside a session. Yoga postures can bring up emotions that have been "stored" in the body in the form of tightness, stress, tension, and pain. Staying mindful in moments when one is confronted with these awakened emotions can build resilience. As van der Kolk and colleagues noted, regular yoga practice helps people "to tolerate physical and sensory experiences associated with fear and helplessness and to increase emotional awareness and affect tolerance."[36] Physiological resilience may also be supported by alternating between postures that the client finds activating and calming.[37]

Yogic relaxation techniques such as savasana may transform self-defeating tendencies by providing deliberate rest, strengthening clients physically, mentally, and emotionally. An experience of equanimity, or living with a resilient system, is similar to a practice of savasana in which the system remains alert but unattached. It is important that there is time for savasana to integrate the session.[38]

Yogic philosophy delineates nine emotions (love, wonder, joy, courage, calmness, anger, sadness, fear, and disgust).[39] *Rasa sadhana* is a practice to temporarily promise oneself to fast/abstain from an emotion in thought, word, and deed.[40] Through this practice, one masters the ability to move away from an emotion, a skill needed for resilience. Other ways to work with emotions are noticing where emotions are found in the body, body scanning, yoga nidra, meditating on emotions, and chanting mantras that connect to the emotions. In addition, *pratipaksha bhavana* is a practice outlined in the *Yoga Sutras* in which negative ways of thinking are transformed through the discipline of cultivating the opposite thought or emotion.

One can sustain resilience by maintaining a consistent yoga practice, making realistic plans, having confidence in abilities, setting up support systems, developing communication and problem-solving skills, and managing strong impulses and feelings. Difficult days on the yoga mat help to cultivate an attitude of deep acceptance that life will include adversity, disappointment, and loss. Resilience comes from knowing that even when external conditions cannot be changed, equanimity can be found within. The discipline of yoga fortifies resilience, which itself is sustained with flexibility, strength, and awareness of internal and external conditions. The challenge of practicing yoga teaches adaptation through novelty and repetition. Yoga requires the brain to problem-solve,[41] which creates new neural connections and makes the system more adaptable to change.[42]

Measuring resilience

In addition to employing their observation skills, yoga therapists can more formally determine clients' levels of resilience by using an assessment such as the Brief Resilience Scale (BRS).[43] This self-reported instrument could be used as part of the intake and re-administered after a number of sessions to measure changes in resilience. Such scales address perceived stress, grit, mental toughness, ability to stay optimistic, learning style, ability to be engaged, flexibility and adaptability, habits, meaning-making, perseverance, self-reliance, equanimity, existential aloneness, self-esteem, and self-confidence.

Building a Safe Container for Experience

One of the first priorities for a yoga therapist interested in facilitating resilience is creating a safe container of practice. Terms encompassing the idea of a safe container include *safe space*, *sacred space*, *positive space*, *sacred container*, and *supportive environment*. Physiologically, when safety is detected in the internal and external environment, the ventral vagal complex supports prosocial behavior and social connection.[44]

The "safe space" came to prominence during the women's rights movement of the 1960s and 1970s. The concept offered "a certain license to speak and act freely, form collective strength, and generate strategies for resistance…not only a physical space but also a space created by the coming together of women searching for community."[45] The safe space has also become an important concept in the LGBTQ communities, where it means:

> a place where anyone can relax and be fully self-expressed, without fear of being made to feel uncomfortable, unwelcome or challenged on account of biological sex, race/ethnicity, sexual orientation, gender identity or expression, cultural background, age, or physical or mental ability; a place where the rules guard each

person's self-respect, dignity and feelings and strongly encourage everyone to respect others.[46]

Violence, harassment, bullying, and hate speech are not tolerated in a safe space.

Safety in yoga therapy

The idea of a safe space in yoga and yoga therapy is a modern Western concept. The related yogic term *suhkha sthanam* means "a place where we feel at ease both internally and externally."[47] In pre-20th century India, becoming a yogi was often an uncomfortable process, including a series of difficult feats or tests to be mastered while maintaining mental equanimity. The yogi pledged devotion to their guru and entrusted that person with their life. In *Autobiography of a Yogi*, young Yogananda swears to follow Sri Yukteswar, who states, "I am hard on those who come for my training…that is my way; take it or leave it…I try to purify only in the fires of severity, searing beyond the average toleration."[48] Training through adversity to find yogic peace is very different from the Western concept of safe space.

"Safe space" has been criticized for being averse to dialogue and difference in perspectives. The term is also difficult to define because what is safe for one person may not be safe for someone else. In contrast, within the yoga framework, one finds the safety within and is not dependent on another person or group. Progressing in yoga therapy can include becoming aware of, working with, and transforming pain and discomfort while finding safety inside oneself.

One definition of the yogic concept *aikyam* and the related Buddhist concept *esho funi* is that "There is a oneness between you and your environment."[49] As the environment changes, the individual changes; as the individual changes, so does their environment. When a yoga therapist sets up a safe environment, the oneness between the client and this environment will influence the client's internal feelings of safety. If the therapeutic container is peaceful, calm, and relaxed, while at the same time productive and engaged, the client is influenced to find these same qualities within themselves. From this position of equanimity, the client's body, mind, and spirit can become relaxed, resilient, and receptive enough to transform and heal.

Yoga therapy has both similarities with and differences from the guru-disciple relationship. Yoga therapists are not gurus who train monastics, create lineage holders, or transmit the teachings to an elite few. A yoga therapist does not demand intense discipline or devotion from clients. Yoga therapy and the guru-disciple relationship similarly require the consistency of practice (*abhyasa*) on the part of the client and aspirant. In contrast to a guru who dictates, proscribes, and requires devotion, however, the yoga therapist is a partner in the process, offering suggestions and possibilities.

Informed consent

As a yoga therapist, it is important to receive informed consent from the client, partly by having them fill out an agreement that includes a waiver before starting the first session. This permission for services may include a description of the yoga therapy services, a confidentiality agreement, fee schedule, and cancellation policy. Establishing a written framework for the therapeutic relationship is part of setting expectations and boundaries, which are important components of a safe container of practice.[50]

The process of securing informed consent involves providing the client with information about the yoga therapy service, evaluating their capacity to understand the information, and obtaining their consent to begin yoga therapy. Informed consent begins the process of communication between the yoga therapist and client. It is the responsibility of the yoga therapist to accurately describe the process, benefits, and contraindications of yoga therapy so that the client knows what they are consenting to.

Whether and how to include touch in sessions, which would be part of any consent discussion, is much debated in the yoga therapy community. Assuming that the therapist has proper training, one modality that might be used therapeutically is long restorative holds with touch. Informed consent is needed before touching. Within any small-group or individual session, the therapist should ask for permission to touch and evaluate why they are touching the client. If a client has been assaulted or raped, touch is contraindicated.[51]

The informed consent process is a time for encouraging the client to ask questions and for discussing alternatives to yoga therapy or to a particular style of yoga therapy. Having the client sign an agreement acknowledges that they have been informed and express their consent to the services being offered.

Foundational work

When a client decides to begin a yoga therapy program, they may understand yoga only from a physical perspective and be unfamiliar with the multiplicity of yoga. The safe relationship between yoga therapist and client starts from the first correspondence, when many therapists explain the completeness of yoga as a vehicle for transformation. Providing a comprehensive intake form for clients to complete in advance lays the groundwork for the holistic experiences they will encounter in a session. As noted by Sullivan et al., "It is when yoga is practiced and understood as a cohesive and comprehensive system that the benefits for self-regulation and resilience may be realized."[52]

When possible, it is important to know the client's profile before the first visit to set up a strategy and to identify biases and blind spots that may arise for the yoga therapist. Does the yoga therapist have another type of relationship with the client (referred to as a "dual relationship" in mental healthcare)? Is their ethnic and religious background the same as the yoga therapist's? Do the client and yoga therapist share the same gender identity? The yoga therapist needs to consider the client's communication styles, values and beliefs, and life experiences (see Chapter 17).

It is the therapist's responsibility to become familiar with a variety of therapeutic orientations and approaches, because one yoga therapy style may not meet the needs of diverse clients. This may include avoiding Sanskrit asana names, replacing yogic mantras with a client's personal or religious affirmations, or incorporating verses from the client's chosen sacred text instead of the yogic canon. Perhaps a different prayer or word for *Aum/Om* when opening and closing the session is needed. Offering alternatives might involve the inclusion of cultural or indigenous healing methods that may differ from the yoga therapist's training; if they feel unprepared to work within the client's framework for healing or it falls outside their scope of practice, referral to a provider who may be a better fit is warranted.

Group or individual sessions usually begin with a check-in, which can be as simple as one word about what the client is hoping to get from the session. It can be beneficial to open and close with the same check-in question so that clients can begin to perceive shifts that took place during the session. Tools like body scans also offer client agency through input into the interpretation. Regularly obtaining feedback provides the opportunity for the yoga therapist to assess and reassess the client's program and goals.

Yogic tools for cultivating safety

Yoga therapy clients need to feel safe and welcomed for the session to be effective. When a client experiences a safe state, they can access the neuroplasticity that allows the brain to retrain habits and make new associations. Their brain is more capable of perceiving and integrating the session, and of engaging with the healing and transformational work that might also include triggers, discomfort, or distress.[53]

In yogic philosophy, physical needs and safety are both characteristics of the root *chakra*, defined as the holder of safety, stability, security, and grounding. A yoga therapist might help clients to access the grounding of *muladhara* chakra by beginning the session with slow deep breaths, emphasizing the elongation of the exhale to move the energy toward *apana vayu*. A grounding mudra such as *bhu* or *adhi* can also be introduced. (See Chapter 4 for a discussion of the *pranavayus* and Chapter 21 on mudra.) Physically, starting a session with savasana or child's pose (*balasana*) can also promote grounding. In addition, cues related to the legs, feet, and body sensation/awareness may facilitate grounding.

The panchamaya system is another excellent framework to use when creating the safe container. On the level of annamaya, it is important to set up a physically comfortable space for the session. This may include blankets, pillows, blocks, bolsters, chairs, and walls. In cases of trauma, straps and ropes are contraindicated. Attending to annamaya includes ensuring that the client has enough props to be comfortable; choosing asana that support the client's body type; modifying postures according to level of fitness, injuries, weakness, and vulnerabilities; and identifying work that promotes *sthira suhkham* (comfort and stillness).

On the level of pranamaya, the yoga therapist can begin the session with an energy-shifting experience by invoking specific rituals—lighting a candle, employing a mudra or mantra, inviting carefully chosen imagery—all "without ever saying, 'It's safe to feel your body,' a concept [the] client's mind may immediately resist."[54] The yoga therapist's goal is to assist the client in staying present throughout the session and working together with whatever surfaces physically, spiritually, and emotionally while remaining within their scope of practice.

On the level of manomaya, a yoga therapist can cultivate an environment of mutual trust, respect, and caring. Each session may begin with a check-in, as described above, that offers an explicit opportunity for the client to express how they are feeling in the present moment. In the therapeutic setting, all emotions are welcomed, even tears. This may include having tissues easily accessible in the space without forcing them on clients (who may think the tissues are a signal to stop crying). Yoga therapist Amy Weintraub writes, "Acknowledging and even honoring tears is an important aspect of setting the safe container."[55] In addition, clients must feel free to share negative emotional responses without fear of judgment.

The therapist may also use practices that focus on working with emotions, such as stair-step breathing with *bhavana* (focus on one image, as taught by Amy Weintraub in LifeForce Yoga), "ha" breath (as taught by Dr. Ananda Balayogi in the Gitananada tradition), yoga nidra (as taught by the Bihar School), rasa sadhana (as taught by Peter Merchand), and pratipaksha bhavana (as taught by Mary and Rick Nurrie Stearns).

The client and yoga therapist can work with vijnanamaya by cultivating a shared sense of ownership of the therapeutic process through mutual engagement in the care plan, co-created therapeutic goals, and shared decision-making—all while practicing non-attachment to outcomes.

At the level of anandamaya, the "bliss body," the yoga therapist offers practices that connect to the client's ability to find joy. This could be a discussion of joyous moments that occurred that day or week, including the client's favorite posture or type of meditation in the session, or something else they enjoy doing. If the client likes drawing, they might be encouraged to draw a picture of a safe space, perhaps with them in it. If they like to write, a journaling practice focusing on everyday experiences, resilience, equanimity, safety, or gratitude might be useful. If the client loves singing or music, mantra chanting or adding sound to asana or meditation could be welcome. A love of nature might inspire a practice outside. Meditations can incorporate the client's favorite imagery, which could also be woven into asana and pranayama. The compassionate caring between client and yoga therapist can bring a further sense of joy to the session. Offering practices that cultivate gratitude, awe, and delight enables the "brain to do better, to be wise and more skillful in...interactions."[56]

The external environment is an important component of a safe space. This is central to upholding the concept of aikyam, that individual and environment are one. Setting up a therapeutic space ideally includes attention to cleanliness, color, availability of windows, presence of nature, furnishing materials, lighting, and room temperature. Potential distractions and triggers in the therapeutic environment include closed-in spaces; clutter; overpersonalization; neglect/lack of maintenance; artwork depicting sadness, violence, or death; and uncomfortable seating or insufficient props. Each session should take into consideration an individual's age, personality, *dosha*, guna, time of day, season, year, and state of mind.

Therapeutic group settings

In the group setting, the first steps in welcoming participants are taking an interest, making eye contact, learning names, playing appropriate music (or none), and having appropriate décor (e.g., flowers, candles, an altar or absence of one). Choices that feel authentic to the yoga therapist and support clients' feelings that they are valued are ideal. Being knowledgeable about cueing, assisting, possible variations in planned practices, and when (and when not) to touch will help create a safe environment.

In a therapeutic yoga class where people share, the group can be asked to formulate agreements to follow, or the yoga therapist can start with their own agreements and ask the group to add to them. This creates an interactive environment and keeps people engaged. When finished, the yoga therapist would verify that everyone is satisfied with the agreements and ask whether there are any more to add. For a longer workshop, the group can revisit the agreements at the start of each day in case something has come up that needs to be addressed with additional agreements.

The yamas and niyamas are a wonderful beginning for establishing agreements within a therapeutic setting. ***Ahimsa*** (non-harming) is an important step for group safety. Everyone in the class or workshop must agree to treat one another with gentleness, kindness, and compassion. No putdowns or abusive language by clients or teachers should be tolerated, nor should unsolicited fixing or counseling.

When a person is called by their name, they feel more valued, respected, and engaged in the conversation, so clients might be encouraged to introduce themselves and to learn one another's names. However, calling students out by name in asana class to criticize or praise them can be problematic. If a student is in an unsafe position, the yoga therapist can go to them and directly and quietly offer a prop or modification. They could also teach the whole group the issue without singling anyone out, as the experience of having one's name said aloud, particularly for those with trauma, can be shaming.[57] When modeling asana, using the most basic version of the posture avoids intimidation. Hands-on assists are contraindicated in trauma-sensitive yoga settings.

Satya (truthfulness) is expressed in asana practice by respecting one's body and not pushing to the point of harm. Offering explicit "permission" to abstain from activities, take breaks, and avoid contributing to a conversation reinforces satya. Encouraging group participants to use "I" statements when sharing beliefs and to share only from personal experience further supports this foundation of safe practice.

Asteya (non-stealing) can be used to form an agreement that when a person is talking, everyone else will listen and not steal their time. A practice of deep listening—to tone, inflection, and inference—supports the intention of asteya.

Bramacharya (appropriate use of one's vital energy) can be explored by agreeing to focus on dignity, decency, mutual respect, and equality for everyone. In addition, "Yoga teachers in a trauma sensitive context might want to dress conservatively to minimize any distractions and to minimize triggers."[58]

Aparigraha (non-grasping) can be used to celebrate abundance and practice gratitude. When the yoga therapist leaves ample time for questions and concerns and are open to suggestions, they reinforce the concept of aparigraha.

In terms of ***shaucha*** (purity), yoga therapist and client alike can keep intentions for the session straightforward, refining as the program goes on.

Keeping the yoga room and personal spaces simple and clean supports shaucha, as does the use of trauma-sensitive language, "which tends to be concrete and gently brings attention to visceral experiences."[59] The yoga therapist can focus on the language of inquiry by using phrases such as "notice," "be curious," "allow," "approach with interest," "experiment," and "feel." They can also use invitational language that promotes choice and control (e.g., "if you wish to," "when you feel ready," "if you like").[60] When using Sanskrit for yoga poses, or Latin or Greek in anatomy, including the lay definitions avoids intimidating those who are unfamiliar with the terms.

Connection to ***santosha*** (contentment) can happen by enjoying the session, but not at the expense of others. Yoga therapists who remain aware of their position in the room when teaching and rarely turn their back to clients create a container for an experience of contentment. "A trauma-sensitive yoga teacher does not move around during the class very much, and students know where to locate her or him (no surprises!)."[61] It may be preferable to keep the room bright, as dim lighting can be more triggering for populations with trauma.[62] Consulting clients when setting up or making changes to the room gives them as much control as possible over the environment,[63] as does offering the option to keep eyes open during savasana or meditation.

Tapas (internal discipline) can be accessed by helping clients to stay engaged. The yoga therapist can encourage the group to do the work presented, challenge themselves, and safely move beyond their comfort zones on and off the mat.

The yoga therapist can work with ***svadhyaya*** (self-study) by encouraging everyone to do the best they can. Svadhyaya is supported by thinking of everything encountered as an opportunity to learn, and by allowing time for self-reflection, journaling, and getting out in nature.

The yoga therapist can work with ***ishvara pranidhana*** (devotion) by seeing everything as a manifestation of the Divine and remembering what a privilege it is to practice yoga. As yoga therapist Nischala Joy Devi said, "Yoga takes us back to the beginning of our journey of becoming human; we spark the memory that we are first and always an aspect of the Divine."[64]

Summary

Often clients come to yoga therapy in search of help in the alleviation of their suffering. Yoga therapy techniques are numerous and diverse depending on the therapist's training, lineage, and worldview. Regardless of the system, a yoga therapist can start the session from a place of empathy and compassion while focusing on providing an environment where the client, often in a vulnerable state, can feel safe. Through the cultivation of suhkha sthanam, a place of internal and external ease, the client in partnership with the therapist can begin the journey toward healing. The concept of aikyam, unity between one and their environment, means that the safety provided in the therapeutic container may be reflected inside the client. From this safe space, resilience, the ability to bounce back from adversity, may be fostered.

The consistent practice of yoga within and outside of the therapeutic session may increase samatvam (upeksha). Through this equanimity, resilience is manifested as clear-mindedness, composure, elation, energy, life purpose, satisfaction, and self-confidence. When the client faces difficult or stressful situations, the techniques practiced in yoga may equip them with the resources to handle the adversity.

The world does not provide a safe container in which to play the game of life. Reality will always include problems, adversity, sadness, disappointment... The more one experiences in life, the more difficulties that may be encountered. As Ramakrishna said, "When the flower blooms, the bees come uninvited." Yoga therapists can listen, advocate, educate, invite, offer, share, nurture, challenge, trust, hold space, and honor clients, but yoga therapists cannot "fix" clients or do the work for them. Building resilience and creating safety is an inside job that begins with a desire, an inner longing to rise out of the mud of whatever adverse circumstances are holding back the blossoming of the lotus of being.

Additional Resource

Ackerman, C. E. (2019). How to measure resilience with these 8 scales. https://positivepsychology.com/3-resilience-scales

Endnotes

1 Hartfiel, N., Havenhand, J., Khalsa, S. B., Clarke, G., & Krayer, A. (2011). The effectiveness of yoga for the improvement of well-being and resilience to stress in the workplace. *Scandinavian Journal of Work, Environment & Health, 37*(1), 70–76.

2 Hahn, T. N. (2014). *No mud, no lotus.* Parallax Press.

3 Sullivan, M. B., Erb, M., Schmalzl, L., Moonaz, S., Noggle Taylor, J., & Porges, S. W. (2018). Yoga therapy and polyvagal theory: The convergence of traditional wisdom and contemporary neuroscience for self-regulation and resilience. *Frontiers in Human Neuroscience, 12*, 67.

4 Bhavanani, A. (2020). Salutogenesis approach to communications. In S. C. Parija & B. V. Adkoli (Eds.), *Effective medical communication* (pp. 235–245). Springer.

5 Friborg, O., Hjemdal, O., Rosenvinge, J. H., & Martinussen, M. (2003). A new rating scale for adult resilience: What are the central protective resources behind healthy adjustment? *International Journal of Methods in Psychiatric Research, 12*(2), 65–76.

6 Sullivan et al., Yoga therapy and polyvagal theory.

7 Sargeant, W. (2009). *The bhagavad gītā* (p. 133). State University of New York Press.

8 Devi, N. J. (2007). *The secret power of yoga: A woman's guide to the heart and spirit of the yoga sutras* (pp. 75–76). Harmony.

9 Raghavendra, B. R., & Singh, P. (2015). Immediate effect of yogic visual concentration on cognitive performance. *Journal of Traditional and Complementary Medicine, 6*(1), 34–36.

10 Vaishnav, B. S., Vaishnav, S. B., Vaishnav, V. S., & Varma, J. R. (2018). Effect of yoga-nidra on adolescents well-being: A mixed method study. *International Journal of Yoga, 11*(3), 245–248.

11 Saraswati, S. N. (2016). *Prana and pranayama* (p. 254). Bihar School of Yoga/Yoga Publications Trust.

12 Zaccaro, A., Piarulli, A., Laurino, M., Garbella, E., et al. (2018). How breath-control can change your life: A systematic review on psycho-physiological correlates of slow breathing. *Frontiers in Human Neuroscience, 12*, 353.

13 Chamorro-Premuzic, T., & Lusk, D. (2017). The dark side of resilience. *Harvard Business Review*, Aug. 16. https://hbr.org/2017/08/the-dark-side-of-resilience

14 Saraswati, S. (2012). *Samatvam: The yoga of equanimity* (p. 5). Yoga Publications Trust.

15 Devi, *Secret power of yoga* (p. 44).

16 Trent, N. L., Borden, S., Miraglia, M., Pasalis, E., Dusek, J. A., & Khalsa, S. B. S. (2019). Improvements in psychological and occupational well-being following a brief yoga-based program for education professionals. *Global Advances in Health and Medicine, 8*. https://doi.org/10.1177/2164956119856856

17 Ramanathan, M., & Bhavanani, A. (2017, June 23). Resilience as an antidote to chronic diseases: Possible role of yoga [Conference presentation]. National Seminar-cum-Workshop on the Role of Yoga in Prevention, Management and Rehabilitation of Chronic Diseases, Pondicherry, India.

18 Posadzki, P., & Parekh, S. (2009). Yoga and physiotherapy: A speculative review and conceptual synthesis. *Chinese Journal of Integrative Medicine, 15*(1), 66–72.

19 Woodyard, C. (2011). Exploring the therapeutic effects of yoga and its ability to increase quality of life. *International Journal of Yoga, 4*(2), 49–54.

20 Ramanathan & Bhavanani, Resilience.

21 Sullivan, M., & Robertson, L. C. H. (2020). *Understanding yoga therapy: Applied philosophy and science for health and well-being*. Routledge.

22 Sullivan & Robertson, *Understanding yoga therapy* (p. 242).

23 Sullivan & Robertson, *Understanding yoga therapy*.

24 Sullivan et al., Yoga therapy and polyvagal theory.

25 Measures that quantify a person's ACEs are sometimes referred to as resilience scores.

26 Sullivan et al., Yoga therapy and polyvagal theory.

27 Sullivan et al., Yoga therapy and polyvagal theory.

28 Telles, S., Gupta, R. K., Yadav, A., Pathak, S., & Balkrishna, A. (2017). Hemisphere specific EEG related to alternate nostril yoga breathing. *BMC Research Notes, 10*(1), 306.

29 Bhavanani, A. B., Udupa, K., & Madanmohan, R. P. (2011). A comparative study of slow and fast suryanamaskar on physiological function. *International Journal of Yoga, 4*(2), 71–76.

30 Daukantaitė, D., Tellhed, U., Maddux, R. E., Svensson, T., & Melander, O. (2018). Five-week yin yoga-based interventions decreased plasma adrenomedullin and increased psychological health in stressed adults: A randomized controlled trial. *PLoS ONE, 13*(7), e0200518.

31 Miyoshi, Y. (2019). Restorative yoga for occupational stress among Japanese female nurses working night shift: Randomized crossover trial. *Journal of Occupational Health, 61*(6), 508–516.

32 Gard, T., Noggle, J. J., Park, C. L., Vago, D. R., & Wilson, A. (2014). Potential self-regulatory mechanisms of yoga for psychological health. *Frontiers in Human Neuroscience, 8*, 770. Cited in Sullivan et al., Yoga therapy and polyvagal theory (p. 11).

33 Sullivan et al., Yoga therapy and polyvagal theory.

34 Sullivan & Robertson, *Understanding yoga therapy*.

35 Weintraub, A. (2016). LifeForce Yoga teacher training, Encinitas, CA.

36 Van der Kolk, B. A., Stone, L., West, J., Rhodes, A., et al. (2014). Yoga as an adjunctive treatment for posttraumatic stress disorder: A randomized controlled trial. *Journal of Clinical Psychiatry, 75*(6), e559–e565 (p. e559).

37 Sullivan & Robertson, *Understanding yoga therapy*.

38 Payne, L., Gold, T., & Goldman, E. (2015). *Yoga therapy & integrative medicine.* Basic Health Publications.

39 Marchand, P., & Johari, H. (2006). *The yoga of the nine emotions: The tantric practice of rasa sadhana.* Destiny Books.

40 Marchand & Johari, *The yoga of the nine emotions.*

41 Raingruber, B., & Robinson, C. (2007). The effectiveness of tai chi, yoga, meditation, and reiki healing sessions in promoting health and enhancing problem solving abilities of registered nurses. *Issues in Mental Health Nursing, 28*(10), 1141–1155.

42 Eyre, H. A., Acevedo, B., Yang, H., Siddarth, P., et al. (2016). Changes in neural connectivity and memory following a yoga intervention for older adults: A pilot study. *Journal of Alzheimer's Disease, 52*(2), 673–684.

43 See, e.g., Smith, B. W., Dalen, J., Wiggins, K., Tooley, E., Christopher, P., & Bernard, J. (2008). The Brief Resilience Scale: Assessing the ability to bounce back. *International Journal of Behavioral Medicine, 15,* 194–200; Connor, K. M., & Davidson, J. R. (2003). Development of a new resilience scale: The Connor-Davidson Resilience Scale (CD-RISC). *Depression & Anxiety, 18*(2), 76–82.

44 Sullivan et al., Yoga therapy and polyvagal theory.

45 Kenney, M. R. (2001). *Mapping gay LA: The intersection of place and politics* (p. 24). Temple University Press.

46 Advocates for Youth. (n.d.). Glossary. Retrieved on March 24, 2012, from https://advocatesforyouth.org/?option=com_content&task=view&id=607&Itemid=177

47 Bhavanani, A. B. Personal communication, Jan. 21, 2020.

48 Paramahansa, Y. (1998). *Autobiography of a yogi* (pp. 119–120). Self-Realization Fellowship.

49 Bhavanani, A. B. Personal communication, Jan. 25, 2020.

50 Carmen, J. (2020). Consent to participate in yoga therapy: Discussing informed consent with clients. *Yoga Therapy Today,* Spring, 22–26.

51 Weintraub, LifeForce Yoga teacher training.

52 Sullivan et al., Yoga therapy and polyvagal theory (p. 13).

53 Graham, L. (2018). *Resilience: Powerful practices for bouncing back from disappointment, difficulty, and disaster.* New World Library.

54 Weintraub, A. (2012). *Yoga skills for therapists: Effective practices for mood management* (pp. 7–8). W. W. Norton & Co.

55 Weintraub, *Yoga skills for therapists* (p. 49).

56 Graham, *Resilience* (p. 23).

57 Emerson, D., & Hopper, E. (2011). *Overcoming trauma through yoga: Reclaiming your body.* North Atlantic Books.

58 Emerson & Hopper, *Overcoming trauma* (p. 127).

59 Emerson & Hopper, *Overcoming trauma* (p. 120).

60 Emerson & Hopper, *Overcoming trauma* (pp. 120–121).

61 Emerson & Hopper, *Overcoming trauma* (p. 127).

62 Emerson & Hopper, *Overcoming trauma.*

63 Emerson & Hopper, *Overcoming trauma.*

64 Devi, *Secret power of yoga* (p. 14).

15

Respecting the Presence of Shakti: Cyclical Wisdom and Menstruality Consciousness in Yoga Therapy for Women's Health

UMA DINSMORE-TULI

All the faces of the Feminine are come to light our way
To a deeper understanding of the changing worlds we are...
So to learn the turning cycles, and to feel the power shift
In the ebbs and flows, and full tides, in the tears and laughing too,
This is all the wisdom of Her. This is every goddess here...
We are all these things together when we step out of the cage
Of attempting to control the flow,
To fix rigidity
Upon the changing faces of our femininity.[1]

This chapter invites recognition or rediscovery of respect for the significance of *Shakti*, the cyclical power of the life force, as an aspect of yoga therapy client intake and co-creative program development. Voices shared from the author's practice illustrate how clients can experience an embodied rediscovery of the nature of Shakti. The healing presence of Shakti can be absent, neglected, or disrespected within yoga therapy, and yoga therapists are called to redress the balance between analytical approaches and the intuitive, nurturing empowerments possible through the respect of Shakti as a primary healing power.

What Is Shakti?

Shakti is a Sanskrit word meaning energy or power. Shakti, or *Shakti Ma*, is also the name given to powers of life personified in the empowered feminine presence of goddesses like *Nidra Shakti* (power of sleep; see Chapter 22), *Kshuddha Shakti* (power of hunger), or *Prana Shakti* (power of life herself). In contrast to *Shiva* consciousness of stillness and pure awareness, Shakti's power is to move and manifest life. She does this in the forms of many *shaktis* that emanate from her core power. There is both Shakti singular—the power of life herself—and plural shaktis, which are both multiple goddess forms and the different ways in which Shakti activates particular functions to support health.

In relation to yoga therapy, these multiple shaktis can be understood as the presence of vital force, or healing energy, moving in cycles. Shakti moves rhythmically and cyclically, in everything that is alive. Healthy human bodily function is an interplay of many interconnecting rhythmic cycles of shaktis—of digestion, assimilation, and elimination; of respiration, sleep, and rest; of menstruation cycles and processes of menopause; and of reproduction (conception, pregnancy, postnatal recovery). Every cycle provides biofeedback to support the rhythmic functioning of health, and each one is an expression of Prana Shakti at work. These physical rhythms of Shakti are not the only cycles; life also dances to rhythms of emotional, psychic, and intuitive cycles of creative process, dreaming, and relating—with one another, with the planet, and with all of life.

Western medicine monitors human health through four vital signs: heart rate, blood pressure, body temperature, and respiratory rhythm. There is also, for female humans, a fifth vital sign: the menstrual cycle. Reconnecting with these rhythmic cycles of life within the body allows the rediscovery of connection with the rhythms of seasonal change, lunar phases, and life stages. To live with full health and vitality is to live in rhythm with the cycles of Shakti, in the context of this habitat, responding to daily and seasonal shifts. When people are out of rhythm with these cycles, health is compromised because of disconnection from the intelligence of Shakti.[2]

Cyclical Wisdom and Yoga Therapy

Cyclical wisdom is a respect for the presence of Prana Shakti's cyclical movements. To cultivate cyclical wisdom is to encourage respect for the embodied presence of internal rhythmic cycles of physiology, emotional response, and intuitive insight in relation to one another and in relation to external, environmental rhythms of daily, seasonal, and lunar cycles. Respect for these interrelating rhythmic cycles as a guidance system for managing wellness is grounded in curiosity, humility, and a willingness to patiently observe patterns over time, learning how Shakti moves through any given individual or group. Cyclical wisdom can be understood to be a form of *svadhyaya* (the *niyama* of self-study), in the sense that the holy text to be studied closely is one's cycles of life.

Living with respect for these cycles promotes interconnection and empowerment, cultivating trust and understanding for rhythms of life as a manifestation of the cycles of Shakti. Indigenous earth-based wisdoms and traditional healing models such as ayurveda and Chinese medicine focus on bodily cycles as indicators of health and integrate all treatment within the contexts of season and place. (See Chapter 4 for an ayurvedic perspective.)

Cultivating respect for Shakti

As Shakti is not always central to yoga therapy, definitions of three key terms crucial to understanding of cycles of Shakti in women's health follow: *Prana Shakti*, *menstruality consciousness*, and the *female siddhis*.

As noted above, Prana Shakti is the power of the life force, which moves in cycles and rhythms through many different systems and dimensions of being. This chapter focuses on cycles of the female reproductive system, exploring how yoga therapy can better support women's well-being when it is founded on respect for Prana Shakti's cycles. These cycles include the menstrual cycle, (peri)menopause, and the experiences of fertility, including pregnancy and postnatal recovery (used here in its inclusive sense of recovery following the end of any pregnancy by any means, including termination, early pregnancy loss, still birth, or live birth). To offer effective yoga therapy to support women's physical, mental, and emotional health in all stages of life requires a willingness to adopt a cyclical approach.

Menstruality consciousness: The fifth vital sign

Menstruality describes the entire female life process. The term was devised by psychotherapist Jane Catherine Severn, who was concerned about the absence of any word to describe what she called the four Ms: menarche, menstruation, menopause, and the mature years.[3] Without a term to describe these related processes, the full power of the female life cycle can be easily ignored or dismissed, so Severn proposed the word *menstruality*. Alexandra Pope and Sjanie Hugo-Wurlitzer introduced this concept through their menstruality education service "Red School" and their book *Wild Power*.[4]

Crucially, there are not one but *four* Ms in the practice of menstruality consciousness. Not only about menstruation, the concept is of immense value throughout the entire life cycle, and relevant to women and girls of all ages, because it includes all cycles and rhythms of women's lives. Experiences of the four Ms can be observed and respected with the same tools used to chart menstrual cycles, with attention to elements like those shown in Figure 15.1.

Menstrual phase (bleed time)

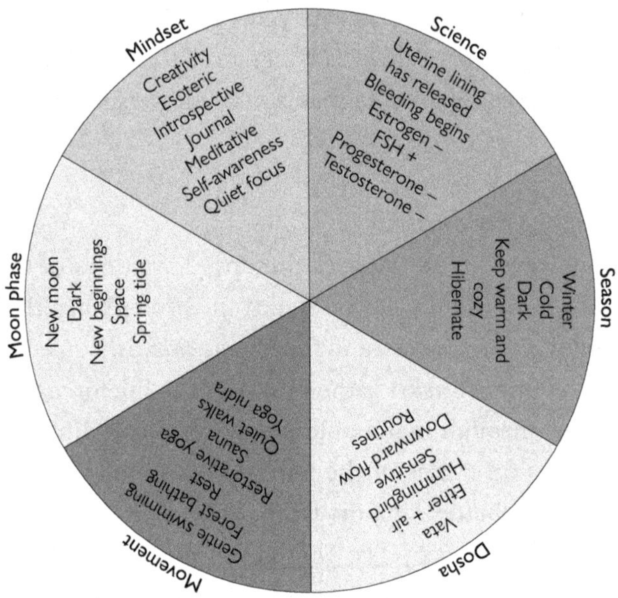

Proliferative follicular phase (preovulation)

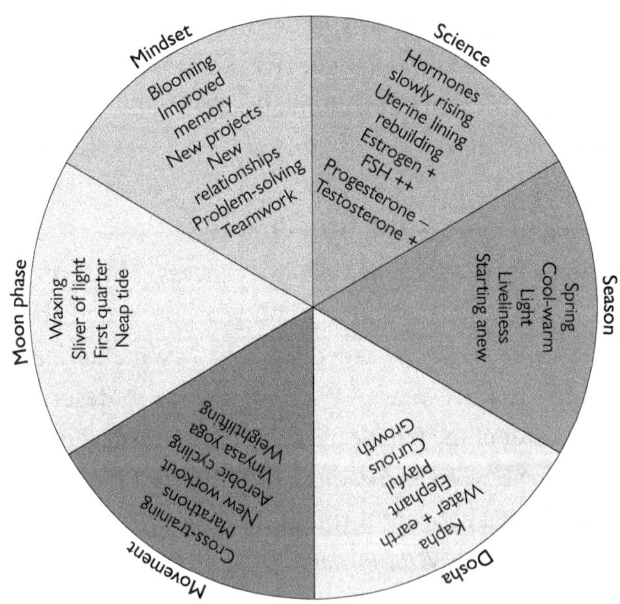

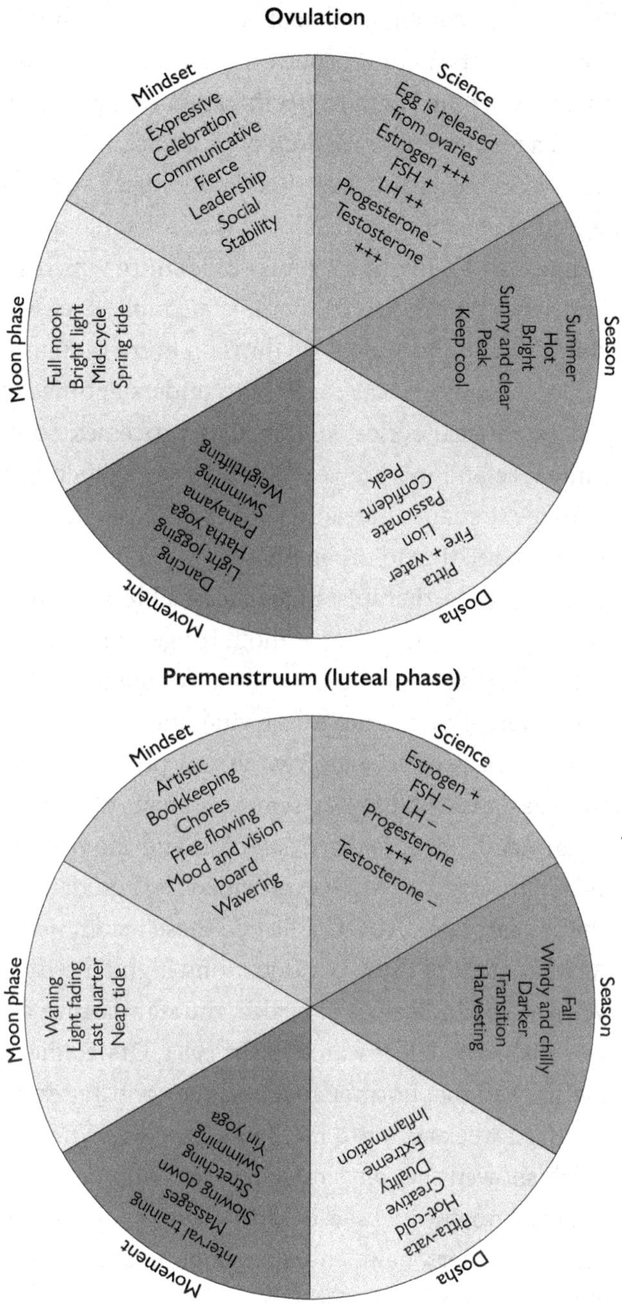

FIGURE 15.1 MENSTRUAL CYCLE MAPPING

Adapted from work by nutritionist, ayurvedic counselor, and yoga teacher Nimisha Gandhi; used with permission.

FSH = follicle-stimulating hormone; LH = luteinizing hormone.

During menstruating years, menstruality consciousness brings awareness to the emotional, physical, and mental rhythms of menstrual cycles so that women and girls (and their male companions, colleagues, and family members) can navigate their lives with respect for this powerful cycle of Shakti. If the menstrual cycle is observed and welcomed with respectful attention, it can be an invaluable biofeedback system, a form of inner wisdom or guidance.

There are many ways to chart cycles. Red School uses a seasonal metaphor which reads the four stages of menstrual cycles as seasonal qualities (see, e.g., those shown in Figure 15.1). Inviting women to identify which season they are in, and to feel into what that means to them, is a simple, accessible method to track the powerful impact of hormonal rhythms on every dimension of women's health. This seasonal metaphor maps easily onto understandings of other cycles, such as lunar phases, diurnal cycles, and creative processes, so it can easily be used during menopause and mature years by inviting women to feel into what seasonal energies they experience in relation, for example, to their vital, emotional, or physical energy or in relation to moon phases.

It is important that yoga therapists have accessible tools to inquire about menstrual and menopausal experiences without triggering feelings of shame and embarrassment. The seasonal model of menstruality consciousness is such a tool to enable the exploration of menstruality as a vital index of well-being.

Many legal and medical professionals have already proposed that the menstrual cycle be recognized as a fifth vital sign in female humans of menstruating age. In 2006, the American Academy of Pediatrics (AAP) and the American College of Obstetricians and Gynecologists (ACOG) provided clear guidance on the value of such charting.[5] Nine years later, ACOG affirmed these recommendations.[6]

More than 50 years before these organizations highlighted the importance of menstrual cycles as key indicators of health, the significance of premenstrual syndrome was established by UK researchers. In 1953, Drs. Katharina Dalton and Raymond Greene showed that hormonal imbalance contributes to premenstrual tension (PMT) in the 2 weeks prior to menstrual bleeding.[7] Dalton and Greene's pioneering research showed that physical symptoms of premenstrual syndrome (PMS), as it became known, include bloating, breast discomfort, headaches and backaches, skin disorders, pain, and a range of mental symptoms including tension, irritability, anxiety, and depression.

Extreme experiences of premenstrual distress are now defined as premenstrual dysphoric disorder (PMDD), which affects an estimated 3 to 8 percent of women of reproductive age.[8] The intensity and life impact of PMDD indicate the need to respect the power of the menstrual cycle to affect mental, emotional, and physical health. Despite increased interest in the effect of the menstrual cycle on women's health, it is still rare for this manifestation of Shakti to be openly discussed without shame, so it is vital to welcome space in yoga therapy to explore what is often unspoken and uncover what has been buried.

Most women under 60 are experiencing either the hormonal effects of menstrual cycles, of (peri)menopause, or other cyclic aspects of female physiology such as pregnancy (or fertility journeys), or some form of postnatal recovery. Women over 60 continue to experience fluctuations in energy and vitality guided by lunar phases and seasonal shifts. To acknowledge that cycles of shakti affect many health issues, for example recurring depression and anxiety, enables women to better understand their own health and yoga therapists to create programs appropriate to the life cycles of all ages of female clients.

Female siddhis

In the context of yoga therapy, it is helpful to understand that menstruation can be seen as one of eight female siddhis.[9] *Siddhi* is Sanskrit for attainment or accomplishment. There are many references to yogic siddhis in the fourth book of Patanjali's *Yoga Sutras*, where they are presented as superhuman or magical powers, manifestations of potent Shakti.[10] Siddhis are also described in tantric texts as the outcome of some practices of Tantra (see Chapter 2 for more information on Tantra). Much of Hatha and Raja yoga has roots in Tantra, which in turn is rooted in shamanism, and the fundamental underpinning of all these systems is a dynamic relationship between Shiva (consciousness) and Shakti (energy).[11]

This relationship between Shiva and Shakti, the dynamic between awareness and energy, is at the heart of a yoga therapeutic response that honors the female siddhis. Human consciousness holds the potential for siddhis when focused awareness aligns with cosmic powers. In Tantra and yoga, siddhis usually enable the practitioner to harness cosmic forces to acquire magical abilities, but these same cosmic forces can also quite spontaneously set the rhythms of women's cyclical life experiences. In the lives of yogis and practitioners of Tantra, siddhis result from intense ascetic yoga practice; the lives of conscious women certainly include naturally arising, intense physical experiences of Shakti that empower specifically female siddhis. The birthing or menstruating woman, or the menopausal woman drenched with sweat in the heat of a raging hot flash, all experience elemental forces flowing unbidden through them; these are fully embodied initiations into the cyclical powers of Shakti. To acknowledge and honor the initiatory power of these experiences in yoga therapy makes possible deep healing.

Initiatory power is the capacity of an experience to shift an individual across a threshold of awareness into another state of being or stage of life. An initiation awakens awareness of other ways of being by opening doors of perception that were previously closed. Major life events, illnesses, and grief all hold the potential of initiatory power if their impact is acknowledged and understood. Absent that respect, the initiatory potential of these experiences can be buried in pain or suppressed in regret, guilt, sadness, or shame; the same can happen to the female siddhis.

Eight biological functions are identifiable as potential female siddhis, and each holds huge initiatory potential: (1) onset of menstruation at menarche, (2) monthly/lunar rhythm of menstrual cycles, (3) female orgasm, (4) pregnancy, (5) pregnancy loss (including miscarriage, stillbirth, and termination), (6) childbirth, (7) lactation, and (8) menopause. Because female siddhis are naturally arising physical experiences, it is important to note the difference between experiencing their physiological aspects as bodily functions and recognizing these experiences as potential siddhis.

Conscious recognition, which transforms physical experience into a siddhi, is crucial to perceive that the hormonal, emotional, and physical experiences of female siddhis have the capacity to be experienced as spiritual initiations. Awareness of female siddhis reveals a radical perspective that women's apparently biological functions can be experienced as a progression of powerful initiations into insight and deep wisdom—embodied knowledge of Shakti's powers of cyclical change and growth.

Sadly, there is little respect for the potent Shakti manifesting in female siddhis. Many of these potentially empowering experiences are reviled, ignored, or suppressed. In many cultures, menstrual blood is considered filthy, and menstruating woman are seen to be so dirty that they are excluded from family homes to prevent them from polluting others. In Nepal, menstruating women are also prevented from touching food or looking at other humans for fear of putting a curse on them. Menstrual shame in Nepali culture is explicit and extreme, although menstrual taboo is prevalent everywhere in the world to different degrees, negatively affecting the well-being of women. Implicit and hidden revulsion for menstruation manifests in Europe, Asia, and across North America, where many churches and temples prohibit entry to menstruating women. Globally, menstruation is generally an unspeakable and hidden source of shame and disgust: Menstrual blood must never be seen; women and girls routinely wrap it up in plastic envelopes, thus turning the blood of life into a toxic biohazard; and women and girls are taught to be so ashamed of female cycles that menstruating and menopausal women endeavor to render evidence of these potential siddhis totally invisible.

Furthermore, menstrual cycles are suppressed through large-scale prescription of hormonal contraceptives,[12] indicating that many female humans rarely experience the rhythmic cycles of normal menstruation. Childbirth is routinely medically managed through rapidly rising levels of labor induction,[13] unnecessary Caesarean sections,[14] and standard use of synthetic hormones to control labor under epidural anesthetic;[15] unmedicated physiological birth is rare in many parts of the industrialized world. Finally, hormone therapy is broadly used worldwide to eradicate the rhythms of menopausal transitions.

In this context, when most naturally arising aspects of Shakti in women's life cycles are comprehensively suppressed, to speak of the potential for specifically female siddhis may seem outrageous or unrealistic. Within the realm of yoga therapy, however, it is possible to honor and recognize these moments of initiatory power as manifestations of Shakti at her most potent.

In the context of yoga therapy, it is important to recognize that if the initiatory potential of any female siddhi has been denied or overlooked in the past, there is always the option to reconnect and honor that siddhi at a later time, for example to heal the pain of a negative menarche experience by acknowledging the experiences of the client at the age she first began to menstruate.

BOX 15.1 A COMPOSITE CASE STUDY

The voices of women speaking about menstruation and menopause are not often heard and rarely dignified by being recorded and shared. This composite case study is woven from the voiced experiences of two individual clients to communicate the intensity of collective suffering caused by disrespect for cyclical wisdom and the personal healing that can occur when women are invited to honor female siddhis as potent initiations into Shakti's cyclical power.

"Anna," 27, was a performer in theater education. She had been experiencing extreme pain and debilitating anxiety during the second half of her menstrual cycle for more than 15 years. General yoga practice gave some pain relief and helped to manage anxiety, but Anna was looking for a more specific approach and sought yoga therapy.

Her first session was in a women's yoga therapy circle, where participants shared the current season of their cycles to help each make wise choices about how to practice that day. Members of that circle referenced *Wild Power* as a key text of menstruality consciousness. After the circle, Anna read the book, and several months later came for individual yoga therapy. She had been using the seasons of the cycle charting method, and on arrival she said,

> Of course! I am not mad after all! What a relief!
>
> This is cyclical! What I've been experiencing all these years is not just general anxiety—it's directly related to my premenstrual experience. It's an "autumn" thing. I can see it clearly now. I was so desperate—I'd been planning to visit the doctor to get antianxiety medications, but I cancelled, because once I realized the feelings were directly related to my menstrual cycle, I recognized what was happening to me. Now I know I can handle this. I feel so relieved. I am not crazy, and I don't need meds. What I need is to pay attention to how I treat myself during different phases of the cycle, so I don't burn out and get super-anxious the week before my bleed. This is natural—and I can handle it.

Anna realized her extreme anxiety was a particular rhythm of Shakti powerfully under the influence of her menstrual cycle, and once she learned to track it, she empowered herself. Through cyclical wisdom she began to know the rhythms of her anxiety. She used daily yoga practices from the women's yoga circle for support, for example practicing *yoga nidra* daily (see Chapter 22) and avoiding more active *asana* in early premenstruum. During that time she focused instead on calming *pranayama* such as Tibetan *bhramari*[16] and psychic alternate-nostril breathing.

Anxiety was only one aspect of Anna's difficulties. She had been diagnosed with severe endometriosis 10 years previously and experienced such intense pain that she was often hospitalized, needing intravenous morphine for pain management. She had undergone three surgeries to remove endometrial tissue between womb and rectum and between bladder and womb.

The endometrial lining of the uterus proliferates and degenerates in response to cycling levels of hormones during different phases of the menstrual cycle. In endometriosis, endometrial tissue is found in places outside the womb. Because all endometrial tissue, wherever found, remains under the control of the endocrine system, this tissue continues to respond to the rhythm of the menstrual cycle, proliferating and flowing like endometrial tissue inside the womb. Unlike endometrial tissue within the uterus, stray endometrial tissue has no way to exit the body during menstruation, instead becoming trapped between organs, potentially adhering to them and causing immense pain. This intolerable pain was another factor that led Anna to yoga therapy.

Anna was also motivated by her desire to conceive: Having recently met the love of her life and wanting to start a family, she had been told by medical doctors that severe endometriosis could prevent conception.

Anna was presented questions intended to raise consciousness of menstruality so this awareness could provide a context for understanding her experience of endometriosis:

- When was your menarche?
- What were you taught as a girl to expect before your first moon?
- What were your early experiences of bleeding?

She answered:

> I was 12. And the only thing my mother said was, "Never, ever let anyone see you are bleeding. Especially keep it totally hidden from Dad and your brothers. Hide the pads and never let anyone see the blood." The main message she gave me was that menstruating was repulsive. There was no place in our family for bleeding. It had to be invisible. I was never allowed to talk about it. I had to pretend I didn't have a cycle.

Many girls receive similar responses at menarche. This kind of menarche experience can cast a long, dark shadow over a woman's health because a central natural function is rendered shameful from the start: Both the siddhi of menarche and a powerful cycle of Shakti are disrespected and suppressed. As she reclaimed dignity for her menstrual cycle, Anna began to feel links between the shame and secrecy surrounding her early experiences of menstruation and the excruciating pain of the endometriosis she had suffered since menarche.

Anna's journey to making peace with endometriosis involved yoga therapy shared in women's yoga circles and individual sessions. More importantly, her yoga therapy care plan involved deep svadhyaya of charting the multidimensional impact of her cycles, noting emotions, feelings, and dreams as well as physical sensations and insights. Through menstruality consciousness she developed a deep respect for the rhythms of her cycle as a siddhi, a source of guidance, and became more compassionate for her body and less fearful of the pain of her premenstruum and menstruations.

Several months after her first women's yoga circle, Anna was in a yoga therapy session practicing "heart-womb breath" (a Yoni Shakti *hasta mudra* [hand gesture]). This practice cultivates love and gratitude in the heart and invites it down into the pelvis so that thankful appreciation can enter the home of the womb.

Before the practice, Anna had spoken about her experiences of endometriosis and was offered this message from Adrienne Egan, a former chair of the Irish Endometriosis Society:

> Endometriosis is not to be underestimated. It can be devastating on all levels, affecting quality of life, ability to work and fertility. In some cases surgery is unavoidable. It's a condition that requires long term care… It is vital to address the health of the body's energetic system, dismantling all blocks to the free flow of energy. It is possible to live well with endometriosis, but it takes effort and a self-care routine that needs to be maintained. The rewards for this effort can be great and deeply healing, reaching further than just the physical level, to how we perceive "the Feminine Principle" within ourselves and its/our place in the world.[17]

Anna nodded, affirming:

> It's as if the endometrial tissue *is* the essence of the feminine principle: That tissue is always changing, always shifting. Very feminine. Every day of the cycle she is changing. She waxes and wanes like the moon. What I feel is this: Endometrial tissue *is* a physical manifestation of the feminine principle. But we can't accept her. So we pretend that she doesn't exist—we don't even give her a home in the womb, and so she ends up in all these other places. The womb is the only place she can thrive, she can grow and flow. I feel how much pain there is when that tissue ends up in other places. It's a kind of exile.

As Anna slid her hands, in *yoni mudra*, down from her heart onto her lower belly, tears filled her eyes and ran silently down her cheeks. She said:

> It's about exile. And this is a homecoming. This is what I need. This is a way to let my womb know she is welcome in my body. Finally. Menstruation is welcome in my body. This heart-womb practice is a "welcome home." All that stray endometrial tissue knows she is welcome, too. She can come home to the womb—because I am sending love into the womb.

Sensing that Anna was in a cycle of very deep healing, the yoga therapist invited her to bring the heart-womb breath into yoga nidra, to co-create a practice that welcomed the heart, the womb, and the movement of awareness between the two as a means to awakening in the *pranamaya* and *annamaya koshas* a warm welcome for the "exiled" tissue of the endometrium.

At the end of the yoga nidra, Anna rested on her side and shared:

> This is so helpful. My womb has been like an exile in my own body. And her tissue too, the endometrium. She has been in exile. She has been exiled from her own home. This is not my fault. When I was told menstruation was disgusting, I suppressed all my feelings and let that belief make my womb a place of shame. And pain. No wonder there is so much pain. Every function of my womb has been exiled and reviled. This tissue has been exiled. And this practice is so healing. It tells the exile she is welcome to return home.

After Anna's epiphany about the exiled endometrium, she decided that she was strong enough to have one last surgery to remove as much of the stray endometrial tissue as possible. She had been seeking to conceive a baby with her new husband, so she agreed to have a pregnancy test just before surgery to ensure it was safe to go ahead. The surgery involved a radical removal of as much endometrial tissue as could be found. Unfortunately, the results of the pregnancy test did not arrive before the surgery went ahead. Only after the operation did she discover that the pregnancy test had been positive.

Anna was devastated, terrified, and 8 weeks pregnant. As she prepared to grieve for the imminent loss of the pregnancy, inside the womb, a tiny embryo buried itself deep within the remaining endometrium.

Sixteen years later, Anna's daughter is a beautiful young woman, and her son, whom she conceived 2 years after the birth of her daughter, is a thriving adolescent. The pain Anna experienced with endometriosis lessened greatly after her two pregnancies.

Anna allows this story to be shared to offer encouragement to women with endometriosis. Although the condition does prevent conception for 30 percent of women who have it,[18] as Anna noted, "It is possible to make peace with this condition by welcoming the cyclical nature of the feminine principle into our bodies, into our lives. When we can welcome her siddhis and cycles of Shakti home, then we can begin to heal."

Summary

Anna's is just one story among many that shows how respect for Shakti is relevant to yoga therapy. From the outset, during client intake, and in the co-creation of yoga therapy plans, a respectful integration of yoga therapy techniques with the cyclical wisdom of menstruality consciousness and an honoring of female siddhis can be very valuable. This approach can uproot years of deep physical pain, but this integration also empowers women to acknowledge the huge power inherent in their bodies.

When the initiations of menarche, menstruation, or menopause go unacknowledged—or are actively disrespected—the Shakti powering these processes can be driven underground and covered with shame, manifesting as serious, long-term health issues that cause harm in every dimension of being.

Anna's story offers an example of how to heal such harm and support women's health with cyclical wisdom and intuitive inquiry that honors the female siddhis. Through the respect for the impact of Shakti's cycles on women's health, yoga therapy can be offered in a manner appropriate to those women's needs. If yoga therapists do not facilitate the integration of menstruality consciousness into women's lives, cyclical patterns of health issues such as anxiety, depression, anger, and dysmenorrhea can be misunderstood and mismanaged.

Menstruality consciousness can be a vital missing piece of the whole picture of client health. Truly integrative yoga therapy can bring this important component into relation with the work of other healthcare practitioners, for example nutritionists and psychotherapists, who may also be part of the client's care team. In the same way as menstruality consciousness can be respectfully integrated into yoga therapy care plans, so too can other healthcare modalities be respectfully integrated within a holistic yoga therapy program.

Every phase of all female life cycles needs cyclically responsive, integrative yoga therapy programs. Invite women to identify their cycles of Shakti in seasonal patterns or, working together with female clients, design seasonally appropriate yoga therapy programs that respect the cycles of their lives. Inquiries into experiences around menarche, menstruation, or menopause, while honoring these threshold times, could also serve as initiations into the presence of Shakti.

Additional Resources

Bennet, J. (2002). *A blessing not a curse: A mother-daughter guide to the transition from child to woman.* Milner Health.

Coburn, T. B. (1991). *Encountering the goddess: A translation of the Devī-Māhātmya and a study of its interpretation.* State University of New York Press.

Delaney, J., Lupton, M. J., & Toth, E. (1988). *The curse: A cultural history of menstruation.* University of Illinois Press.

Dinsmore-Tuli, U. (2006). *Mother's breath: A definitive guide to yoga breathing, sound and awareness practices during pregnancy, birth, postnatal recovery and mothering.* Sitaram and Sons.

Hendrickson-Jack, L. (2019). *The fifth vital sign: Master your cycles & optimize your fertility*. Fertility Friday Publishing.

Knaapen, L., & Weisz, G. (2008). The biomedical standardization of premenstrual syndrome. *Studies in History and Philosophy of Biological and Biomedical Sciences, 39*(1), 120–134.

Northrup, C. (2009). *Women's bodies, women's wisdom: The complete guide to women's health and well-being*. Piatkus.

Pope, A., & Bennet, J. (2008). *The pill: Are you sure it's for you?* Allen and Unwin.

Rako, S. (2003). *No more periods? The risks of menstrual suppression and other cutting-edge issues about hormones and women's health*. Harmony.

Saraswati, S. (2008). *Srī Saundarya-Laharī: The descent*. Yoga Publications Trust.

Vostral, S. L. (2008). *Under wraps: A history of menstrual hygiene technology*. Lexington Books.

Endnotes

1 Extract from Dinsmore-Tuli, U. (2019). Thirty nityas dancing in the phases of the moon. www.youtube.com/watch?v=Kyo7qJnelaE

2 Much of the suffering of female humans who navigated childhood and puberty as girls is rooted in the experience of "femaleness," regardless of whether they currently choose to identify as women. Many who presently choose to identify as women may not have encountered any of the experiences described, so the approaches presented in this chapter may feel neither appropriate nor necessary.

This work is of specific service to humans who began to menstruate during or after puberty, and although reference is made to "women and girls" because that is how those described in this chapter choose to identify themselves, these techniques can resonate for humans of all genders. Some female humans never menstruate, but they still grow up as girls under patriarchy and therefore share many experiences with those who did menstruate at puberty. Some females who menstruate do not identify as women, some humans who identify as women do not menstruate, and in the author's experience all of these humans (including some who identify as men and have never menstruated) have found these inquiries into Shakti's cycles to be helpful.

Life's cycles and rhythms move through all beings, of all genders. Yoga therapy that acknowledges cycles of Shakti in women and girls can empower all humans to live with respect for Prana Shakti and to restore respect for the cycles of the power of life—for the benefit of all humans and the Earth herself.

3 See, e.g., What Is Menstruality? (2018). Luna house. www.lunahouse.co.nz/conscious-menstruality

4 Pope, A., & Hugo-Wurlitzer, S. (2017). *Wild power: Discover the magic of your menstrual cycle and awaken the feminine path to power*. Hay House.

5 American Academy of Pediatrics Committee on Adolescence, American College of Obstetricians and Gynecologists Committee on Adolescent Health Care, Diaz, A., Laufer, M. R., & Breech, L. L. (2006). Menstruation in girls and adolescents: Using the menstrual cycle as a vital sign. *Pediatrics, 118*(5), 2245–2250.

6 ACOG Committee Opinion No. 651: Menstruation in girls and adolescents: Using the menstrual cycle as a vital sign. (2015). *Obstetrics and Gynecology, 126*(6), e143–e146.

7 Greene, R., & Dalton, K. (1953). The premenstrual syndrome. *British Medical Journal, 1*(4818), 1007–1014.

8 Halbreich, U., Borenstein, J., Pearlstein, T., & Kahn, L. S. (2003). The prevalence, impairment, impact, and burden of premenstrual dysphoric disorder (PMS/PMDD). *Psychoneuroendocrinology, 28*(Suppl. 3), 1–23.

Others give a lower prevalence estimate: Gehlert, S., Song, I. H., Chang, C. H., & Hartlage, S. A. (2009). The prevalence of premenstrual dysphoric disorder in a randomly selected group of urban and rural women. *Psychological Medicine, 39*(1), 129–136. For an illustration of the potentially extreme effects of hormonal symptoms, see Biden, L. (1981, Dec.). British legal debate: Premenstrual tension and criminal behavior. *New York Times*. www.nytimes.com/1981/12/29/science/british-legal-debate-premenstrual-tension-and-criminal-behavior.html

9 The concept of female siddhis is introduced in *Yoni Shakti*, which humbly invokes the protection of each siddhi by powerful shaktis known as the ten great wisdom goddesses (*Dasa Mahavidyas*). A respectful exploration of these shaktis is beyond the scope of this chapter; for more information on these wisdom goddesses and their relationship to female siddhis and women's health, see Dinsmore-Tuli, U. (2020). *Yoni shakti: A woman's guide to power and freedom through yoga and tantra.* YogaWords.

10 See, e.g., Hartranft, C. (2003). *The yoga-sutra of Patanjali: A new translation with commentary.* Shambhala; Satyananda, S. (1976, 1989). *Four chapters on freedom: Commentary on yoga sutras of Patanjali.* Yoga Publications Trust; Stiles, M. (2002). *Yoga sutras of Patanjali.* Red Wheel/Weiser.

11 These ideas are elucidated in many places, including Dinsmore-Tuli, *Yoni shakti.*

12 Among women who use contraception, an estimated 30.8 percent in the United Kingdom (26% worldwide) take hormonal birth control (via injection, implant, or pill). United Nations, Department of Economic and Social Affairs, Population Division. (2019). *Contraceptive use by method* [Data booklet ST/ESA/SER.A/435].

13 In the United Kingdom, where the author lives, 31.6 percent of labors were induced in 2018. UK National Health Service, NHS Digital. (2018). Summary. https://digital.nhs.uk/data-and-information/publications/statistical/nhs-maternity-statistics/2017-18

14 A total of 32.7 percent of US births are by Caesarean, and global rates of C-sections have doubled since 2003. World Health Organization. (2018). WHO recommendations: Non-clinical interventions to reduce unnecessary Caesarean sections. www.who.int/reproductivehealth/publications/non-clinical-interventions-to-reduce-cs/en

15 Seventy-one percent of all US births between 2009 and 2014 were under epidural or other spinal anesthesia. Butwick, A. J., Wong, C. A., & Guo, N. (2018). Maternal body mass index and use of labor neuraxial analgesia: A population-based retrospective cohort study. *Anesthesiology, 129*(3), 448–458.

16 The Tibetan form of this practice "washes" the practitioner with their own sound: The palms move up over the face, scalp, and head, returning to the heart during the humming. See Dinsmore-Tuli, *Yoni shakti.*

17 Quoted in Dinsmore-Tuli, U. (2010–2020). *Yoni shakti well woman yoga therapy course manual.* Sitaram and Sons.

18 Fadhlaoui, A., Bouquet de la Jolinière, J., & Feki, A. (2014). Endometriosis and infertility: How and when to treat? *Frontiers in Surgery, 1*, 24.

16

Understanding the Role of Interoception

KAREN SOLTES

The appreciation of interoception as a key process in the field of yoga therapy has increased steadily since the early 2010s. Although the understanding of interoception and how it represents a complex interaction of the body, mind, and emotions is still relatively new, its importance is becoming clearer. This chapter defines interoception, discusses it as a key ingredient in yoga therapy (including meditation practices), and examines how yoga therapists can both develop their own skills and support clients in developing interoceptive connection.

Given an increasing understanding that the mind and body are not separate but instead vitally interwoven, interoception is the key that links body and mind. In the simplest definition, interoception is the "felt sense" of the body—feeling not from the conceptual mind or from memory, but from direct, present-moment, first-hand experience.

The broad definition of interoception as the sense of the internal state of the body includes both conscious and non-conscious sensing.[1] It encompasses the neurological process of integrating signals relayed from the body in a variety of subregions of the brain (e.g., brainstem, thalamus, insula, and somatosensory and anterior cingulate cortices) to allow for a representation of the body's physiological state. Interoception is involved in many different physiological systems, including cardiorespiratory, gastrointestinal, nociceptive, endocrine, and immune function.

The body's components, including heart, bladder, lungs, and skin, as well as signals such as hormones, can be felt on both the gross and subtle levels. Interoception connects an individual to virtually every functioning part of the physiological body.

Interoceptive signals are communicated to the brain via a diversity of neural pathways, allowing for the sensory processing and prediction of internal bodily states. Misrepresentations of internal states—or a disconnect between the body's signals and the brain's interpretation and prediction of those signals—have been suggested to underlie some mental disorders such as anxiety,[2] depression, panic disorder, anorexia nervosa, bulimia, posttraumatic stress disorder (PTSD), obsessive compulsive disorder (OCD), autism spectrum disorders, and somatic symptom disorder (see Chapter 12).

The earliest definition of interoception focused on the viscera (the heart, lungs, stomach, bladder, and other internal organs in the trunk of the body), but the definition has been broadened to include the brain and skin. Interoception encompasses visceral transmission of sensation and all the tissues that relay signals to the central nervous system about the current state of the body.[3]

There has been a dramatic increase in interest about the role interoception plays in psychological and physical health: In 2000, approximately 50 research publications referenced interoception; by 2015, that number had increased to more than 300. This increase could be attributed to growing attention on and understanding of the mind-body connection and accompanying efforts to scientifically study the complex links.

Background for Yoga Therapy

In a broad sense, interoception is what connects the body and mind and is essential to any process of mind-body healing approaches such as yoga therapy. This connection is vitally important to surviving and thriving. The ability to perceive and feel the complex sensations of the body can be potent, if not essential, for well-being, the ability to meet psychological and physiological challenges, and bouncing back after setbacks.[4] Interoception helps to fuel resilience, supporting the sense of safety and well-being (see Chapter 14).

When a person turns their attention toward sensations in the body, they have access to information that helps, first and foremost, in survival. Hunger, for instance, is a basic survival message that fuels the need to seek food and nourish the body. Hunger might first arrive as a rumbling in the stomach, or a sense of tiredness as one's blood sugar starts to drop. Arising bodily sensations that register intuitively as hunger signal the need take action to nourish the body. The need to drink, sleep, and the infinite variety of functions necessary to survive arrive initially as sensations in the body; registering and attending to these most basic messages is vital.

The same can be said of psychological and emotional states, which arrive as bodily sensations before the mind labels them. Anxiety may show up as a knot in the stomach, tightness in the chest, or some other sensation. The thinking mind then assigns a label or name to that sensation. Happiness and joy might show up as a flutter in the heart with an accompanying smile on the lips.[5] Science now has the capacity to measure the time between the first experience of a physical response in the body and the mind's tendency to label that experience (through *ahamkara*'s processing; see Chapter 11). For example, about 500 milliseconds after a sensation of contraction in the stomach, the mind labels the feeling "I am hungry." Bodily sensations give the mind the information it needs to actively respond to basic physical and psychological needs.

Those basic human needs include feeling safe and having a sense of trust. The five senses continually take information into the system (exteroception) to alert one to the surrounding world and assess safety. In the yogic perspective, this instinct of risk assessment is associated with the first chakra.

Long before the development of language to describe experience, a newborn perceives and responds to the world through interoception. Hunger, temperature, tiredness, frustration, and the range of human experience are registered first as bodily sensation. Infants subsequently learn mechanisms to announce their needs to the world (see Chapter 9).

As children develop, they are further conditioned by the environment, which includes families, caregivers, and culture. Children learn to look toward external cues and complex relationships to label experiences. These interactive relationships may or may not facilitate accurate labeling of interoceptive experience. If experience is not understood and reflected accurately back to a child, they may have difficulty trusting their felt experience as a guide to meeting basic needs. For example, if a child is told she is tired when in fact she is hungry, she learns to override and mistrust the wisdom and intuitive sense of her own body. If children feel unaccepted sadness or anger, they might learn to deny these important messages or use other means to self-soothe feelings and emotions as they appear. External mislabeling of experience may negatively affect a child's development, leading to distrust of their own felt sense of the world. This mislabeling can also affect confidence in the ability to meet one's own needs.[6]

Conversely, as an individual learns the skills to re-attune to a felt sense of the body and to trust the information arriving via interoceptive listening, they open the potential of responding appropriately to meet their needs. Yoga therapists can offer a range of skills that enable a person to reestablish trust in the wisdom of the felt sense of the body and to build a sense of agency in the world.

Polyvagal theory

Polyvagal theory has been largely informed by the work of behavioral neuroscientist Stephen Porges. Current ideas about the role of the vagus nerve in human experience and response have significantly increased understanding about regulation of the autonomic nervous system (ANS).[7] One of the mediating interfaces between the brain and body is the vagus nerve. Vagal response is vital for establishing and maintaining a sense of safety and well-being.

The ANS can be thought of as a personal surveillance system, always on guard.[8] Porges coined the term *neuroception* to describe ANS processing of cues of safety, danger, and life threat. This continual assessment of safety, which includes interoceptive and exteroceptive input, happens below awareness, outside of conscious control.

The two main branches of the ANS, the sympathetic nervous system (SNS) and parasympathetic nervous system (PNS), respond to sensations via three pathways ("neural platforms"), each with a characteristic pattern that serves survival.

The SNS response prepares one for action in the face of a perceived threat by mobilizing the body for defense or fleeing—the fight/flight response. The immobilization response is activated when the other functions are overwhelmed in the face of potentially life-threatening situations.

In the PNS, the two main vagal stress responses are the dorsal vagal and ventral vagal pathways. The dorsal vagal response elicits immobilization ("freeze") behaviors or shut down when one's life is threatened and taking action is no longer an option. The ventral vagal response, in contrast, is linked to social communication, safety, connection, and self-soothing behaviors.

Through the process of interoception, one can recognize the body's subtle signals as they first arrive. A sense of tension, anxiety, stress, etc., can be felt before the response accelerates to the point of overwhelm and the activation of fight/flight/freeze responses. The ability to sense tension before it mounts to anxiety or panic, or irritation before it explodes as rage or anger, enables a range of responses. Having more available choices can support the maintenance of social connection and safety in the face of external events that activate strong feeling states.

"Vagal tone" is a measure of stress vulnerability and reactivity that can be strengthened through yoga therapy practices. Even everyday stresses can leave people overreacting as if there was a threat on life. Slow *asana* such as standing postures that offer a sense of stability, calming forward bends, and restorative practices incorporating breath and relaxing postures may increase vagal tone and activate the PNS relaxation response.

The various vagal responses can be viewed through the lens of the *gunas* (see Chapter 3). When the system is more *rajasic*, with qualities of energy, action, change, and movement, it is similar to an activated SNS state. An extremely *tamasic* system, marked by darkness, inertia, inactivity, and materiality, is similar to the PNS freeze response. Yoga therapists can support clients to establish a state of *sattva*, with the accompanying qualities of harmony, balance, joy, and intelligence, by offering practices that restore a healthy PNS response. In a sattvic state, with its quality of safety and connection, clients may be more open to new learning.

Diaphragmatic breathing and practices that extend the length of the exhalation can activate the vagus nerve and improve vagal tone, which, in turn, may improve heart rate variability (HRV).[9] Greater HRV (higher vagal tone) is associated with better health and increased emotional resilience; diaphragmatic breathing with a pause at the end of the exhale has been shown to have an even greater impact on improving vagal tone and resilience.[10] (See Appendix 16A for an example practice.)

An aid to focus and non-judgmental awareness

Focusing, a practice born in the field of psychotherapy, is based on the work of Eugene Gendlin (see Chapter 13). Gendlin theorized that it is not the therapist's technique that determines the success of psychotherapy, but rather the patient's ability to intuitively focus inside, on subtle bodily awareness—a "felt sense" that contains information that, if attended to and inquired into, holds the resolution to their problems.[11]

A yoga therapist can play a key role in holding the container of attention to those inner states with non-judgmental listening as a client explores their inner terrain. Open-ended questions communicate this intent (see Box 16.1). Reflecting back the client's exact words as they describe experience can also be helpful in developing an ability to hold attention on the present sensation. The yoga therapist is "congruent" by being authentic and genuine with the client. Congruence between one's internal and external experiences fosters a sense of trust and is an essential ingredient in the therapeutic relationship (see Chapter 13).

BOX 16.1 SAMPLE OPEN-ENDED QUESTIONS TO SUPPORT INNER EXPLORATION

- What is present for you in this moment?
- Is there a sensation in the body that is most calling for your attention?

- What are you noticing now?
- Can you say more about that? Or can you describe the sensation more fully?
- To the degree that you can, stay with the sensation that is present. Can you describe the sensation you are feeling now?
- Are you okay to stay with this sensation or feeling? (Allow the client to choose.)

Self-practice for yoga therapists

Although yoga therapists are not providing psychotherapy, staying present in one's own experience while supporting the interoceptive experience of clients is within yoga therapy's scope of practice. While offering the safety of unconditional positive regard for clients, it is important for yoga therapists themselves to be able to note and feel their own reactions to whatever material emerges. The yoga therapist can "bracket" their own reactions, taking them back into personal practice or sessions with their supervisor. For example, when working with a client who has experienced trauma, anger, or helplessness, the yoga therapist may connect with their own history of similar experiences in the session. The task of the yoga therapist is to offer a congruent response of support to the client while noting to themselves what might be triggered in their own experience. The therapist's internal experience might include discomfort with what the client is presenting, a sense of helplessness, or identification with some other aspect of the client's experience.

The personal practice of attuning to one's own body with a sense of curiosity and welcoming acceptance is essential to the yoga therapist's effectiveness with clients. Cultivating one's own interoceptive sense through *pranayama*, asana, and meditation enables modeling of these skills for clients. As yoga therapists authentically know themselves, they can see what might be their own needs versus what will serve the client best. The process of interoceptive introspection helps to illuminate where one's own agenda—e.g., the impact of past history, the need to be right or to be liked—is being activated. Ultimately, the yoga therapist's job is to make themselves expendable, supporting the client to trust their own wisdom so that they function independently or in collaboration with care providers.

Cultivating Interoceptive Processes

When a person can deliberately turn toward sensations in the body, they shift from the "default mode network"—thought to represent, in part, the self-referential me/my identification with sensations—to the "present-centered" network. The present-centered network opens one to the world of infinite possibility in which new perceptions and solutions may emerge. Here, someone in physical or psychological pain may also have the opportunity to experience themselves as more than the experience.[12]

Yoga therapy facilitates clients' fundamentally important reconnections and attunement to the body's messages. Yoga therapists must begin this work with the belief and understanding that each person has the capacity to find the solutions for themselves. Although the yoga therapist can offer a toolbox of practices and skills, ultimately the client has to try these on for themselves, sensing what feels right, what is helping, and where their resistances may lie as they learn to trust their own bodily sensations as guideposts to information and healing.

Guiding clients in a way that enables them to cultivate the skills and attention required to access the body's messages through interoception supports agency and autonomy. Given this ability, people are able to act on their own behalf from the deeper knowing and wisdom of their own bodies and experiences. This helps to establish trust in an innate felt sense of the right action or decisions that lead to an increase in feelings of safety, security, and well-being.

A yoga therapist's role is not to identify what is wrong or tell the client how to fix it, but rather to inquire into what is important and find out how to help. This approach ensures client agency over their priorities. The yoga therapist can offer skills that may help a client to meet their own needs and concerns, and the client can then essentially "run their own experiments" to see what is most beneficial.

The value of intuition

Connecting to one's interoceptive sense affords more access to the intuitive process. Intuition has been defined as the ability to acquire knowledge without recourse to conscious reasoning.[13] Different writers give the term a great variety of meanings, ranging from direct access to unconscious knowledge, unconscious cognition, inner sensing, and inner insight to unconscious pattern recognition and the ability to understand something instinctively. The common thread to these definitions of intuition is an inner sensing, conscious or not, that bypasses the thinking mind. Yoga therapists use a combination of well-honed skills as well as intuition to discern what tools or practices might be useful to the client.

In the philosophy of Samkhya (see Chapter 2), access to information can come from perception (*pratyaksha*), inference (*anumana*), or the word or testimony of reliable sources (*shabda*). Interoception is a vehicle that enables connection to one's perceptions as they arise in the body via the five senses; the ability to infer meaning from that information offers the possibility of more harmony. Given a foundational ability to observe without reactivity, increased awareness of interoceptive signals may enable profound healing as well as clearer messages around right action.

Therapeutic relationship

Everyone has a fundamental need to feel seen, heard, and connected, and a sense of belonging. When these qualities are absent in an interaction, one cannot be fully open to new learning or experiences. (As described above, the sense of safety is intimately connected to neuroceptive processing that is always on alert.) When a yoga therapist is able to feel into their own authentic experience and support the same in the client, the door opens for the client to find solutions to challenges.

"Projection," a term that comes from the world of psychodynamic psychotherapy, occurs when an individual assigns to others their own feelings. The more intimately a yoga therapist knows themselves, developing comfort via interoception, the less likely they are to project their needs onto the client, drawing a clearer boundary between the experiences of the two.

Tools for Developing Interoceptive Skills

Meditation

Meditation practices that include attention to the body's ever-changing gross and subtle sensations help to develop the sense of interoception. The body scan that is included in practices such as mindfulness and iRest yoga nidra help to redirect attention from thoughts, away from past- and future-oriented thinking, to present-moment sensations. (Appendix 16B offers a method for introducing a body scan.) Just the act of shifting attention from thinking about the body or visualizing it to direct sensation slows the thinking mind.

Taking attention to bodily sensations disrupts the mind's tendency to preconditioned responses that come from memory. Another byproduct of body sensing is that simply feeling the body may enable it to relax without "trying to relax" (an endeavor that can have the opposite effect). Body sensing offers practitioners an anchor of security that is directly accessible, cultivating a sense of safety and agency.

Body scanning systematically directs attention to specific areas, especially those with the highest neural density. The mouth, hands, feet, and genitals offer the most intensity of sensation, as they have the highest concentration of nerve endings, which is why body scans often start with or focus on the mouth, hands, and feet. Although the genitals may offer intense sensation, for most populations one would not focus on that area.

Accessing grosser feelings in the body, such as vibrations in the finger, lays the groundwork for accessing more subtle emotional states. According to the *panchamaya kosha* model (see Chapter 3), attention to sensation in *annamaya kosha* opens the doorway to accessing the felt sense of the remaining four koshas.[14]

BOX 16.2 BODY SENSING AND EMOTIONAL REACTIVITY: CASE NOTE

As the skill of sensing bodily sensations develops, an emotion may be felt before it moves a person to action or reaction. For example, a client at the Veterans Health Administration (VHA) had sudden rages he could not understand, that seemed to erupt from nowhere. He experienced these explosive emotions as though he were moving from 0 to 60 mph without knowing how he got there.

This client participated for about a year in a regular iRest practice that featured consistent body scanning/sensing, moving from head to feet along a predictable pathway. The primary instruction was to simply feel what was present, not visualizing but feeling the firsthand immediate experience of sensations. As he shifted attention to sensation in the body, he could notice areas of tension or contraction that he recognized as irritation. He developed the awareness to be able to detect when he was feeling irritated, whereas in the past he might ignore these sensations until they increased to the point of rage: "When I feel irritation, I realize that I have a range of options of responding before it escalates into rage."

It is important to note that when supporting a person in meeting challenging, difficult, or unwanted emotions or sensations, one need not take the hardest one out of the box. If deep grief is present, one could first work with meeting sadness or disappointment. Just as a new weightlifter would not start with the heaviest weight but rather build and strengthen their capacity, allowing clients to move at a pace that feels ideal for them builds capacity over time.

Asana

Physical movement can be a direct highway to awakening the felt sense in the body. Rather than acting on the body in a prescribed manner, asana practice provides opportunity to "become the body" and to reconnect to and investigate the infinite world of sensation.[15] When yoga therapists offer postures or practices with an accompanying inquiry into the felt sense of the body, they are helping to develop interoception. (See Appendix 16C for example questions to begin a practice of interoceptive inquiry.)

Unless someone is at risk of injuring themselves, yoga therapy is less concerned with the outside form than with directing attention to the internal experience. The physical practice of yoga is another vehicle to open to the present-centered network, and to direct moment-to-moment experience, as well as the world of infinite possibility and solutions that might not be accessed through the thinking mind alone.

Pranayama

Breath practices can be incorporated into yoga therapy to increase interoception. The felt sense of the movement of breath in the body is one of the most direct experiences of sensation available.

Intentional breath practices, such as lengthening the exhale (e.g., 1:2 breath ratio), alternate-nostril breathing, or simply exhaling deeply, have the potential to calm the body. Pranayama can also increase the potential for interoceptive awareness by stilling the body. Research demonstrates that breath practices calm the nervous system by shifting it from sympathetic toward parasympathetic dominance.[16] Additionally, pranayama practices have been shown to help increase vagal tone and HRV, in turn increasing nervous system resilience.[17]

One can use the breath as a pointer to body sensation by simply feeling the movement of respiration. Yoga therapists should be cautious about pranayama to "breathe out" tension, anxiety, etc., as using breath to get rid of an experience bypasses the opportunity to learn from the internal state that is present. Rather, one can use the breath to settle the body and activate the PNS to establish a safe base for exploring sensation.

Sound and mantra

Studies have shown that chanting the mantra *Om* can stimulate the vagus nerve, calming the brain's limbic system.[18] Electrical stimulation of the vagus nerve has been used as a treatment in depression and epilepsy and has a positive effect on settling the reaction of the amygdala, the part of the brain that initiates the fight/flight response in the face of perceived danger.

Chanting has the potential to also awaken sensation in the body as one attends to the vibration of sound. Practices such as *brahmari* (bee breath), which combine breath with sound, could be effective alternatives for clients who are not comfortable with chanting or incorporating Sanskrit words into their practices.

Regardless of the practices chosen, inquiry focuses on feeling sensation rather than "doing to" the body-mind.

Supporting Challenged Clients

Some clients have difficulty turning toward physical sensations. For example, someone who has been challenged by pain may turn away from sensations in the body in an attempt to distract from or override what is unpleasant. The yoga therapist can offer experiences that gradually invite the client toward the ability to feel, perhaps starting with areas of the body, such as the hands or feet, that may be easier to access due to a higher concentration of nerves and, often, less emotional charge.

For example, a client with chronic back pain may discover that even when there is pain in an area of the body, other areas are not painful. If the client is feeling sadness, watching subtle moment-to-moment emotional shifts may eventually enable them to stay with challenging states. As one dives into the direct sensorial experience of an emotion, it becomes less solid and more fluid and changeable. One might discover that there are moments in which the sadness is not present, or that even amidst deep grief come moments of happiness, joy, or at least a feeling of being okay.[19]

BOX 16.3 BODY SENSING AND CHRONIC PAIN: CASE NOTE

In a VHA class, one student who had served three tours in Vietnam was struggling with crippling arthritis that left him unable to walk without the assistance of a cane. When he first started learning body sensing via iRest sessions, the instructions were simply to feel each part of the body, moving slowly from head to feet systematically. Students were asked to notice and feel whatever sensations were present and reassured that some places may have a lot of sensation and others very little. The instructor also noted, "There is no way to do this wrong." At the end of the third practice, the student commented, "I get what you are trying to get me to do...you are trying to get me to FEEL my body. I have been trying for 40 years NOT to feel it. When I got home from Vietnam, I had to just suck it up."

Over the course of months of sessions that each offered a body scan, coupled with additional daily practice by recordings at home, the tensions this student had been "sucking up" began to release. His arthritic pain began to abate, allowing him to relinquish his cane. For him, simply taking attention to the body, noticing and feeling sensation, increased relaxation without the strain of trying to relax.

Some people who have been in consistent pain, often over years, might report that they are numb, or that they cannot feel anything. They may confuse the absence of pain with not feeling anything because they are so accustomed to feeling and attending to pain that its absence is experienced as nothing. One might then inquire "What does nothing or numbness feel like?" as that is itself a unique feeling.

For many people, feeling the vast array of physical sensations does not come naturally. Many yoga therapy clients have also turned away from their bodies for any number of reasons, including trauma, military service, eating disorders, and chronic or acute pain. Those with developmental challenges, such as autism-spectrum or sensory-processing disorders, may be oversensitive to bodily sensation or unable to sense what is arising until the sensations have magnified to proportions that overwhelm the system and lead to behavioral reactions.[20] Even in the absence of more overt and identifiable challenges, in a culture that values thinking as a primary method of living in the world and for problem-solving, focusing on body sensation is not often valued.

In addition to body scanning and the other practices outlined above, progressive relaxation may also support the ability to feel sensations. This systematic tensing and releasing of specific muscle groups has also been shown to create relaxed states.[21]

Cultural and psychological influences

When teaching body sensing to a group of enlisted soldiers on an Army base, the discussion turned to bringing attention to sensations in the body. One man, who was likely speaking for the majority of the group, pointed to his chin, saying, "We don't go below here."

Military communities provide one example of people who are oriented toward following directions from superiors. In combat situations, following external directions and *not* stopping to feel the experience in the present moment may be essential to survival. Cultivating an interoceptive sense of signals as a way to inform action is not highly valued in this setting, particularly in a combat setting.

When working with any individual or group that has difficulty feeling sensation, one can start with the grossest level of feeling, such as feeling of the points of contact on the surface on which they rest or noticing sensations in the hands or feet.

Other groups or individuals may be challenged by sensing their bodies, such as people who address emergency situations (e.g., emergency medical personnel, firefighters, police, or other emergency response professionals). Cultural values might also prioritize the ability to process experience with thoughts, overriding physical signals.

In these settings or groups, it is especially important to respect the reasons behind a person's capacity to feel their body. Offering consistent practices, such as a body scan that is repeated over time in the same sequence, can help clients to gradually relax their nervous systems, gaining more access to the interoceptive sense.

As noted above, children and young adults with developmental challenges or sensory-processing disorders may be hypersensitive to stimuli, but they may also be unable to identify and label feeling states. Additionally, for some people with learning and other developmental challenges, including autism, levels of anxiety may be high. The sense of not feeling safe in the world can interfere with the capacity to turn attention inward, as the system is constantly scanning the environment on high alert.[22] Repeated practices of body scanning, with explicit and predictable directions that turn attention away from the incoming stimulus of the outside world and into the felt sense of the body, may reduce anxiety.

The effect of trauma

One of the hallmarks of trauma is dissociation, or disconnecting from body sensations and essentially taking leave of the body. Varying degrees of dorsal vagal shutdown are a natural response when the body and mind are overwhelmed with challenging situations. Although a dissociative state can help someone to survive horrific experiences, in the long term they might have difficulty accessing the body and a persistent tendency toward dissociation even when there is no immediate threat to survival.

At least one research study also suggests that trauma history negatively affects interoceptive ability.[23] One pathway to healing from traumatic events or circumstances is to gradually befriend the sensations of the body, developing greater interoceptive skill and (re)learning to trust the body's wisdom.

Coordination with other healthcare professionals

As healthcare professionals weave practices that utilize interoception into their work, yoga therapists can provide guidance regarding specific practices and methods of inquiry to support patients. As an increasing number of healthcare professionals receive yoga training, education as to how to incorporate those practices more specifically into standard treatment can be valuable. Conversely, yoga therapists might serve as a referral option for mental health professionals. Healthcare professionals may offer yoga therapists valuable information about a client's capacity to make use of therapeutic practices. Respectful collaboration between professionals to augment the understanding of each can be of great benefit.

Yoga therapists who do not have training as mental health practitioners should develop collaborative relationships with other professionals who can serve as consultants and referral options. It is also important to recognize when a client has significant mental or physical health challenges that exceed the scope of practice of yoga therapy. The yoga therapist's own interoceptive sense of discomfort with a particular client is one clue as to whether the yoga therapist has the ability to address the needs of that client. Yoga therapists have an ethical responsibility to note when challenges are outside their scope of practice (e.g., a client with severe depression and suicidal ideation who has not consulted a licensed mental health provider).

Summary

It is important for yoga therapists to continue to track the newest research in the field. An understanding of interoception as a tool for survival and self-care is also essential for the cultivation of a personal practice that enables the successful integration of skills and intuition. The ability to deeply sense and feel the infinite world of messages coming from the physical body is the essential link to healing in a mind-body approach. Yoga therapy supports self-agency through inquiry that develops clients' discernment of what is right for them.

Additional Resources

Ceunen, E., Vlaeyen, J. W., & Van Diest, I. (2016). On the origin of interoception. *Frontiers in Psychology*, *7*, 743.

Dunn, B. D., Galton, H. C., Morgan, R., Evans, D., et al. (2010). Listening to your heart: How interoception shapes emotion experience and intuitive decision making. *Psychological Science*, *21*(12), 1835–1844.

Farb, N., Daubenmier, J., Price, C. J., Gard, T., et al. (2015). Interoception, contemplative practice, and health. *Frontiers in Psychology*, *6*, 763.

Füstös, J., Gramann, K., Herbert, B. M., & Pollatos, O. (2013). On the embodiment of emotion regulation: Interoceptive awareness facilitates reappraisal. *Social Cognitive and Affective Neuroscience*, *8*(8), 911–917.

Miller, R. C. (2015). *The iRest program for healing PTSD: A proven-effective approach to using yoga nidra meditation and deep relaxation techniques to overcome trauma.* New Harbinger Publications.

Pearson, N. (2019). Interoception: A nuanced look within. *Yoga Therapy Today*, Winter, 24–26.

Sullivan, M., & Robertson, L. C. H. (2020). *Understanding yoga therapy: Applied philosophy and science for health and well-being* (pp. 143–153). Routledge.

van der Kolk, B. (2015). *The body keeps the score: Brain, mind, and body in the healing of trauma.* Penguin Books.

Appendix 16A: 1:2 Breath Practice for Calming the Autonomic Nervous System and Activating the Parasympathetic Nervous System

1. Sit upright, with eyes open or closed.
2. Inhaling, sense the breath moving down, expanding the diaphragm in all directions.
3. Exhaling, sense the diaphragm contracting and moving up, as the breath moves up and out.
4. Repeat this several times, turning attention to the sensations of the breath in the body. On the exhalation, gently contract the belly to release as much breath as possible without strain.
5. On the next exhalation, slow the exhalation so that it becomes longer than the inhalation. If it is helpful, count the length of the inhale and exhale, for example inhaling for 3 and exhaling for 5 or 6.
6. Continue to breathe, extending the exhalation so that there is 1:2 ratio of inhalation to exhalation. To the degree that you can, add a pause at the end of the exhale. Notice the effect on your body and mind as you continue this breath ratio.

When teaching *pranayama* practices, it is important to go slow enough to enable clients to gently guide the breath rather than straining to do so. The focus is on the felt sense of the breath in the body and on the client noticing the effects so that they can assess for themselves what is helpful.

Appendix 16B: Introducing a Body Scan

Instructions should be given slowly, allowing 10–15 seconds between each invitation.

1. Sit or lie down, with eyes open or closed. Settle the body into the feeling of the support underneath you. Take a few breaths, exhaling as fully as you can without strain.
2. Now take attention to the palm of the right hand. Notice what sensations are present—a sense of heat or coolness, a tingling, a pulse, a vibration, an effervescence of sensation...allowing whatever is there with a sense of welcoming curiosity.
3. As you feel the right palm, you might notice if your eyes are visualizing the hand. To the degree that you can, let the visual image of the palm dissolve or fade. Notice how sensation may change. Perhaps the sensation feels even more alive.
4. Notice what happens to the thinking mind as you take attention to the hand.

(Note: One could add other areas of the body if time allows. As we take the visual image away, our attention becomes even more alive to the subtle sensations in the body. Thoughts often slow down, with more space between them.) Richard Miller offers a variety of body sensing/body scan practices that can be incorporated into work with clients.[24]

Appendix 16C: Questions to Begin Interoceptive Inquiry

These simple directions can start the process of exploring sensation with oneself or with clients. Take time with each step and linger as long as you like.

With eyes open or closed, feel the surface you are sitting or lying on, noticing the sense of the body touching the surface.

- Direct attention to the breath. As you inhale, feel the sensation of breath as it moves from the nostrils, into the throat, down into the lungs. Notice the expansion of the belly. Notice any other sensations that accompany the movement of breath. As you exhale, feel the sensation of breath as it moves up through the chest, into the throat, and out through the nose (or mouth). (This can be repeated several times so that each cycle of breath serves to awaken the felt sense of the breath moving in the body.)

- Sense the beat of the heart. Notice whether it is slow and steady or more rapid.
- Notice sensation in the hand. (Closed eyes may enable stronger perception of sensation, whereas open eyes may be more useful when dealing with fear or rumination.) Allow your attention to rest there. Sense if there is a warmth or heat, a vibration, or other sensations. Rest attention there for a few more seconds, and notice how sensation may come more alive as you notice what is present.
- If other sensations arise in the exploration, you can offer the invitation to explore whatever is present. If there is pain, you might suggest that the person turn attention *toward* the area that has strong sensation to the degree to which they are able. It can be useful to substitute the word "sensation" for "pain." Explore the sensation: How tight is it, does it have a shape, a temperature, a texture? Is there an outer boundary to this sensation? You might also invite the person to notice what areas of the body are more comfortable or where the sensation is less intense.
- If an emotion is showing up, you might invite the person to notice where they feel that emotion most strongly in the body. "As you feel this sensation, how might you describe it? Does it have a temperature, a texture, a size, a shape? Are there any other words that might describe this sensation?" We are always giving the client a choice about whether to stay with what is present, and for how long.

Endnotes

1 Khalsa, S. S., & Lapidus, R. C. (2016). Can interoception improve the pragmatic search for biomarkers in psychiatry? *Frontiers in Psychiatry*, *7*, 121.

2 Paulus, M. P., & Stein, M. B. (2010). Interoception in anxiety and depression. *Brain Structure and Function*, *214*(5–6), 451–463.

3 Cameron, O. G. (2001). Interoception: The inside story—A model for psychosomatic processes. *Psychosomatic Medicine*, *63*(5), 697–710.

4 Haase, L., Stewart, J. L., Youssef, B., May, A. C., et al. (2016). When the brain does not adequately feel the body: Links between low resilience and interoception. *Biological Psychology, 113*, 37–45.

5 Gazzaniga, M. S. (1998). *The mind's past.* University of California Press.

6 Hayes, S. C., Strosahl, K. D., & Wilson, K. G. (2012). *Acceptance and commitment therapy: The process and practice of mindful change* (2nd ed.). Guilford Press.

7 Sullivan, M. B., Erb, M., Schmalzl, L., Moonaz, S., Noggle Taylor, J., & Porges, S. W. (2018). Yoga therapy and polyvagal theory: The convergence of traditional wisdom and contemporary neuroscience for self-regulation and resilience. *Frontiers in Human Neuroscience, 12*, 67.

8 Dana, D. (2018). *The polyvagal theory in therapy: Engaging the rhythm of regulation.* W. W. Norton.

9 HRV refers to the heart rate's natural fluctuations when the PNS is dominant; see, e.g., Sullivan, M., & Robertson, L. C. H. (2020). *Understanding yoga therapy: Applied philosophy and science for health and well-being* (p. 140). Routledge: "In this resting state, the heart rate naturally increases on the inhale and decreases on the exhale. In a sympathetically dominant state, this variability decreases or disappears."

10 Minassian, A., Maihofer, A. X., Baker, D. G., Nievergelt, C. M., et al. (2015). Association of predeployment heart rate variability with risk of postdeployment posttraumatic stress disorder in active-duty Marines. *JAMA Psychiatry, 72*(10), 979–986.

11 Gendlin, E. T. (2007). *Focusing.* Bantam Books.

12 Miller, R. (2018). *Integrative Restoration iRest yoga nidra meditation training manual* (v. 5). Anahata Press.

13 Aurobindo, S. (1996). *The synthesis of yoga* (pp. 479–480). Sri Aurobindo Ashram Trust.

14 Mahler, K. (2015). *Interoception: The eighth sensory system.* AAPC Publishing.

15 Fahri, D. (2003). *Bringing yoga to life: The everyday practice of enlightened living.* HarperCollins.

16 Chen, S., Sun, P., Wang, S., Lin, G., & Wang, T. (2016). Effects of heart rate variability biofeedback on cardiovascular responses and autonomic sympathovagal modulation following stressor tasks in prehypertensives. *Journal of Human Hypertension, 30*(2), 105–111.

17 Russell, M. E., Scott, A. B., Boggero, I. A., & Carlson, C. R. (2017). Inclusion of a rest period in diaphragmatic breathing increases high frequency heart rate variability: Implications for behavioral therapy. *Psychophysiology, 54*(3), 358–365.

18 Kalyani, B. G., Venkatasubramanian, G., Arasappa, R., Rao, N. P., et al. (2011). Neurohemodynamic correlates of "OM" chanting: A pilot functional magnetic resonance imaging study. *International Journal of Yoga, 4*(1), 3–6.

19 Brewer, J. A., Worhunsky, P. D., Gray, J. R., Tang, Y. Y., Weber, J., & Kober, H. (2011). Meditation experience is associated with differences in default mode network activity and connectivity. *Proceedings of the National Academy of Sciences of the United States of America, 108*(50), 20254–20259.
Raichle, M. E., MacLeod, A. M., Snyder, A. Z., Powers, W. J., Gusnard, D. A., & Shulman, G. L. (2001). A default mode of brain function. *Proceedings of the National Academy of Sciences of the United States of America, 98*(2), 676–682.

20 Kalyani et al., Neurohemodynamic correlates.

21 US National Center for Complementary and Integrative Health. (2016). Relaxation techniques for health. https://nccih.nih.gov/health/stress/relaxation.htm

22 Mahler, *Interoception.*

23 Schaan, V. K., Schulz, A., Rubel, J. A., Bernstein, M., et al. (2019). Childhood trauma affects stress-related interoceptive accuracy. *Frontiers in Psychiatry, 10*, 750.

24 See, e.g., Miller, R. C. (2015). *The iRest program for healing PTSD: A proven-effective approach to using yoga nidra meditation and deep relaxation techniques to overcome trauma* (pp. 62–79). New Harbinger Publications.

17

Bridging Cultural Gaps in Yoga Therapy

ROBERT H. STUCKY

Healing is experientially transcultural. The challenge for yoga therapists working with clients from other traditions is to be able to bridge the gap between terminology and understanding in ways that respect the client's tradition without requiring a dilution or distortion of the therapist's medium. In this necessarily mutual endeavor, the client may better receive the full benefit of the yogic insights offered, and the therapist may have their own experience and understanding reinforced and enlarged by the exchange.

Articulating what is meant by specific terminology is essential to bridge cultural gaps. Yoga therapists may assume that a client who has chosen specifically a *yoga* therapist may have some inclination toward spirituality, even if that may be only vaguely defined. That inclination may create conflicts between the client's notions of the yogic traditions and their cultural upbringing. As the American Sufi Sam Lewis pointed out, "The concept of spirituality has nothing to do with spirituality—it has to do with concepts. That's an entirely different subject."[1] In the United States, even the concept of spirituality is frequently misperceived as a foreign or "new age" religion that threatens or contradicts the Judeo-Christian values underpinning mainstream culture.

Religion and Spirituality

Religion and spirituality are not synonymous. Religion is the structural offshoot of spirituality. Religion provides a frame of reference in which to understand, share, and nurture life's noetic[2] spiritual experiences while providing an applicable sense of meaning and higher purpose. At its worst, religion becomes a tool of manipulation based on rewards and punishments, using intimidation and fear that confuses conformity of belief, practice, or behavior with universal recognition and acceptability of experience.

Institutional religion can be self-contradictory, becoming exclusive rather than inclusive, thereby driving the individual away from the unitive experience it professes rather than toward it.[3] Spirituality, on the other hand, like the very breath it implies, is integral to all human life and knows no cultural or institutional boundaries.[4] Nevertheless, if misunderstood, an emphasis on spirituality can encourage escapism and indulgence in fantasy that frustrates the individual's ability to function in the world. (When used to avoid addressing difficult or unpleasant aspects of oneself or one's environment this imbalance becomes "spiritual bypassing.")

Many people turn to clergy or psychotherapists to sort out the sometimes confusing relationship between these two powerful shapers of life experience. Unfortunately, regardless of their tradition, those who are presumed to facilitate noetic experience and its integration into everyday life may be untrained and inexperienced in the inner experiential "mystical" dimension. Neither seminaries nor graduate schools teach the subtleties of spiritual practice and experience, and some even deem them heretical threats to both psychological and religious orthodoxy. The clergy and psychotherapists, through no fault of their own, may end up being rather like the blind men asked to describe the elephant standing before them, each one describing the part they touch as if it represented the whole. Those who purport to be religious leaders, spiritual teachers, or healers run this risk regardless of institutional or lineage affiliation.

Multifaceted Spirituality in the Context of Healing

Such cognitive dissonance may constitute a subconscious or even unconscious element in therapeutic encounters and therefore needs to be acknowledged and understood. To get a full picture of spiritual reality as it pertains to health and healing, exploring more than one perspective can be helpful for both yoga therapist and client. The corrective lens of each perspective can shed light and clarity on the other without compromising the integrity of either.

One of the Latin titles of the Bishop of Rome (the Pope) is *Pontifex Maximus*, generally translated as Supreme Pontiff, but meaning literally "the greatest bridge-builder." It is worth contemplating the nature of bridge-building. From an engineering standpoint, it is necessary to understand the strength and stability of each shore, as well as the depth and nature of the gulf to be crossed. Obviously, the wider and deeper the apparent chasm, the more difficult the challenge and the more important it is to understand the ground of being on which the bridge is built. This is as true psychospiritually as physically. In the Gospel of Matthew (7.24–27), for example, Jesus exhorts his followers to apply his teachings to their lives on the solid ground of understanding to avoid the hazards of building their lives on a faulty foundation of sand.

Applying the metaphor to the field of yoga therapy, the yoga therapist must understand the client's background and their own. A yoga therapist who is unfamiliar with the religious beliefs and practices of the client (even if that person is more culturally conditioned than observant) may miss essential clues and opportunities for helping that person to gain a deeper understanding of healing. Given the propensity for spiritual teachers to speak in parables and teach anecdotally, becoming familiar with folklore, teaching stories, and accounts of masters and saints from many different traditions can be illuminating and helpful.[5] The well-documented history of master-disciple relationships as an experiential mode of learning is a therapeutically fruitful subject to explore.[6] In examining the phenomenology of basic practices and beliefs, it is quickly apparent that archetypes and parallels run through all recorded traditions.[7]

It is essential to avoid confusion by seeming differences in terminology or praxis; although a variety of words can describe these experiences, most of those words have direct equivalents in other languages. *Rice*, *chawal*, *riz*, and *arroz* all connote the same thing to different people, no matter how they may season it, and human beings tend to experience things in similar ways, no matter where or when they live, what language they speak, or what they believe. The dynamics of basic human motivators—desire, love, hunger, fear, the need for belonging—have been consistent throughout history, as is clear in world literature, art history, and archeological evidence.

Universal Phenomena

Viewed from the Darwinian evolutionary perspective, behaviors that have survived for millennia hold some positive value for survival or they would presumably have died out eons ago. Although the constituents may vary, it is no accident that there are behaviors and practices common to all religious and spiritual traditions, as discussed below.

All religious traditions and schools of spiritual practice also share the idea that there exists something greater than the individual self. That Something, by whatever name or names it is called, influences people's lives and contributes context and meaning to them. It is, moreover, presumed that it is possible in some meaningful measure for the individual to be in "right relationship" and experience oneness with that greater being, finding fulfillment in that mystical union.

The very etymology of the word *religion*—from Latin *re-ligare*, to tie again—implies an original experiential union between the individual and the Absolute that has somehow been severed but can be rejoined by deliberately yoking the individual's awareness to that higher understanding. The word *yoga* (from the Sanskrit root *yuj*, to join together) and the English word *yoke* (as of oxen) share the same root meaning and spiritual implications. Consider this quote ascribed to Jesus, the West's ultimate guru figure: "Take my yoke [yoga] upon you, and learn from me; for I am gentle and humble in heart, and you shall find rest for your souls" (Matthew 11.29).

The case can be made that Jesus' teachings are a path of yoga.[8] In Sanskrit, the term *yoga* means both the state of union between the individual and the Absolute Consciousness and the means by which that union is achieved. The parallelism of Jesus' exhortation suggests that seekers contemplate what might be considered universal yogic principles; these unitive practices form connecting threads in the tapestry of human spirituality depicting the *imago Dei*, the human being created in the image and likeness of God (Genesis 1.27).[9]

The purpose and effects of several powerful yogic practices seem to be transcultural: chant, prayer, meditation, ritual, sacrifice, the study of sacred texts and teachings, and apprenticeship to a spiritual master; selfless service and compassion for the suffering, the needy, the poor, the hungry, widows, orphans, and those in mourning; purity of thought, body, and action; right livelihood; moral values such as humility, honesty, justice, mutual respect, and compassion; and, arguably, reverence for the environment entrusted to human stewardship. These behavioral guidelines ensure social stability. These tenets are also fundamental to both individual and collective human fulfillment and well-being. They appear in one form or another in every tradition throughout history (e.g., the *yamas* and *niyamas* of Raja Yoga, eightfold path of Buddhism, *mitzvot* of Judaism, injunctions of Christian catechism). Understanding their proper application (orthopraxy) is fundamental to optimal outcomes.

The phenomenon of liturgy in Christianity provides an example. Liturgy (from the Greek *leitourgia*, "the work of the people") is the consciousness-transforming exercise of the rituals and content of public worship. For example, Christians of Catholic tradition (Roman, Eastern Rite, Coptic, Maronite, Lutheran, or Anglican) follow a specific shape and sequence of prayers, gestures, chants, and scriptural readings designed to prepare, purify, and lead worshippers to a unitive experience with the Divine in the act of holy communion. Through the blessing and ritual consumption of the bread and wine representing the body and blood of Christ, the deity literally enters the worshipper and they become one, empowering the faithful to lead a life of right relationship with God, neighbor, and self.

Likewise, in Judaism, congregants engage in rituals that include the reverential covering of the head, touching or kissing the sacred Torah scrolls, *davening* (reciting) prayers, chanting scripture and listening to commentary exhorting a life of righteousness, singing hymns in praise of the Almighty and in recognition of humanity's dependence on the Divine will, and the ritual sharing of food and drink.

Muslims doing daily *salat*, whether alone at home or in community in the mosque, engage in a specific series of gestures and postures, from the *Adhan* calling them to the purifying ablutions and prayer to bowing the head to the ground, denoting humility and surrender to Allah while reciting Qur'anic prayers, listening to the chanting of sacred texts by the Imam, and reflecting on the text's or sermon's applicability to daily life.

Hindus remove their shoes, entering the temple with hands folded in reverence, *pranaming* (bowing the head to the ground), devoutly touching the feet of the sacred *murtis* (statues), chanting hymns of praise in *arati* as lights and incense are waved, honoring the divine presence in the image in the sanctuary, coming forward to receive *prasad* (blessed food), and sitting in meditation to silently imbibe the wisdom presumed to emanate from that holy space.

The patterns of all of these acts, and their infinite variations, are designed to bring the individual's heart and mind into focus, put the body at receptive rest, and open the worshipper to a transcendental experience of connectedness, not only with the Divine, but also with fellow worshippers, all creatures, and the whole of creation. From Neolithic times to the present, ritual has played an essential role in cementing social bonds from generation to generation, granting a glimpse of the transcendence that humanity is hard-wired to seek and inspiring the term *neurotheology* as a scientific descriptor.[10]

Invitations to Harmony in Clinical Practice

Worship originally meant "to endow with worth." Historically, worship has been both an individual and communal means of valuing life and honoring its source. Liturgy, properly engaged and understood, is a regular invitation to and evocation of restorative harmony. Why are certain gestures, sights, sounds, and symbols consistently pressed into transcultural service to elicit positive changes of consciousness? Why does their repetition strengthen the experience of those changes? The subjective answers to these questions can best be explored experientially through practice.

For example, a Christian client who resists not being in charge in daily life may discover experientially the principle of *ishvara pranidhana* (attunement or surrender to the Absolute) in the "yogic" act of bowing to the ground, or making a full prostration, even though the practice may initially feel uncomfortable. With understanding, the same person might recognize a similarity to the rituals of genuflecting or kneeling before an altar and find it liberating to discover the gift of humility and submission to higher wisdom in such gestures. A devout Jew who puts on a *tallis* (prayer shawl) before prayer might feel put off by a yogini wrapping herself in a *dupatta* before meditation, yet discover that they both instinctively surround themselves in a protective covering that symbolically intensifies, internalizes, contains, and privatizes their following actions, setting them apart from the chaos and distractions of life outside this personal sanctuary.[11]

Yoga therapists can make use of such actions to invite clients to a deeper reflection that is integral to healing and wholeness. (It is worth noting that the English words *wholeness* and *holiness* share a common etymology. The pursuit of holiness is in fact the pursuit of wholeness—the experiential perfection of health, both physical and metaphysical.)

Yoga therapists who are able to recognize cultural parallels between traditions may also help clients awaken to understanding their own traditions in new and enlightening ways that have direct bearing on their healing. For a Christian, Jew, or Muslim brought up on Bible stories and parables, the "idolatrous" world of yoga may appear exotic and alien—until they discover the Biblical and Qur'anic similarities to the yogic tradition. Because experiential learning is often more powerful than text- or lecture-based learning, the yoga therapist has available persuasive tools to elicit positive changes in clients' awareness.

Psychological breakthroughs can often be triggered when the mind's defenses are lowered or caught off-guard. Ironically, the very foreignness of yogic practice to the average Westerner can prove to be an asset rather than an impediment. The yoga therapist can assure clients that every experience has a useful teaching for practitioners who are alert to the possibilities.

For example, playing recordings of chanting, from any tradition, and asking the client to listen attentively while observing how and where the sounds affect them may open doors of perception and emotional connection that can inform yoga therapy work. Listening to a repetitive chant like *Om Namah Shivaya* and asking the client to pay attention to what is happening in the body as the chant goes on, taking note of any pain, release, or flow of energy, is a powerful tool. The client might also be asked to observe the mind's reactions to the chant: Does the mind grow calmer, or perhaps more agitated? What does that suggest to the client about what is really going on inside?

This exploration can become even more powerful if the client is able to actually join in the chant,[12] as the impact is likely multiplied by connecting breath to sound. When the client's own body is the resonator, they can feel a chant's vibrations on a deeper internal level than listening allows. Using this technique, along with the practice of self-inquiry and self-observation, *svadhyaya*, offers clients agency for self-discovery. Interestingly, sacred chants from all traditions often use similar intervals and patterns of sound, and, anecdotally at least, chanters report similar experiences of the benefits of the practice regardless of language, faith, or cultural tradition. Neuroscience supports these experiences through scans indicating the effects of chant on the brain.[13]

Yoga therapists who are well-versed in the catalog of mystical experiences[14] and the phenomenology of spiritual awakening possible through yogic practices can help clients recognize similarities with their own experiences. Such recognition can elicit insights into what is going on internally and interpersonally in a client's life. It can be reassuring and comforting for the client going through an intense period, perhaps with powerful experiences they find disorienting, to know that these experiences place them within a long history of people undergoing spiritual awakenings and transformations. Moreover, the physical and contemplative tools of yoga can offer clients a view of their own background and world with clear, less judgmental eyes, no matter the practices of their family of origin. This in itself may be a healing experience, particularly if someone is dealing with past trauma.

Seeing all experiences as part of a continuum is fundamental to the yogic understanding of *karma* (action) (see Chapter 2). Such a view helps to convert action from something that binds one to its consequences to a liberating force. Showing clients that this is a universal concept can also be powerfully affirming. Jesus saying, "As you sow, so shall you reap," is the summary of the law of karma, as is Rabbi Hillel's injunction, "That which is hateful to you, do not do to your fellow. That is the whole Torah; the rest is commentary; go and learn" (Shabbat 31a, Babylonian Talmud). The Qur'an, the Buddha, Confucius, and Lao Tze all said as much.

Summary

To enable them to serve clients with integrity it is incumbent on every yoga therapist to redouble their own yogic practice and become conversant in its parallels with other traditions. That, too, is *sanatana dharma*, the universal teachings. Working with clients to make judicious use of what is culturally familiar fulfills the definition of yoga as skill in action.

As we come full circle, it is worth keeping in mind that, etymologically, *therapy* implies a curing, healing, or service done to the sick. Building a bridge of understanding that allows the client and therapist to cross comfortably and safely from one worldview and frame of reference to another is an enormous service. Moreover, when one of those worldviews is the treasury of knowledge and experience implicit in the word *yoga*, traversing that bridge offers clients both the theoretical and experiential means to heal old wounds and discover an inner balance that supports lasting well-being. Being sensitive not only to the yogic wisdom and tools being offered, but also to the personal and cultural history through which the client may view them, is most likely to bring about optimal therapeutic outcomes.

BOX 17.1 BEING WITH THE DYING AS A YOGA THERAPIST

JENNIE LEE

When a soul embodies in human form, a process of identification as a physical being begins. Over a lifetime, through the many stages of human development well-documented in traditional psychology, this identity evolves. At the end of each lifetime, when the physical body dies, those who have known themselves *only* in this way suffer greatly, believing in the annihilation of self.

Yogic philosophy, as expounded in the Vedic and post-Vedic literature such as the *Yoga Sutras* and the *Bhagavad Gita*, offers more about who embodied beings truly are. These sources explain true nature as spiritual in essence, part of the One, all-pervading consciousness or energy, manifest and unmanifest in the Universe. The goal or purpose of yogic *sadhana* is to expand awareness into this eternal, non-physical identity, reuniting soul with Spirit and disidentifying Self with limited mortal nature. Those who achieve this higher state of understanding would be expected to experience far less, if any, suffering when the physical body passes away.

With modern pain management interventions available to relieve the discomforts of a dying body, suffering in relation to death is often more psychological than physiological. Like long-caged birds habituated to confinement, most people are reluctant to leave the bodies to which they have become accustomed. Even if the body is aged, broken, or diseased, there remains an attachment to it and a forgetfulness of one's omnipresence and freedom.

In the *Yoga Sutras*, Patanjali describes this forgetfulness with which all incarnate beings struggle. He termed the five aspects of forgetfulness *kleshas*, or coverings over the divine being. As described in Chapter 3, the kleshas are

- ***avidya:*** individual delusion (ignorance)
- ***asmita:*** ego, or the body-identified state of the soul
- ***raga:*** attachment to what one likes (desire)
- ***dvesha:*** aversion to what one does not like
- ***abhinivesha:*** body attachment or fear of physical death

These difficulties are experienced throughout life, and suffering occurs as a result of the perceived separation from one's spiritual essence. As death draws near, however, this suffering may come to a dramatic climax. A primal psychological fear of death exists, related in people to fear of leaving the "I" or personal identity, the ego's body-circumscribed human nature. Added to this are the fear of and aversion to physical pain, concerns for those being left behind, attachments to known places and to loved ones, relationships left unresolved, and other regrets.

How yoga therapy may help

In support of those transitioning through death, yoga therapists need to bring less technical acumen and more simple humanity. Therapeutic skills such as deep listening and holding compassionate space are essential. The end of life is not a time for providing solutions or imposing personal perspectives, beliefs, or desires.

Yoga therapists must be present at a feeling level with clients, attempting to understand and empathize with whatever arises. They must also face their own fear of death and other limiting beliefs about what comprises true being.

"When this 'I' shall die, then will I know who am I," wrote Paramahansa Yogananda.[15] This teaching affirms that the more one practices disidentification with and non-attachment to the body, seeking instead to know the eternal nature of Self, the less fear and suffering will accompany both life and the time of death. The return from individual expression of being to the expansive state of pure unified consciousness can indeed be easeful.

Useful practices

The first and most important aspect of any yoga therapy session is to provide clients with a compassionate space in which they can explore what is arising internally. Open-ended questions enable people to examine their thoughts and beliefs and address their fears.

Creating loving, non-judgmental space for clients to explore their spiritual experience can allow much healing and integration. Useful aids are inclusive language rather than religion-specific terminology and an understanding that yogic philosophy honors the divinity within all creation.

Examples of helpful questions include

- Do you believe you are more than this body?
- Would you like to talk about your spiritual beliefs?
- Do you believe in something greater than self, and if so, what do you believe is the nature of it?
- What do you believe happens after you die?
- Are you afraid?
- What brings you a sense of peace?
- How can I help?

As in any yoga therapy setting, practices that calm the mind and the nervous system, appropriate to the client's physical capacities, should be offered. A gentle *pranayama* like *sama vritti* (rhythmic, balanced breathing) is usually possible and helps to regulate emotional states of fear and anxiety.

Repetition of mantra or the invocation of peace through simple affirmations can also soothe a troubled mind. Again, words or phrases that align with the client's religious or spiritual beliefs are essential.

To assist clients in attuning with the transcendent essence of their being, yoga therapists can direct the inner awareness to the third eye as one might in meditation. If a person is unable to concentrate there, a gentle caress to the center of the forehead, when possible, may help. This point is considered a portal to expanded awareness, and focusing energy there relaxes the mind in the same way that concentrating on the breath eases the body.

Perhaps most important is reassuring the person of the continuity of life beyond the physical dimension in accordance with yogic teachings. In these simple yet profound ways, yoga therapists can convey deep truth combined with gentle care to clients as they exchange physical form for the unlimited, eternal Self.

Additional Resources

James, W. (2016). *The varieties of religious experience*. CreateSpace.

Maharaj, V. T. (1980). *Devatma shakti (kundalini): Divine power* (5th ed.). Yoga Shri Peeth Trust.

Malki, S., & Stucky, R. H. (2014). *Reductionism, globalization and faith: The challenge and opportunity*. New Impact Publishers.

Occhiogrosso, P. (1997). *The joy of sects: A spirited guide to the world's religious traditions*. Image.

Smith, H. (2009). *The world's religions*. HarperOne.

Stucky, R. H. (2017). *The tantric Jesus: Christ as god, guru, and self*. Eastcliff Editions.

See also the works of Karen Armstrong, Diana Eck, Elaine Pagels, Mircea Eliade, and Louis Dupré.

Example sources for aphorisms, parables, and teaching stories

The Wisdom series from New Directions Publishing.

The works of Idries Shah on Sufism, e.g., the World Tales books and *The wisdom of the idiots* (Isf Publishing, 2018).

Endnotes

1 Cohn, A. (Dir.) (1973). *SunSeed—The journey* [film]. FilmFreeway.

2 From the Greek *noēsis/noētikos*, meaning inner wisdom, direct knowing, or subjective understanding. As defined by the philosopher William James in 1902, *noetic* refers to "states of insight into depths of truth unplumbed by the discursive intellect. They are illuminations, revelations, full of significance and importance, all inarticulate though they remain; and as a rule they carry with them a curious sense of authority": James, W. (1929). *The varieties of religious experience: A study in human nature* (p. 371). The Modern Library.

3 See, e.g., the records of the Holy Office of the Inquisition (Archive of the Congregation for the Doctrine of Faith [ACDF] in the Vatican Library); Erhman, B. D. (2011). *The orthodox corruption of scripture: The effect of early Christological controversies on the text of the new testament*. Oxford University Press; Pagels, E. (2004). *Beyond belief: The secret gospel of Thomas*. Vintage; and more recent data from the Pew Research Center on Religion & Public Life (www.pewforum.org).

4 The Latin Vulgate Bible, originally translated by St. Jerome in the late 4th century CE, interchangeably uses the term *spiritus Dei* as both the breath and Spirit of God, as does the Hebrew original *ruach Elohim*. The spirit is thus the force that endows people with life and connects them to the Creator, and spirituality is the practices that promote and enhance that unitive experience of life.

5 See, e.g., Shah, I. (2018). *The wisdom of the idiots*. Isf Publishing; Prakashananda, S. (1995). *Don't think of a monkey and other stories my guru told me*. Sarasvati Productions; Evans-Wentz, W. Y. (2002). *Tibet's great yogi Milarepa: A biography from the Tibetan*. Pilgrims Publishing; and Buber, M. (1995). *The legend of the Baal-Shem*. Princeton University Press.

6 As noted in Chapter 1, however, this relationship embodies a potential for abuse that cannot be ignored.

7 See, e.g., the classic Smith, H. (2009). *The world's religions*. HarperOne; the works of mythologist Joseph Campbell; and Malki, S., & Stucky, R. H. (2014). *Reductionism, globalization and faith: The challenge & opportunity*. New Impact Publishers.

8 For a detailed exploration of the historical, theological, and experiential basis for this contention, see Stucky, R. H. (2017). *The tantric Jesus: Christ as god, guru, and self.* Eastcliff Editions.

9 The notion of humans' participation in divinity is echoed by the sage Shankara in the *Brahma Jnanavali Mala*: "Brahma satyam, jagat mithya, jivo brahmaiva naparaha" (Brahman is real, the universe is mithya [it cannot be categorized as either real or unreal], the jiva is Brahman itself and not different." This can also be translated as "Brahman (the Absolute) is Truth, the world is illusion, the individual self (jiva) is nothing other than the Absolute Self" (20). Sanskritdocuments.org (n.d.). *Brahmajnanavalimala.* https://sanskritdocuments.org/doc_z_misc_shankara/brahmajna.html

10 The term *neurotheology* was first coined by writer Aldous Huxley, and humans' instinctive search for transcendent experience has subsequently been explored in the work of neuroscientists like Andrew E. Newburg, Michael A. Persinger, Benjamen Shapero, and Gaëlle Desbordes. The use of magnetic resonance imaging (MRI) of the brains of people during experiences of spiritual upliftment has led Harvard researchers, for example, to conclude that meditation has a measurably positive effect on the brain and health. See, e.g., Hölzel, B. K., Carmody, J., Vangel, M., Congleton, C., et al. (2011). Mindfulness practice leads to increases in regional brain gray matter density. *Psychiatry Research, 191*(1), 36–43; Lutz, A., Dunne, J., & Davidson, R. (2007). Meditation and the neuroscience of consciousness: An introduction. In P. Zelazo, M. Moscovitch, & E. Thompson (Eds.), *The Cambridge handbook of consciousness* (Cambridge Handbooks in Psychology) (pp. 499–551). Cambridge University Press; and Cahn, B. R., & Polich, J. (2007). Meditation states and traits: EEG, ERP, and neuroimaging studies. *Psychological Bulletin, 132*(2), 180–211.

11 The *Laya Yoga* practice of systematically and intentionally withdrawing the senses from their outer objects, or Jesus' exhortation to inner prayer (Matthew 6.6), makes clear the purpose and rewards of such a practice.

12 To counter the excuse of not having a "good enough voice to chant," and thereby missing out on the practice's full benefits, Swami Muktananda used to tell his devotees, "If you have a bad voice, sing louder! God should know what He's done to you!"

13 Gao, J., Leung, H. K., Wu, B., Skouras, S., & Sik, H. H. (2019). The neurophysiological correlates of religious chanting. *Scientific Reports, 9*(1), 4262.

14 See, e.g., this catalog of the psychospiritual and physical symptomology pursuant to spiritual awakening: Maharaj, V. T. (1980). *Devatma shakti (kundalini): Divine power* (5th ed.). Yoga Shri Peeth Trust.

15 Yogananda, P. (2007). *The yoga of the Bhagavad Gita* (p. 42). Self Realization Fellowship.

Section IIIB Yoga Therapy Tools

This section introduces specific tools and approaches within the vast traditions and practices of yoga therapy. In each chapter, the authors discuss a specific component of yoga and how it might be applied within a therapeutic context. In some cases, this homes in on particular strategies, whereas in others the tools are discussed more broadly.

The section begins at the grossest level of *annamaya kosha* with a discussion of *asana* and how it might be made more accessible to diverse clinical populations, and ends with the application of yoga's ethical tenets applied to self-inquiry and spiritual growth. In between are chapters on *pranayama*, ayurvedically informed yoga tools, *mudra* and *bandha*, yoga nidra, and meditation.

Although the available tools are far broader than this section can present, these chapters allow a deeper dive into the real and varied work of practicing yoga therapists around the world today. Readers are advised to deeply consider how they might apply some of these strategies with yoga therapy clients and how to discern when each approach might best serve the established goals and challenges within each therapeutic relationship. In fact, many of these tools may deepen yoga therapists' own *sadhana* and allow them to better serve clients with authenticity, understanding, and grace. Ultimately, this section encourages critical thinking about the application of yogic tools in yoga therapy practice.

Steffany Moonaz

18

Accessible Asana

JIVANA HEYMAN

Asana is the most popular, and one of the most powerful, tools available to yoga therapists working in Western settings. A paradox inherent in contemporary practice lies in the fact that asana, generally understood to be yoga's physical postures, is simultaneously accessible yet out of reach for many clients. Asana's obvious practicality can make it feel very accessible: The idea that the body can be moved into different shapes to enable the experience of immediate, tangible results is compelling. Unfortunately, contemporary asana teaching often equates advanced yoga with gymnastic ability, diminishing its accessibility.

Ironically, yogic practices that many would consider to be more obviously spiritually oriented, for example meditation and mantra, can feel esoteric and ethereal; practitioners may find them too subtle and complicated. But these practices, if taught in simple ways, may actually be more accessible, because they don't rely on physical ability. Exploring this tension between subtlety and accessibility is essential in making these practices more available to all clients.

This chapter offers techniques for making asana, and, in turn, potentially the entirety of yoga practice, accessible. Most people in the West are initially drawn to yoga because of the physical practice, so it is imperative that yoga therapists have a clear understanding of how to make the practice inviting, safe, and effective for all clients.

Accessibility is an orientation, not an achievable goal. It is impossible to create a single yoga class that is accessible to everyone. In fact, sometimes people's needs are at odds, as when one client's condition requires a warm room and someone else needs a cold room. Similarly, an instruction that works for one person may be wholly ineffective for another, or a practice that supports one client is contraindicated for another.

In one-to-one yoga therapy, the therapist has time to investigate an individual client's needs and abilities. In the context of group classes, appropriate individualization is more complicated. Helping clients to find the variations that work for them is an important skill for yoga therapists, one that stems from the ability to offer practices as a spectrum of possibilities rather than a finite objective.

Bringing in the Yoga

Before focusing on adapting practices, one must consider the purpose of asana practice and of yoga in general. This clarity is the foundation of effective teaching. The yoga therapist's job is not only to give people an experience of yoga; it is also helping them to understand the nature of yoga and to make yoga a part of their lives.

To make asana accessible, the outer form of a pose may need to be released to enable clients to connect to internal experience. Ironically, connecting to the inner energetic experience is a more advanced way to practice. To adapt asana, yoga therapists actually need to take clients into the subtler, and in many ways more advanced, aspects of the practice.

The physical practices in a yoga therapy session may not be immediately identifiable as asana: A chair yoga class might look like a chair exercise class to an outside observer. Questions around what makes a particular physical movement or shape yoga are worth exploring. Is the external form or the inner experience the goal of the practice?

BOX 18.1 WHAT IS ADVANCED YOGA?

Reflect on the following questions:

- If a long-time yoga practitioner gets into an accident and becomes completely paralyzed, can they still practice yoga?
- Can they still practice asana?
- Is there a certain age at which one has to stop practicing yoga?
- Or an age at which one has to stop practicing asana?
- If a senior can still practice asana, but the poses they do become more limited and subtle, does that mean they are less advanced than when they were younger and practiced more physically advanced poses?
- How is "advanced" defined in yoga?

In striking a balance between tradition and innovation, it is possible to connect deeply to the underlying purpose of a practice while the external form changes. For this reason, it is essential that yoga therapists consider some of the basic principles of yoga philosophy when attempting to share yoga in these modern times.

Answering any of the questions posed in Box 18.1 first requires that one look to the yoga teachings to understand what yoga practice is. In Yoga Sutra 1.13, Patanjali explains that "Practice is the effort towards steadiness of mind."[1] This clear and simple definition emphasizes steadiness of mind, or focus, as the way to practice yoga.

Focusing the mind becomes an essential theme in the *Yoga Sutras*. Patanjali explained that the way to practice yoga is by calming the mind, which allows an experience of one's true nature. Yoga is therefore practiced by learning to calm and focus the mind. Asana offers a variety of potential focal points: sensations, breath, *drishti* (a focal point inside or outside the body), a mantra or other meditative technique. Patanjali emphasized the essence of the practice rather than the specific technique; as discussed in Chapter 2, texts describing asana in detail came much later.

This point is specifically addressed in the discussion of asana in three sutras in chapter 2 of the work. After defining asana as a steady, comfortable pose (2.46),[2] Patanjali explained that the way to practice asana is by lessening the mind's natural tendency for restlessness and meditating on the infinite. This sutra (2.47)[3] is essential in understanding the mental component of asana practice. Patanjali described the inner experience of asana—working with the mind to become steady and expansive—rather than focusing on an outward form.

When adapting asana, the practice's element of mental focus must be retained. This intention is the means by which yoga can be brought into a class that may lack the outward appearance of most studio classes. This is also how asana can be practiced if the body has limited movement; a subtler practice of asana can be found on a mental level. The clearer the yoga therapist's understanding of these essential teachings, the more they can integrate yoga into their work in subtle and profound ways.

BOX 18.2 SUN SALUTATIONS IN THE MIND

Lie in *savasana* or another comfortable position, and take a few breaths to ground and relax. Without moving the body, see if you can practice three rounds of sun salutation in your mind. Do your favorite form of the practice, and rather than observing yourself practicing from the outside, see if you can embody the *feeling* of doing the practice. Try breathing the way you do when you practice, and imagine your body moving as it usually does. See if you can stay focused for three full rounds. Then come back to the feeling of lying where you are and notice sensations. Does it feel like you just did your sun salutation practice?

Adapting Asana

Creativity is a key element in adapting asana. Given an understanding of the essential purpose of the practice, variations on the theme can be developed for the person in front of us. Careful attention to language is essential. Words like asana "modification" may subconsciously imply "less than"; more positive or neutral terms like "variation" or "adaptation" can be helpful. Supporting clients' agency over their own bodies, and to discover what works or does not work for them at any given moment, is empowering.

Agency, or the power to make decisions, is an important subtext in a yoga therapy session. The yoga therapist/client power dynamic can create an unconscious bias that leads the client to avoid questioning authority, instead simply doing what they are told. The use of conscious language is the most potent tool for undoing this tendency. Asking questions and offering options, rather than simply giving step-by-step instructions, can lead to a feeling of choice, control, and power.

Often, teachers and therapists tell clients to "find their own version of a pose," but this tactic may fall short, especially in clinical populations. Rather than simply leaving clients to find their own way, offering a selection of options is a more generous approach. Another problem with asking clients to find their own version of a pose is that many will tend to focus on the pose's outer appearance and structure rather than considering the benefits or underlying purpose. The challenge for yoga therapists is to understand the purpose and benefit of a practice and to find ways to offer clients who are practicing at different levels similar benefits, working from the inside out, and inspire them to find their own practice.

When adapting asana, yoga therapists obviously need to keep clients safe while supporting them to explore their own limits and potential. Limiting transitions from floor to chair and chair to standing, understanding common contraindications (e.g., inversions with uncontrolled hypertension), and not judging one form as better or more advanced than another are all helpful points to bear in mind.

The underlying purpose of the term *alignment* in asana practice is also worth considering. Does use of this term mean there is an ideal way to be in a pose?

Is "ideal" alignment a useful concept for bodies that look and move differently, such as in people with disabilities, amputees, seniors, or those with larger bodies? Alternatively, is alignment actually a question of safety? Of energy flow? If the latter are true, alignment will shift and change according to what is safest for the individual client in a particular moment.

Curiosity, creativity, and collaboration

The most important aspects of adapting asana are the attitude of the yoga therapist and the relationship between therapist and client. Approaching the client as a collaborator in an exploration of possibilities can make the therapeutic process more rewarding for everyone involved. Often clients will think of pose variations that the yoga therapist never dreamed of; much can be learned from them, particularly when the yoga therapist remembers that each individual is the leading expert on their own body. Of course, the priority is to keep the client safe, but yoga therapists would also do well to explore whether they can balance their knowledge and experience with the freedom that clients find in their own personal explorations.

Dissect the pose

When offering specific asana to clients, generally it is helpful to begin by considering the benefits of the pose, and to explore why it has been practiced as it is. The pose can then be broken down into elements so that clients can investigate the portions of the pose that are accessible to them. For example, *vriksasana* (tree pose) involves many different actions: balancing, strengthening the supporting leg, externally rotating the hip of the raised leg, shoulder and chest opening according to the arm position, the energetic experience of standing tall in an open position, and more.

To make the pose accessible, the yoga therapist can support the client in experiencing the elements that they can perform and remove those that are inaccessible. For example, using a wall for support in tree pose decreases the element of balance so clients can focus more on the experience of standing on one leg.

Similarly, a client practicing a chair variation of tree pose could potentially get the benefit of strengthening the hip extensors and external rotators and lengthening the adductors from the position of the raised leg and shoulder and chest expansion from the raised arms. From there, the client can be led inward to explore lifting and lengthening like a tree, even in a seated position. This is the inner energetic, subtle experience essential to practicing asana. The yoga therapist may want to consider *why* they are including a particular asana, which will guide the elements of the pose they retain.

Beyond simply adapting a pose to a person's body, variations of poses can be used to offer specific benefits to clients. For example, if someone is working on improving their balance, this aspect of a pose can be either supported or challenged by the chosen variation. If they are practicing tree pose at the wall, they can use the wall to support balance; if they are practicing tree pose in a chair, their balance can be challenged in some other way, maybe by sitting forward in the chair, or by balancing a block in either hand or on top of the head. Adaptions of poses not only fit a person's body but also have specific purposes.

Use props

Props offer ways of adapting the space around the client to fit their individual needs. Props can raise the floor, connect parts of the body, add or relieve pressure, offer support for balance, build structure in the pose, and more. For example, a blanket under the hips when sitting cross-legged, such as in *sukhasana* (easy seated pose), can raise the floor and lower the knees by creating space to anteriorly tilt the pelvis and release hip-flexor tension, making the pose more comfortable.

Props can also change the relationship between parts of the body. A strap around the extended foot in a seated forward bend like *janu sirsasana* (head-to-knee pose) can help a client relax into the pose and avoid straining the lower back. In this example, the strap also creates an energetic structure for the pose. Rather than reaching out into space with the hands, holding a strap connected to the foot can offer a grounded feeling that allows the body to release and let go.

Change orientation/effects of gravity

Another way to adapt an asana is to change the body's orientation in space, thereby changing the way in which gravity affects the body. For example, for someone with tight hamstrings, a seated forward bend such as *paschimottanasana* (westward bend) can be challenging. If the person is straining to sit upright in *dandasana* (staff pose), they are working against gravity to lift and lengthen the spine and therefore may not be able to sufficiently engage the spinal erectors to counteract gravity's effects and move forward without compression. Instead, *uttanasana*, a standing forward bend, offers the help of gravity to move into the pose. Alternatively, *supta padangustasana* (supine hand-to-foot pose) offers a forward bend with the spine completely supported.

Make it dynamic

Sometimes approaching an asana in a different way can make it more accessible. Moving into and out of a pose with the breath dynamically can be a gentler experience than holding a pose in a more static way. For example, coming into *bhujangasana* (cobra) on an inhalation and coming out on an exhalation can be a useful way of exploring the practice and building strength.

Use inner experience

When a form of a pose that works for a client cannot be identified, they might be invited to imagine the pose in their mind. On the one hand, this can feel like an inadequate solution, but on the other hand visualization is an opportunity to explore the inner experience of an asana and offers an opportunity to strengthen concentration in a meditative way. Visualizing a pose or exercise is a subtle and powerful way to practice.[4] Many of the benefits of a pose can be experienced by performing it mentally. Additionally, practicing only in the mind can offer an opportunity to explore the energetics of yoga. The experience of a pose can be felt in the body even as one imagines it.

Integrated Accessible Group Sessions

One essential skill in offering effective group yoga therapy sessions is being able to address individual differences within one session, a key step toward true inclusion of people with disabilities into group classes. Although making an asana work for every client in a group session may seem impossible, therapeutic groups in which people share a common condition or life circumstance are one way to increase yoga therapy's accessibility—and one reason yoga therapy groups should be kept small.

Teaching practices in an integrated manner means teaching to all clients at the same time rather than teaching one level of the practice to one group of clients and then another (usually more gentle) version to a different group of clients. The latter creates a segregated experience in which some clients may think or feel that they are more advanced than the others, and other clients may think or feel that they are less advanced. Ultimately, the goal is to create a unified experience in the group class even when it appears from the outside that clients are all doing different things. This integration creates a powerful feeling of equality rather than hierarchy in the group and enables clients to access the benefits of a community of practice.[5]

It can be especially challenging to teach poses in an integrated manner when some clients are on mats and some are in chairs. Chair yoga, however, offers safe and effective alternatives to asana that may otherwise be inaccessible.

One technique for teaching asana in an integrated manner is to divide the instructions for a pose into three parts to create a moment where all clients are practicing at the same time rather than separately. Cues can be categorized as follows:

1. prepare
2. practice
3. release

The *prepare* portion of the pose is taught at different levels, allowing for separate, clear instruction. If some clients are in a chair and some are on a mat, those in chairs would be instructed to prepare in one fashion, and then those on mats would prepare another way. The yoga therapist would then work to find the right words to teach the *practice* portion in a universal way that applies to all. Finally, the yoga therapist would decide whether clients can all *release* together or instead require separate instructions for coming out of the pose.

This method represents a question of pedagogy—how yoga therapy practices are taught. The general approach and style of teaching are keys to yoga therapy's accessibility and have less to do with the specific asana being taught than with *how* they are being taught. That said, some poses are easier to translate to different levels of practice than others. Generally, simpler practices translate better, such as cobra, tree, seated twist (e.g., *matsyendrasana* variations), *utkatasana* (chair), seated forward bend, sidebending, *navasana* (boat), etc.

A number of poses are difficult to do in chairs. In particular, asana that call for hip extension are challenging to practice in a chair because the sitting posture creates hip flexion. When integrating chair and mat practices, a yoga therapist might therefore avoid poses such as *shalabhasana* (locust), *urdvha dhanurasana* (upward bow), and deep back bends that involve the legs. Consider instead the energetic intention of a deep back bend and determine whether other techniques—a cue in meditation, a mudra—can produce a similar result.

Chair yoga is not always easier, and some practices require significant strength and flexibility to execute in a chair. Speaking about chair yoga in a way that shows respect for the practice, rather than categorizing it as less than, creates an inclusive environment and may foster clients' sense of self-efficacy. Chair practices can also be combined with standing/wall work or bed yoga. These kinds of variations are important for clients who have challenges getting down on the floor. It is essential to avoid pushing people to practice on a mat if there is any chance that they will not be able to easily get back up after class or if they are not ready to address fears related to doing so. However, teaching clients how to transfer from floor to chair is tremendously beneficial in case they fall when they are alone (see Box 18.3).

BOX 18.3 TRANSFERRING FROM FLOOR TO CHAIR

One of the most useful tools for seniors or people with disabilities to learn is how to transfer from floor to chair independently. This skill can release clients from the fear of falling and being helpless. There are many different techniques for making this transfer, and the choice depends largely on where the client has strength or weakness in their body. One method follows.

Find the sturdiest chair you can crawl to. If possible, have the back of the chair against a wall. Crawl to the front of the chair, with padding under the knees if needed. Decide which leg is stronger and step the foot of that leg forward just in front of the chair. Place the forearms on the seat of the chair and lean the body's weight forward, pushing into the foot of the front leg. Try to swivel the opposite hip onto the seat of the chair. It may be helpful to hold on to the arms or back of the chair to help with pulling the body up (although care must be taken not to pull the chair forward off its back legs). Once the hip is on the chair, rotate so the buttocks come fully onto the seat of the chair.

Summary

It is essential for yoga therapists to have a clear understanding of how to make asana accessible to all clients in both individual and group settings. These skills allow clients to get the most out of their yoga therapy experience and offer the gift of yoga to people who previously thought that it was not for them. Understanding the intention behind yoga practice in general, and individual asana specifically, enables yoga therapists to effectively adapt poses and exercises for a range of clients. Tools for creating useful variations include considering individual benefits of poses (e.g., balance work, arm strengthening, confidence-building, energetic effect), using props creatively, changing the pose's orientation or teaching it dynamically, and employing inner experience rather than outward form.

Beyond simply helping people to feel welcome, yoga therapists can work toward active inclusion of marginalized populations and proactively share yoga with communities that are currently not being served. This work begins with the way in which yoga is marketed and used by commercial interests.

The imagery of young, thin practitioners doing physically complex poses sends a powerful message to the general public about what yoga is and who can do it. Consciously using diverse imagery that represents people of different abilities and backgrounds practicing asana can slowly shift this misrepresentation. The language used to market yoga therapy services also speaks volumes about who is welcome or invited into the practice. Pricing is another essential consideration, as yoga therapy may be an expense that many low-income people cannot afford; offering integrated group practices is one way to begin to address this type of inequity.

To be inclusive of people with disabilities, the theory of universal design is a useful way to consider whether yoga is being offered in an accessible fashion. Universal design considers the entire life of a person with a disability when looking at whether a specific service or activity is accessible. For example, is public transportation available to the location of the offerings? Is the building physically accessible, and has its layout considered the needs of people who use wheelchairs or are deaf, blind, or have other disabilities? The many variables mean that it may be best to consult with people with different disabilities, ideally asking them to come to the location and experience it themselves and giving feedback on their experiences.

The benefits of making asana accessible extend beyond the individual to allow yoga therapy to reach communities that are generally excluded from yoga practice. This work is at the heart of sharing yoga in an equitable fashion, expanding the reach of the practice so it can touch the lives of everyone who is interested in releasing stress and connecting with their own heart.

BOX 18.4 YOGA THERAPY WITH AMPUTEES

MARSHA THERESE DANZIG

Amputation is the removal, through surgery or accident, of a limb or limbs. The loss is multilayered, from the physical difference of the musculoskeletal system to the psychosocial differences of body and emotions one experiences within their community. Working therapeutically with amputees requires sensitivity to the whole person rather than a specific focus on issues such as phantom pain or neuromas.

Most people who have had amputations are looking for better balance, range of motion, flexibility, and strength; reduced pain; and a renewed sense of physical competence. They often face fear—fear of falling, injury, stigmatization, limitation, loss of control, or additional health problems. A therapeutic approach of moment-by-moment awareness of sensation and breath can work to soothe those fears, helping amputees to feel more in control of their experience. Yoga therapists must leave limiting thoughts about the capabilities of amputees at the door and focus on possibility. Independence is paramount for an amputee's sense of self.

An estimated 30,000 to 40,000 amputations are performed each year in the United States.[6] Nearly 2 million people in the country live with limb loss, with the number of amputees predicted to double by 2050, largely as a result of increased diabetes prevalence.[7] This means yoga therapists may well have clients who are amputees.

The most common reasons for amputation are diabetes, vascular disease, cancer, accident, congenital limb difference, and sepsis caused by infection. Any yoga therapy practice for an amputee must also address the reasons for the amputation as well as the client's personal preferences and goals.

Amputees are categorized by the level and type of limb loss.

Leg amputations include the following types:

- *below-knee* (transtibial)
- *above-knee* (transfemoral)
- *below-knee single* (unilateral), which is the most common amputation
- *ankle, knee, or hip disarticulation* (an amputation surgery that preserves the joint): These have the advantage of keeping all the tissue surrounding the joint, which allows for more muscle to be preserved for better limb function.[8]
- *hemipelvectomy:* This is an amputation that removes the entire hip and often the ischial tuberosity (sit bone).

Arm amputations include the following types:

- *below-elbow* (transradial)
- *above-elbow* (transhumeral)

- *wrist, elbow, or shoulder disarticulation*
- *forequarter* (including shoulder, clavicle, and entire arm)

Within the amputee population are those who have lost one limb (*unilateral*), two limbs (*bilateral*), three limbs (*trilateral*), and four limbs (*quadrilateral*).

Within these groups, in turn, are variations such as amputees who use wheelchairs, crutches, or prosthetics. The value of a physical yoga practice can be directly affected by the quality and stability of the particular prosthesis or mobility device, which is the result of cost/insurance or the actual fit of the prosthesis or type of mobility device. It should also be noted that amputation of a digit or digits will likewise affect a client's *asana* practice, potentially significantly, and that congenital limb absence or difference can also substantially affect one's practice.

Combining all these factors, working with amputee clients starts with five main concepts:

1. Clients are whole, and all aspects of the practice are designed to help amputees re-remember their wholeness. The yoga therapist adapts to the amputee, rather than the other way around.
2. Focus on the body they do have, not on the missing limb(s).
3. Move from the center to the periphery in all poses, as described below.
4. Help the amputee client develop strong core muscles for better stability and support in transitioning between frontal, transverse, and sagittal planes.
5. Phantom pain, the sensation of pain in the missing limb, can affect up to 80 percent of amputees. Teaching meditation, *pranayama*, and visualization can alter the perception of pain, although preemptively mentioning phantom pain if the client does not bring it up is not recommended.[9]

Setting up the physical practice

The floor, walls, chairs, yoga blocks, and straps all provide necessary feedback for amputees, whose proprioceptive experience and relationship to the physical world will differ from those of four-limbed people.

Most leg amputees wear shoes that are more like an extension of their leg, as the prosthetic is often aligned to the height and direction of the shoe. This means that the ritual of taking off shoes before asana practice may have to change. If a leg amputee is barefoot, that person is often on the ball of the prosthetic foot. Such a position requires tremendous balance as well as an extra measure of care when transitioning between poses; leaning back can have serious consequences for the posterior knee of a below-knee amputee. In such cases, static poses may be more beneficial, with support such as a foam wedge behind the prosthetic heel. Prosthetic feet can be slippery, so if barefoot it may be helpful for the leg amputee to wear non-slip socks or wrap non-skid tape around the ball and heel of the prosthetic foot (as long as the tape will not damage the prosthesis).

Some with lower-extremity amputations will practice without their prostheses. If they are using a wheelchair or crutches, consider those mobility devices as extensions of the client. They may or may not want to incorporate them into their practice. Most importantly, if an amputee is practicing without a prosthesis, they *must* be able to confidently and safely transition from standing to sitting to the floor if the practice involves these level changes. If they are new to transitioning from one surface or orientation to the next, that may require extra work with their physical therapist or with a yoga therapist and an assistant to build the most accessible path to the floor. In general, if an amputee is working without a prosthesis they will use a chair and the floor. Over time, prolonged single-leg standing is not healthy for the remaining limb.

Arm amputees will often work without a prosthesis, as they can be cumbersome. Some prosthetics, which look similar to plungers, have grip and stability that make it possible to put full body weight on the prosthesis without harm to the residual limb or undue pressure on the remaining arm; not all amputees will be able to fully weight-bear on a prosthetic arm.

Falling is one of the main concerns for amputees,[10] so clients may prefer to practice near a wall or two corners for better balance. Have at least one sturdy chair nearby on a non-slip surface such as a yoga mat or wedged against a wall.

When working with an amputee wearing a prosthesis, remember that the prosthesis is extremely expensive and uniquely adapted to the amputee's residual limb. Work around the prosthesis but avoid pressing directly on it when possible. For example, placing a hand directly above or below the prosthetic knee of someone with an above-knee amputation may collapse the setting of the prosthesis or torque the pelvis in the prosthetic socket. Collaborate with the client to find out how they feel about having their prosthesis touched; remember that like any other body part, the client has total agency over the prosthesis. As with any touch, always ask whether it is okay to touch the prosthesis or residual limb.

Assessment

An amputee wanting to practice yoga can arrive with any fitness level. An active athlete may value independence and collaboration with the yoga therapist, whereas a less active, new, or physically ill amputee will have different needs. Assessment is crucial to determine the appropriate focus. For example, an amputee with addiction, posttraumatic stress disorder (PTSD), and phantom pain should have the challenge they perceive to be the most acute addressed first.

As for any client, assessment should begin with range of motion, balance, ease of transition from one plane to another, lifestyle habits, support network, and emotional concerns. Next, whether working with someone who has had an upper- or lower-extremity amputation, look to the hips. For example, is one hip pressed forward, tilted up, dipping down? There are many possible reasons behind such findings, such as arthritis in the hip, a socket misalignment, or a prosthetic foot and ankle that do not bend. Pelvic position provides key information on how the amputee is managing their alignment.

Note that *alignment* is always a relative term, but especially after limb loss as the body adapts with its own interpretation. Adaptations may include scoliosis, arthritis, compensatory injuries, repetitive movement tension, weight gain, and fit of the prosthesis, which is influenced by any changes in the structure of the body and by wear and tear. Still, practices must always be designed for the whole person rather than being prescriptive and reductionist.

Practice suggestions

One of the best gifts a yoga therapist can give an amputee is clear, step-by-step directions with adaptations prepared in advance. Amputees spend their waking hours adapting to everything, so a mental vacation with caring guidance is usually most welcome. Mental fatigue is an often unnoticed, unreported reality for amputees.[11] Although a co-created practice is still the aim, offering extra cues that offer the mind a break supports independence. Visualizations on ease and grace in daily living may also alleviate mental fatigue.

Many amputees develop their own methods of mindfulness and become quite skilled at listening to their bodies' cues about balance, pain, and stiffness.

Related to the desire for independence and concerns about falling or losing control, those with amputations may want to practice balance, such as variations on crescent lunge, tree, warrior II, chair, and mountain pose.

It is recommended that yoga therapy practices for those with limb loss include easily accessible, uncomplicated pranayama. Three-part *dirgha* and belly breath are relatively easy to master, whereas a practice like *anuloma viloma* (alternate-nostril breathing) can be more challenging.

Nearly everyone can perform spinal movement in the six planes of motion to some degree, whether in a chair or on the floor. This practice promotes spinal health and mobility and teaches amputees to move from their center. Additional poses that teach movement from a stable center to the periphery include five-pointed star, wide-leg forward bend, seated wide angle, locust, and plank variations.

Core work is extremely important, as those with amputations may need specific support for strengthening to perform daily tasks such as getting out of bed, sitting on a toilet, getting dressed, or getting in and out of a car.

In restorative poses like *savasana* (corpse pose), comfort is important. Because so many amputees have learned to adapt to daily discomfort, they may not indicate when they are uncomfortable in relaxation. Not every amputee will be comfortable lying supine, especially if they are wearing a full shoulder prosthesis or above-knee prosthesis that digs into the groin. Lying on the side, inviting the amputee to take off their prosthesis if able to, or sitting in a chair may be better.

Consider asking clients what language they prefer but avoid being overly worried about wording or unusually sensitive to a client's emotional state. As with any other client, an amputee is the yoga therapist's peer, one who can offer a unique reminder of what it means to be a whole person.

Additional Resources

Bondy, D. (2019). *Yoga for everyone: 50 poses for every type of body*. Alpha Publications.

Danzig, M. T. (2018). *Yoga for amputees: The essential guide to finding wholeness after limb loss for yoga students and their teachers*. Sacred Oak Publishing.

Heyman, J. (2019). *Accessible yoga: Poses and practices for every body*. Shambhala Publications.

Yang, I., & Fahey, K. (2020). *Adaptive yoga*. Human Kinetics.

Endnotes

1 Satchidananda, S. (2012). *The yoga sutras of Patanjali* (p. 19). Integral Yoga Publications.

2 Satchidananda, *Yoga sutras* (p. 152).

3 Satchidananda, *Yoga sutras* (p. 154).

4 Slimani, M., Tod, D., Chaabene, H., Miarka, B., & Chamari, K. (2016). Effects of mental imagery on muscular strength in healthy and patient participants: A systematic review. *Journal of Sports Science and Medicine, 15*(3), 434–450.

5 Davis, A., Taylor, J., & Cohen, E. (2015). Social bonds and exercise: Evidence for a reciprocal relationship. *PLoS ONE, 10*(8), e0136705.

6 Hanyu-Deutmeyer, A. A., Cascella, M., & Varacallo, M. (2020). Phantom limb pain. StatPearls. www.ncbi.nlm.nih.gov/books/NBK448188

7 Ziegler-Graham, K., MacKenzie, E. J., Ephraim, P. L., Travison, T. G., & Brookmeyer, R. (2008). Estimating the prevalence of limb loss in the United States: 2005 to 2050. *Archives of Physical Medicine and Rehabilitation, 89*(3), 422–429.

8 Baumgartner, R. F. (1979). Knee disarticulation versus above-knee amputation. *Prosthetics and Orthotics International, 3*(1), 15–19.

9 Dijkstra, P. U., Geertzen, J. H., Stewart, R., & van der Schans, C. P. (2002). Phantom pain and risk factors: A multivariate analysis. *Journal of Pain and Symptom Management, 24*(6), 578–585.
Hanyu-Deutmeyer et al., *Phantom limb pain.*

10 Geurts, A. C., Mulder, T. W., Nienhuis, B., & Rijken, R. A. (1992). Postural reorganization following lower limb amputation: Possible motor and sensory determinants of recovery. *Scandinavian Journal of Rehabilitation Medicine, 24*(2), 83–90.
Miller, W. C., Deathe, A. B., Speechley, M., & Koval, J. (2001). The influence of falling, fear of falling, and balance confidence on prosthetic mobility and social activity among individuals with a lower extremity amputation. *Archives of Physical Medicine and Rehabilitation, 82*(9), 1238–1244.

11 Bhuvaneswar, C. G., Epstein, L. A., & Stern, T. A. (2007). Reactions to amputation: Recognition and treatment. *Primary Care Companion to the Journal of Clinical Psychiatry, 9*(4), 303–308.
Sinha, R., van den Heuvel, W. J., & Arokiasamy, P. (2011). Factors affecting quality of life in lower limb amputees. *Prosthetics and Orthotics International, 35*(1), 90–96.

19

Pranayama

SUNDAR BALASUBRAMANIAN

Pranayama, one of the traditional eight limbs of yogic practice, involves the regulation of the breath as a way to influence the body and the mind. Empowering the physical and emotional/mental systems is a historically perceived benefit of pranayama. The voluntary regulation of one's breathing—explicitly connecting body and mind and possibly serving as a gateway to meditation—is intended to increase vitality and may thereby create the capacity for behavior change.

The South Indian Siddha tradition, which likely began during the Indus Valley Civilization (see Chapter 2), includes numerous literary works by yogis collectively called *Siddhars* (those who attained *siddhis*, or great heights/powers). Siddha philosophy includes four paths to physical and emotional well-being and spiritual growth: (1) *sariyai* (performing one's duties); (2) *kiriyai* (rituals, also called *kriya*); (3) *yogam* (the practice of various types of yoga, including the eight-limbed Ashtanga Yoga, Pariyangi Yoga, Kesari Yoga, etc.); and (4) *jnanam* (the path of wisdom that involves contemplation and self-inquiry).

Pranayama is a tool common to all four of these pathways. Tirumular, a contemporary of Patanjali (both were said to be disciples of Nandhi), indicates the use of pranayama in over 285 verses of the *Tirumantiram*, a poetic work that explains Siddha philosophy.[1] Although the yogic Siddha literature has not yet been fully understood or translated from its original Tamil, this inclusion emphasizes the value of breathing regulation in all four routes to spiritual growth.

According to Siddha philosophy, breathing is the physical process that allows the circulation of life force in ten different forms of awareness of the air, or winds (*vayu*). Of those ten forms, the one called *prana* feeds life specifically via inhalation. Pranayama as a whole deals with voluntary alteration of overall respiration to mindfully modify the awareness of these ten forms of air, including prana. Contemporary yoga largely ignores awareness of the ten vayus, devoting practices mainly to inhalation and exhalation.[2] This chapter draws on a perspective of this broader Siddha tradition.

As breathing can be regulated through a number of methods depending on the school of practice, and individual, time, and other factors, the effects of pranayama on the human system cannot be generalized. For instance, fast-paced breathing exercises may be geared toward increasing the activity/energy level, whereas a slower pace tends to relax the body-mind through cardiovascular and autonomic effects.[3] Even among slow-paced practices, the effects could conceivably vary depending on whether the focus is on the lower or the upper respiratory tract (see Box 7.1).

Biological Mechanisms

Although distinctions among pranayama exercises might appear to hinder efforts to elucidate clear biological mechanisms, the diversity of the techniques provides a range of opportunities to design exercises to target individual systems. For instance, *sheetali pranayama* (rolled-tongue "cooling" breathing)[4] is a slow exercise that may be useful in reducing hypertension,[5] whereas *bhastrika* (bellows breath) is a fast exercise practiced to improve ventilatory functions of the lungs.[6] The biological mechanism(s) behind these two exercises are distinct, with the former decreasing blood pressure and increasing heart rate variability and the latter improving vital capacity and ventilatory volume to improving lung function (see Box 7.1). Vigorous practice of bhastrika along with shoulder/trunk movement is also thought to strengthen trunk musculature.

Initial studies on yoga therapy largely involved a combination of *asana*, pranayama, and meditation to mirror a typical yoga session. Consequently, the results were not attributable to a specific component of yoga. Subsequent studies evolved with the advancement of specific disciplines, for instance meditation with neuroscience, asana with kinesiology, and pranayama with respiratory biology, and mechanistic reviews are now available.[7] Studies in the areas of pulmonary medicine and neuroscience provided important clues as to pranayama's effects, but are limited because of the combinatorial exercises involved. Quantitative analysis of pranayama in human systems remains an underdeveloped area of study.

Novel mechanisms: The salivary induction pathway

Work by Balasubramanian et al. sheds light on the mechanisms behind pranayama's effects by linking the practice with biomarkers.[8] Breathing regulation alters salivary stimulation, and the saliva thus produced exhibits differential expression of biomarkers relevant to normal physiological functions.

Siddha texts suggest that the practice of breathing regulation stimulates "milk" or "nectar" in the body, increasing longevity. Studies on pranayama methods from the *Tirumantiram* showed that the practice stimulated salivation and the following alterations in the salivary biomolecules:

- increased levels of nerve growth factor (NGF)
- induction of immunoglobulin-class molecules, mucin and other glycoproteins, and tumor suppressors
- reduction in proinflammatory cytokines[9]

Based on existing literature on the transport and bioavailability of molecules, these alterations in salivary expression could be linked to changes in overall biological functions, including immune system regulation and neurological health.

Saliva has been recognized to contain several key biomolecules,[10] which include peptides (amino acid chains) and proteins with biological and therapeutic properties. Given the effect of salivary and biomarker stimulation noted above, it is reasonable to conclude that regulating the breathing through the various available pranayama methods can alter biological responses.

Neurological Mechanisms

In addition to the effects on the physical system, the emotional aspects of pranayama are only beginning to be reported in the literature. Studies have found that the effects of pranayama cannot be explained solely by altered blood gas levels (e.g., oxygen and carbon dioxide). Instead, the effects of pranayama could be mediated through the involvement of neural elements and emotion.[11] This notion is supported by alterations in nerve circuits and activities:

- The pre-Bötzinger complex (an area of the brainstem thought to generate respiratory rhythm) contributes to higher attention, cognitive function, and memory; slow breathing may connect this group of neurons to the locus coeruleus (also in the brainstem and key to the physiological stress response) to affect those higher-order brain functions.[12]
- Nasal but not oral breathing is involved in memory consolidation, memory embedding, and memory retrieval; this could be because olfactory bulb neurons are activated by nasal breathing.[13]

- Activation of the default mode network pathway through nasal breathing could in turn activate the hippocampus (part of the limbic system and important for memory) through the piriform cortex ("association cortex").[14]
- Adult neoneurogenesis that occurs in the olfactory bulb and hippocampus, an indicator of neuroplasticity,[15] again suggests the importance of nasal breathing in neuronal pathways.
- Mindful breathing could influence the limbic brain,[16] largely responsible for emotion and memory, rather than the neocortex, which is activated by outward attention.

These points argue that breathing regulation is a potential regulator of the neuronal systems. The influence of breathing on the mind is well-explored in yogic scriptures. The *Tirumantiram* (v. 564), for instance, says that the mind travels on the horse of respiration:

The [mind] is the master of senses five;
He is the head of the body habitat;
There is a steed he rides to his destined goal;
The masterly one the steed carries,
The feeble one it throws away
—That steed the Prana breath is.[17]

Clinical Applications

Pranayama is a tool to alter mind and body—one who wants to control their system should control their breathing. Because of this unique feature, clients who are non-ambulatory or fatigued due to underlying disease or treatment procedures could potentially benefit substantially from pranayama. This possibility is illustrated below using several examples.

Cancer

Cancer may include a number of comorbidities, including anxiety, depression, fatigue, and distress (see Box 7.4). Apart from the physical challenges, the emotional burden can aggravate the overall experience to be overwhelming—irrespective of disease severity and site. Such effects are heavily influenced by socioeconomic factors, including age, gender, ethnicity, living conditions at home, and other demographic features of the patient.[18]

Pranayama was used in a clinical trial among breast cancer patients, showing improvement in symptoms including fatigue and anxiety.[19] Another study involving kriya and pranayama showed an increase in natural killer cells in peripheral blood, indicating improved immune function.[20] However, no large-scale studies in other cancer types, treatment choices, or effects of individual exercises have to date been done. The author's research team conducted a quality-improvement study in participants, consisting of both cancer patients in active treatment and their caregivers.[21] These weekly 20-minute sessions included five pranayama exercises designed to address distress, anxiety, fatigue, and breathing difficulties (Box 19.1).

BOX 19.1 SAMPLE PRANAYAMA PRACTICE WITH CANCER PATIENTS

Bhramari (bee breath), 4 minutes

Sit comfortably or take another position suggested by the yoga therapist. Close or soften your eyes, and look toward the middle of your forehead. Inhale slowly and deeply through the nostrils. Make a humming sound from the base of your abdomen as you exhale as completely as possible. Repeat with long inhalations and exhalations, humming (perhaps experimenting with different tones) on the exhale, for up to 10 minutes. (Humming can be replaced with chanting Om.)

Anuloma viloma (alternate-nostril breathing), 5 minutes

Sit comfortably or take another position suggested by the yoga therapist. Close or soften your eyes, and look toward the middle of your forehead. Fold the index and middle fingers of one hand toward the palm and extend the other fingers. With your thumb (or ring and little fingers), close your right nostril and breathe in slowly and fully through your left nostril. After complete inhalation, close the left nostril with your little and ring fingers together (or thumb) and exhale through your right nostril. At the end of the exhalation, inhale through the right nostril. After the complete inhalation, close the right nostril and breathe out through the left nostril. Inhale through the left nostril. Exhale through the right nostril. Continue this cycle.

Tirumular pranayama, 5 minutes

During tirumular pranayama (a form of *nadi shodhana*), the inhalation-hold-exhalation cycles are measured using a combination of chanting and counting with the fingers. Mentally chant a mantra (e.g., "Om Namashivaya,"

"I'm beautiful") two times (inhalation), eight times (hold), and four times (exhalation). Then, (1) close the right nostril and inhale through the left nostril for two chants; (2) close both nostrils so no inhaled air escapes and hold the breath in this position for eight chants; and (3) open the right nostril and exhale as completely as possible to a count of four chants. Repeat steps 1 to 3. (If you cannot keep up with the timings, inhale fully, hold as long as you can comfortably, and exhale completely.)

Sheetkari (hissing breath), 3 minutes

Sit comfortably or take another position suggested by the yoga therapist, with closed or softened eyes. Bring your teeth together lightly and pull the lips back, just like you are smiling. Inhale slowly and deeply, allowing the air to pass through your teeth with a hissing sound. After complete deep inhalation, close your mouth and exhale slowly and as completely as possible through the nose. This completes one round. Repeat for 3 minutes or longer, as long as you are comfortable.

Ujjayi (ocean-sound or victorious breath), 3 minutes

Gently constrict the throat muscles to make a soft hissing sound with the mouth closed. The yoga therapist will explain how to produce this sound (similar to fogging a mirror with your breath). Inhale and exhale slowly, hearing this sound with eyes closed or softened.

After a single session, patients and caregivers reported that the exercises decreased stress, improved mood, and helped them with relaxation. Moreover, the feedback suggested that the participants would like to continue the exercise if it were provided in a convenient location for a length of time they deemed appropriate.[22]

Scleroderma

Scleroderma, or systemic sclerosis, is a rare autoimmune disease affecting approximately 300,000 people in the United States.[23] This condition is characterized by autoantibodies, skin abnormalities (especially tightening), and multi-organ failure, largely due to fibrosis. Disease progression varies after diagnosis, and the 5- and 10-year mortality rates are 15 percent and 29 percent, respectively.[24]

Although a rare condition, it has been included here because as with other autoimmune conditions, physical limitations may prevent scleroderma patients from attending traditional yoga asana classes; simple, gentle practices that consider the whole person rather than the specific disease state apply across a range of populations. The author therefore started providing gentle chair yoga and pranayama to scleroderma patients through state and national patient education conferences.[25] Practices consisted of 30 minutes of asana (eye movements; wrist, shoulder, and neck rotations; cat-cow; standing locust backbend; forward bend; head-to-knee pose; and spinal rotation) and 30 minutes of pranayama similar to the protocol outlined above for cancer patients.

Respiratory illness

Traditionally, pranayama has been prescribed and used for improving respiration among clients with impaired lung function. Consistent practice of pranayama is thought to prolong longevity.[26] Distinct pranayama exercises might be used to address the effects of different lung conditions. For example, chronic obstructive pulmonary disease (COPD) results in dyspnea (shortness of breath) and decreased exercise tolerance. In a small double-blind randomized controlled trial, three-part *dirgha* (long) pranayama improved exercise tolerance in COPD patients, possibly because of facilitated lung emptying and relaxation.[27]

Acute disturbances to the upper respiratory system on exposure to allergens or due to hyperresponsiveness to other physiological challenges (e.g., cold temperatures) could potentially be managed or prevented using sustained pranayama because the practices may attenuate cytokine induction. Asthma, for example, results in dyspnea, decreased exercise tolerance, and impaired exhalation. This condition causes inflammation and increased mucus in the airways. Symptoms can be worsened (or present only) during exercise, allergic reactions, or illness like a cold or flu virus. A systematic review of yoga and/or pranayama in childhood asthma concluded that a pranayama regimen consisting of deep breathing coupled with fast breathing exercises like bhastrika and *kapalabhati* (skull-shining breath) may have an adjunctive role in the treatment of childhood asthma by improving pulmonary functions.[28]

Some viral infections, such as COVID-19, primarily affect the respiratory system. Multiplication of this virus (SARS-CoV2) and the initial immune response cause inflammation of the respiratory tract. Inflammation can lead to the accumulation of fluid containing active viral particles, metabolic wastes, and tissue debris in the alveoli. As a result, these functional units of the lung cannot perform gas exchange, whereby oxygen is delivered and carbon dioxide is removed from the body through respiration. Because the nasal and oral passages are major routes of SARS-CoV2 entry, boosting mucosal immunity, as in the respiratory tract, may help with prevention, symptom management, and healing. The governments of India and Tamilnadu have recommended bhastrika and bhramari pranayama for the prevention and management of COVID-19.[29] Bhastrika, when included in a pranayama and kriya regimen (not in isolation), promoted anti-apoptotic and prosurvival genes in immune cells.[30] Bhramari involves humming, which has been shown to stimulate nasal nitric oxide production;[31] nitric oxide is increasingly recognized for its ability to improve antiviral, immune, and vascular function.[32]

Pranayama in Yoga Therapy Practice

Choosing tools

Pranayama can be a key adjunctive practice in chronic disease management when chosen correctly and delivered effectively. Tailoring the exercises for individual or group needs, partly through a thorough analysis of existing literature related to any disease conditions (including organ systems affected) and identification of potentially helpful themes, is important to success. Also, from the more than 50 different pranayama exercises practiced today in traditional Siddha schools, yoga therapists should be able to offer a rationale for which exercises should be attempted, in which order, and for what duration.

The above cancer and scleroderma examples, for instance, used a similar soothing yet revitalizing regimen consisting of breath awareness, alternate-nostril breathing, breath retention, and cooling breath that together encouraged improved breathing function. In the case of scleroderma, the physical component was included to offer gentle movements that could promote circulation and alleviate some of the musculoskeletal ailments. However, care must be taken to avoid physical exertion when clients experience pain or fatigue because of disease severity, hospital visits, etc. To support prevention of a virus such as COVID-19, bhastrika and bhramari might be included to promote sinus clarity and to exercise both the upper and lower respiratory tracts.

The following aspects are important considerations in the success of therapeutic pranayama:

- client characteristics (type of disease, age, affected domains, ability to perform the exercise)
- delivery approach (in-person, group, virtual; the yoga therapist's experience)
- pranayama details (type, dose, intensity, duration, frequency, order of practice)

- availability of additional client support (caregivers, additional educational resources, motivation to sustain the practice)

Delivering interventions

It is important to assess the type of pranayama being recommended and the benefits, risks, and contraindications for each exercise-condition combination. Considerations include any underlying pathology, the client's prior experience with breathing exercises, their normal breathing pattern, and potential difficulties. In addition, the mechanism for individual pranayama exercises, although not fully elucidated by the literature, should be taken into consideration for contraindications.

A few general guidelines are helpful:

- Suggest that clients practice on an empty stomach or at least 2 hours after a meal so that the parasympathetic nervous system is not occupied with digestive processes and feelings of fullness or bloat do not interfere with comfort. Adequate hydration is necessary, and avoiding the influence of drugs or alcohol is recommended.
- Comfortable seating, with adequate back support and the sitting bones higher than the knees, frees the abdomen to facilitate breathing. For clients who cannot be seated upright, gentle slow breathing such as bhramari or ujjayi may be most appropriate.
- Introduce lessons with patience, and clarify any doubts. Pranayama can be confusing for people learning it for the first time. Provide sufficient background information and mechanistic details, avoiding unfamiliar mythological stories, and introduce practices slowly. Offer modifications appropriate to client needs and ability.
- Obtain feedback. Watch how clients perform the exercise, offer refinements, and ask how they felt and whether they have any questions. Give sufficient detail in home practice plans.
- Address adverse effects. Make sure clients tolerate each exercise at the dose, frequency, and intensity delivered.

The advent of telehealth or virtual visit approaches has improved healthcare access in recent years. As pranayama is particularly suited to such approaches, distance delivery may be an option.

Measuring outcomes

Apart from measurable biological molecules, self-reported outcome measures are key to defining what therapeutic options work best for each client.[33] Scales for various patient population groups are available as standardized instruments. For example, validated health-related quality of life questionnaires are critical in understanding patient perception. Similarly, standardized and validated scales for measuring depression, stress, and other psychological parameters may be useful for tracking effects.

Summary

Pranayama is an ancient practice supported by information from the Siddha and other traditions and, increasingly, contemporary scientific literature. Regulated breathing practices impact the body and mind and could play a key role in well-being and healing processes. Alterations to the emotional system are evident in several disease conditions, and these psychological effects may correlate with poor prognosis. Similarly, imbalances in physiologically relevant biomarkers could indicate chronicity or illness severity. Pranayama may influence both the emotional and physical bodies through cardiovascular, neural, and other physiological mechanisms.

Effective use of pranayama has been demonstrated in several disease conditions, and owing to the ease of practice, pranayama can be an effective adjunct in integrative healthcare. Judicious use of pranayama in yoga therapy is possible given awareness of existing methods, details of relevant client conditions, potential interactions of intervention and subject (i.e., the knowledge of how a pranayama can affect health), delivery methods that can sustain the practice, and possible adverse reactions and contraindications. Developing and delivering a pranayama adjunct and measuring the outcomes will strengthen the evidence base for this unique integrative health modality. Understanding the mechanisms of pranayama is important to move this field forward. Literature from the Siddha tradition is a largely untapped source for new pranayama methods.

Additional Resources

Ganapathy, T. N., & Arumugam, K. R. (2004). *Yoga of Siddha Tirumular: Essays on the Tirumandiram*. Kriya Yoga Publications.

Muktibodhananda, S. (1998). *Hatha Yoga Pradipika* 2.1–21, 2.40–78. Yoga Publications Trust.

Saraswati, S. N. (2010). *Prana and pranayama*. Yoga Publications Trust.

White, D. G. (1998). *The alchemical body: Siddha traditions in medieval India*. University of Chicago Press.

Endnotes

1 Saint Tirumular. (n.d.). Tirumantiram: English translation of the Tamil spiritual classic by Saint Tirumular. www.himalayanacademy.com/media/books/tirumantiram/Tirumantiram.pdf
See also Anand, G., & Ganapathy, T. N. (2014). Sivavakkiyam: Songs of a spiritual rebel. https://archive.org/details/SivavakkiyamSongsOfSpiritualRebel

2 Yoga Sutra 2.50 refers to pranayama as the regulation of the inhalation, exhalation, and suspension of the breath, with manipulation of the inhalation and exhalation ultimately serving to lengthen the pause of the suspension; it is said that when the breath is still, the mind is still. Unlike the *Yoga Sutras*, which begin with the ethical practices of *yama* and *niyama*, the medieval *Hatha Yoga Pradipika* recommends asana and pranayama as purifying preparations for achieving transcendent states through deeper meditative practices. According to the *Hatha Yoga Pradipika*, pranayama "is not merely breath control, but a technique through which the quantity of prana in the body is activated to a higher frequency": Desikachar, T. K. V. (1999). *The heart of yoga: Developing a personal practice* (pp. 181–182). Inner Traditions, Muktibodhananda, S. (1998). *Hatha yoga pradipika* (p. 149). Yoga Publications Trust.

3 Nivethitha, L., Mooventhan, A., & Manjunath, N. K. (2016). Effects of various prāṇāyāma on cardiovascular and autonomic variables. *Ancient Science of Life*, *36*(2), 72–77.

4 For the method, see Balasubramanian, S. (2019). *Mind your breathing: The yogi's handbook with 37 pranayama exercises.* Notion Press.

5 Shetty, P., Kiran Kumar Reddy, B., Lakshmeesha, D. R., Shetty, S. P., Kumar, G. S., & Bradley, R. (2017). Effects of sheetali and sheetkari pranayamas on blood pressure and autonomic function in hypertensive patients. *Integrative Medicine*, *16*(5), 32–37.
Thanalakshmi, J., Maheshkumar, K., Kannan, R., Sundareswaran, L., Venugopal, V., & Poonguzhali, S. (2020). Effect of sheetali pranayama on cardiac autonomic function among patients with primary hypertension—A randomized controlled trial. *Complementary Therapies in Clinical Practice*, *39*, 101138.

6 Budhi, R. B., Payghan, S., & Deepeshwar, S. (2019). Changes in lung function measures following bhastrika pranayama (bellows breath) and running in healthy individuals. *International Journal of Yoga*, *12*(3), 233–239.

7 Melnychuk, M. C., Dockree, P. M., O'Connell, R. G., Murphy, P. R., Balsters, J. H., & Robertson, I. H. (2018). Coupling of respiration and attention via the locus coeruleus: Effects of meditation and pranayama. *Psychophysiology*, *55*(9), e13091.
Saoji, A. A., Raghavendra, B. R., & Manjunath, N. K. (2019). Effects of yogic breath regulation: A narrative review of scientific evidence. *Journal of Ayurveda and Integrative Medicine*, *10*(1), 50–58.
Zaccaro, A., Piarulli, A., Laurino, M., Garbella, E., et al. (2018). How breath-control can change your life: A systematic review on psycho-physiological correlates of slow breathing. *Frontiers in Human Neuroscience*, *12*, 353.

8 Balasubramanian, S., Mintzer, J. E., & Wahlquist, A. E. (2015). Induction of salivary nerve growth factor by yogic breathing: A randomized controlled trial. *International Psychogeriatrics*, *27*(1), 168–170.

9 Balasubramanian, S., Janech, M. G., & Warren, G. W. (2015). Alterations in salivary proteome following single twenty-minute session of yogic breathing. *Evidence-Based Complementary and Alternative Medicine*, *2015*, 376029.
Twal, W. O., Wahlquist, A. E., & Balasubramanian, S. (2016). Yogic breathing when compared to attention control reduces the levels of pro-inflammatory biomarkers in saliva: A pilot randomized controlled trial. *BMC Complementary and Alternative Medicine*, *16*, 294.

10 Edgar, W. M. (1992). Saliva: Its secretion, composition and functions. *British Dental Journal*, *172*, 305–312.
Zhang, A., Sun, H., Wang, P., & Wang, X. (2013). Salivary proteomics in biomedical research. *Clinica Chimica Acta, International Journal of Clinical Chemistry*, *415*, 261–265.

11 Kuntsevich, V., Bushell, W. C., & Theise, N. D. (2010). Mechanisms of yogic practices in health, aging, and disease. *Mount Sinai Journal of Medicine*, *77*(5), 559–569.
Melnychuk et al., Coupling of respiration.
Nivethitha et al., Effects of various prāṇāyāma.
Zaccaro et al., Breath-control.

12 Yackle, K., Schwarz, L. A., Kam, K., Sorokin, J. M., et al. (2017). Breathing control center neurons that promote arousal in mice. *Science*, *355*(6332), 1411–1415.

13 Arshamian, A., Iravani, B., Majid, A., & Lundström, J. N. (2018). Respiration modulates olfactory memory consolidation in humans. *Journal of Neuroscience, 38*(48), 10286–10294.

14 Noble, D. J., & Hochman, S. (2019). Hypothesis: Pulmonary afferent activity patterns during slow, deep breathing contribute to the neural induction of physiological relaxation. *Frontiers in Physiology, 10*, 1176.

15 Derby, C. D. (2007). Why have neurogenesis in adult olfactory systems? The Presidential Symposium at the 2006 AChemS Conference. *Chemical Senses, 32*(4), 361–363.

16 Froeliger, B., Garland, E. L., & McClernon, F. J. (2012). Yoga meditation practitioners exhibit greater gray matter volume and fewer reported cognitive failures: Results of a preliminary voxel-based morphometric analysis. *Evidence-Based Complementary and Alternative Medicine: eCAM, 2012*, 821307.

17 Saint Tirumular, *Tirumantiram* (p. 134).

18 American Cancer Society. (2017). Breast cancer facts & figures 2017–2018. www.cancer.org/content/dam/cancer-org/research/cancer-facts-and-statistics/breast-cancer-facts-and-figures/breast-cancer-facts-and-figures-2017-2018.pdf

DeSantis, C. E., Ma, J., Goding Sauer, A., Newman, L. A., & Jemal, A. (2017). Breast cancer statistics, 2017, racial disparity in mortality by state. *CA: A Cancer Journal for Clinicians, 67*(6), 439–448.

19 Niedzwiedz, C. L., Knifton, L., Robb, K. A., Katikireddi, S. V., & Smith, D. J. (2019). Depression and anxiety among people living with and beyond cancer: A growing clinical and research priority. *BMC Cancer, 19*(1), 943.

20 Dhruva, A., Miaskowski, C., Abrams, D., Acree, M., et al. (2012). Yoga breathing for cancer chemotherapy-associated symptoms and quality of life: Results of a pilot randomized controlled trial. *Journal of Alternative and Complementary Medicine, 18*(5), 473–479.

Kochupillai, V., Kumar, P., Singh, D., Aggarwal, D., et al. (2005). Effect of rhythmic breathing (sudarshan kriya and pranayam) on immune functions and tobacco addiction. *Annals of the New York Academy of Sciences, 1056*, 242–252.

21 Balasubramanian, S., Warren, G. W., Sterba, K. R., & Wahlquist, A. H., unpublished data.

22 This information resulted in the incorporation of these pranayama exercises as a key component of the Survivors' Fit Club, a 10-week program for breast cancer survivors provided by the Wellness Center at the Medical University of South Carolina.

23 Varga, J. (2016). Etiology and pathogenesis of scleroderma. In G. S. Firestein, R. C. Budd, S. E. Gabriel, I. B. McInnes, & J. R. O'Dell (Eds.), *Kelley and Firestein's textbook of rheumatology*, Vol. II (10th ed., pp. 1400–1423). Elsevier.

24 Denton, C. P., & Khanna, D. (2017). Systemic sclerosis. *Lancet, 390*(10103), 1685–1699.

25 Structured feedback collected from more than 4 years of these workshops indicated that the practices were acceptable to scleroderma patients, and a clinical trial is currently underway.

26 Stern, E. R., Grimaldi, S. J., Muratore, A., Murrough, J., et al. (2017). Neural correlates of interoception: Effects of interoceptive focus and relationship to dimensional measures of body awareness. *Human Brain Mapping, 38*(12), 6068–6082.

27 Kaminsky, D. A., Guntupalli, K. K., Lippmann, J., Burns, S. M., et al. (2017). Effect of yoga breathing (pranayama) on exercise tolerance in patients with chronic obstructive pulmonary disease: A randomized, controlled trial. *Journal of Alternative and Complementary Medicine, 23*(9), 696–704.

28 Das, R. R., Sankar, J., & Kabra, S. K. (2019). Role of breathing exercises and yoga/pranayama in childhood asthma: A systematic review. *Current Pediatric Reviews, 15*(3), 175–183.

29 See, e.g., Ministry of AYUSH, Government of India. (n.d.). Guidelines for yoga practitioners for COVID 19. www.ayush.gov.in/docs/yoga-guidelines.pdf

30 Sharma, H., Datta, P., Singh, A., Sen, S., Bhardwaj, N. K., et al. (2008). Gene expression profiling in practitioners of sudarshan kriya. *Journal of Psychosomatic Research, 64*(2), 213–218.

31 Weitzberg, E., & Lundberg, J. O. (2002). Humming greatly increases nasal nitric oxide. *American Journal of Respiratory and Critical Care Medicine, 166*(2), 144–145.

32 Stefano, G. B., Esch, T., & Kream, R. M. (2020). Potential immunoregulatory and antiviral/SARS-CoV-2 activities of nitric oxide. *Medical Science Monitor: International Medical Journal of Experimental and Clinical Research, 26*, e925679.

33 Outcomes of an adjunctive pranayama intervention can be both subjective and objective. Pranayama generally targets stress, so stress biomarkers such as cytokine levels in blood and saliva are often measured. Standardized biomarkers such as HbA1c and C-reactive protein have been used in clinical diagnosis, but

their utility has not been fully tested in pranayama. However, patient-reported outcomes are generally more convenient to collect and analyze compared to biological markers. Self-reported outcomes such as pain scales may also be more dependable than the measure of pain biomarkers; see, e.g., Younger, J., McCue, R., & Mackey, S. (2009). Pain outcomes: A brief review of instruments and techniques. *Current Pain and Headache Reports*, *13*(1), 39–43.

20

Ayurvedic Asana and Pranayama Interventions

SARAJEAN RUDMAN

Yoga therapists who understand how to assess from an ayurvedic lens gain additional perspectives for creating unique client interventions. This is not to suggest that yoga therapists are ayurvedic practitioners, only that an understanding of the ayurvedic perspective can inform the delivery of yoga therapy.

Assessing from the ayurvedic perspective includes consideration of the ten pairs of opposites and the way these combine to create elemental energies. The elemental energies, in turn, combine into *doshas*, or constitutional types, that form the person's *prakruti* (birth constitution or nature) and *vikruti* (how the prakruti has become imbalanced), which are considered alongside *kala* (time of day, year, and life).

Employing ayurvedic assessment tools for the grosser sheaths of *annamaya* and *pranamaya kosha* is a useful way of incorporating this wisdom tradition into yoga therapy while remaining within scope of practice. Applying the information from these observations to inform specific *asana* and *pranayama* can further help to individualize these interventions. For work with the subtler *panchamaya* sheaths, clients should be referred to a trained ayurvedic practitioner. Additionally, it is important to consider the whole client for contraindications prior to creating the plan of care.[1]

Prakruti-Informed Interventions

As discussed in Chapters 3 and 4, ayurveda classifies people into ten constitutional types that tend to remain stable throughout life.[2] These doshas, as mentioned above, are combinations of elemental energies that comprise the entire cosmos.

Vata is composed of the subtlest of the elements, ether and air, which means that this constitution is the least stable. *Pitta*, composed of fire and water, is considered to be hot and mobile but a more stable constitution. *Kapha*, earth and water, is the most stable but also the most likely to stagnate.

The doshas combine to form unique birth combinations, prakruti. The most common prakruti are the single presentations of vata, pitta, and kapha and the dual doshas of vata-pitta, vata-kapha, pitta-kapha, pitta-vata, kapha-pitta, and kapha-vata; occasionally an individual's birth constitution may be *tridoshic* (an equal blend of vata-pitta-kapha).

When a person with a dual prakruti of vata and pitta doshas is moving through a vata season, they may experience excess qualities of vata (air and ether), which then creates an imbalance (too much air and ether creating greater instability). Likewise, when that person moves through a pitta season, they may experience an excess of the pitta energies (too much heat and mobility, which could lead to inflammations or angry outbursts). Such excesses are the individual's vikruti, or seasonal presentation—the way their unique constitution responds to the pressures of the seasons and the world around them.

Below are asana and pranayama practices recommended according to ayurvedic principles for each of the three main doshas. These practices can be applied by considering a client's nature, or prakruti; their current presentation, or vikruti; and the season or time of day, kala. As with any asana or pranayama practice, the specific needs of the individual client (body, mind, and spirit) must be taken into account before considering including any of the example interventions suggested here.

Seasonal considerations are important generally for all clients. Vata practices are useful for all constitutional makeups during the vata time of year (late fall to early winter in the Northern Hemisphere), pitta practices are useful for all constitutions in the pitta time of year (summer and early fall), and kapha practices are useful for all constitutions in the kapha time of year (late winter to spring).

For example, the client with a pitta prakruti (original nature) would probably benefit from a pitta-appropriate practice, especially in the summer, a pitta time of year. Likewise, a client with a pitta vikruti (presentation, an excess of the qualities involved in pitta dosha) may benefit from a pitta practice to help to restore them to their original state.

All of these considerations together—nature, imbalance, and time of day/year/life—can become complicated, so returning to the *gunas*, or qualities, and evaluating what might be out of balance in the moment may be useful. Working with opposite gunas to bring them back into balance can be a more approachable mechanism for recommending practices. (Consider revisiting the gunas for each of the doshas in Chapter 3.) Ayurvedic practices are meant to oppose the gunas of the dosha they are assigned to balance.

Another consideration for presenting interventions involves the senses through which each dosha imbibes the world. Vata is said to engage with the world through the skin and ears, so sound and touch are important for interventions intended to return vata to its original state. This may mean they crave aural stimulation and touch or, if in an aggravated state (as may happen with a vata type in a vata season, where too much of one dosha is present), sound and touch may irritate them.

Kapha is said to engage with the world through the nose and tongue, so scent and taste are important. As with vata, a choice could further their access to self-healing or irritate them if the kapha dosha is in an aggravated state: a cup of sweet tea and incense burned to perfume the air before a session could be welcome or annoying.

Pitta engages with the world through the eyes, so being able to see what is going on matters to the pitta personality. Again, in hot seasons, when pitta is the dominant dosha, those with pitta prakruti may be aggravated and benefit from cool darkness.[3]

Vata asana

Poses and sequences for vata prakruti should be done slowly and rhythmically, so the client can literally sense their way into the practice. It might seem logical to ask the vata-imbalanced person to sit still, but this can work as a pressure cooker, causing restlessness. Vata dosha needs to move.

Rhythmic and gentle *surya namaskara* (sun salutations) provide a wonderful way to warm up vata. Vata dosha is cold and erratic by nature, and slow, rhythmic sun salutations can help to alleviate both of these qualities by balancing with opposites. This is calming to the mind and the body of vata, relieving anxious thoughts as a sort of meditation in motion. Linked breath and movement anchors the attention, especially with focus on the sensation of the breath in the nostrils, potentially making erratic and anxious thoughts easier to manage.

Vata dosha may also benefit from strength-building poses in which both hands and feet are on the ground, like *adho mukha svanasana* (downward dog), *phalakasana* (plank), and work in hands-and-knees tabletop position. Additional strength-building poses like *virabhadrasana* (warrior), *tadasana* (standing mountain), *vriksasana* (tree), and *utkatasana* (chair) may also be helpful.

Poses that allow breath to get into the seat of vata, the colon area, such as *bhujangasana* (cobra) are also useful. *Malasana* (yogic squat), *pavanamuktasana* (knee-to-chest wind-releasing pose), and *prasarita padottanasana* (wide-angle forward fold) stimulate *apana vayu*, or downward-moving energy (discussed in Chapter 4 and below). *Viparita karani* (legs up the wall), *savasana* (corpse pose), *supta baddha konasana* (reclining cobbler), as well as *sukhasana* (easy pose) are all appropriate poses with which to end vata-balancing practices. (As with any practice, the individual's experience is primary: Corpse pose and reclining cobbler, for example, can feel unsettling and vulnerable to those who are anxious or hypervigilant, especially in cases of trauma history. Consider the use of a weighted blanket for savasana and eyes open for those with a history of trauma.)

Music should be simple and without lyrics. Absolute silence can make those with a vata-dosha imbalance nervous. Ideally, colors in the room should be warm, such as deep red and warm yellow, and the temperature of the room should be warm as well. The *drishti* (focal point) for balancing vata energy is toward the earth to ground the elements of air and ether.

Vata pranayama

Breathwork that warms the body and stimulates circulation while inviting a sense of groundedness will help to pacify vata. *Nadi shodhana* (*anuloma viloma* alternate-nostril breathing with retention after the inhale and sometimes exhale), *ujjayi* (victorious breathing), *dirgha* (three-part diaphragmatic breathing), and box breathing (equal-ratio inhalation, internal pause, exhalation, and external pause) are good pranayama options for vata dosha. Vata-presenting clients can be encouraged to close their eyes if comfortable, or to find a soft gaze with drishti on the earth.

Pitta asana

Poses and sequences for pitta should be straightforward and simple. It is important to keep pitta types aware and in their physical bodies. Pitta prakruti can be "hot-headed," as the element of fire predominates. Pitta types must remain non-competitive but also need to be challenged. Yoga therapists might consider challenging pitta clients to practice at 75 percent capacity instead of at their end range in every asana. A straightforward approach is recommended: Offer appropriate challenges that avoid encouraging competition and that promote strength while avoiding overly descriptive or flowery cues; basic and specific instructions will often earn the respect of pitta types. For example, when cueing sun salutations, "Inhale and raise the arms overhead, exhale and fold down toward your toes" would be preferred over "Inhale and raise your arms joyfully overhead, exhale like a bird diving through the clouds down to your beautiful toes." Direct cues will keep pitta's attention.

Any pose that bows the head below the heart will serve pitta dosha, such as *uttanasana* (standing forward fold), seated forward folds such as *paschimottanasana*, wide-angle forward fold, and *balasana* (child's pose); *setu bandhasana* (bridge) and *ardha sarvangasana* (half shoulderstand) are ideal inversions and should be done with the eyes closed if possible.[4] Twists that target the small intestine, liver, and kidney areas will also serve pitta; *parivrtta parsvakonasana* (revolved side angle pose), *parivrtta utkatasana* (revolved chair), and *ardha matsyendrasana* (seated half lord of the fishes pose) are ideal choices and can be modified for any movement limitations. *Chandra namaskara* (moon salutation) offers a cooling alternative to the heating sun salutation and can be used in its place for warming the body at the start of a practice.

Plenty of time to settle down in savasana serves pitta dosha well. Guide them into relaxation with the breath and allow them to stay for as long as they like after the session is over, but also offer a container with a start and end time—and a rationale for practicing savasana; the strong pitta person may feel they do not need the rest if it is presented as an option.

No music is ideal during pitta-balancing sessions, as it can annoy the fiery dosha. Colors in the room should be cooling, like deep blues and greens, and the temperature should be cool or moderate, never hot. Drishti for pitta types is out on the horizon so they can remain level with the world.

Pitta pranayama

The pranayama of *sheetali* (performed with a rolled tongue) and *sheetkari* (with teeth touching, lips parted, and tongue to the upper palate) are ideal, cooling breaths for pitta. A regular practice of victorious, three-part diaphragmatic, and alternate-nostril breathing will also serve to balance pitta types and relax the fight/flight mode their focused and busy lifestyles may engender.

Kapha asana

Because the qualities of kapha include cold, heaviness, dullness, and stability, working with opposites would indicate warm, light, sharp, and mobile practices.

Kapha-balancing practices can begin standing up, perhaps using mantra or deep, sighing exhales. The practice should start off slow and pick up speed. Think of attempting to move a heavy boulder: Running full speed into it to get it to move would be fruitless; instead, slowly nudging it little by little would be more likely to overcome its inertia and get it rolling.

The seat of kapha is the stomach and lungs, so twists and lateral flexion are appropriate poses to include. Balance poses that create a sense of instability for kapha are also ideal. Sun salutations that get the blood flowing and heart pumping help to lighten and warm up the heavy and cold kapha dosha. Warrior I and II both help to build heat, and *viparita virabhadrasana* (reversed warrior) builds heat while targeting the ribs and lungs as well. Downward dog can offer kapha types a much-needed new perspective on the world and their physical bodies. For those who are physically able, flowing between downward dog and plank helps to build heat and movement; a sequence from *chaturanga dandasana* (four-limbed staff pose) into *urdvha mukha svanasana* (upward dog), and back to downward dog—or more accessible variations of any of these poses based on the unique individual in session—is also appropriate for kapha. Supine, seated, and prone twists as well as core work will help to wring out the heavy dampness of kapha.

Balancing kapha dosha requires variety; offering changing practices and keeping these clients on their toes is key to warding off excess of the dosha. The music for a kapha client can be fun and lively, the colors should be bright and exciting (e.g., yellows and pinks), and the room should be warm. Drishti for kapha is toward the sky, as this promotes a sense of airy and ethereal freedom that stuck kapha types can embrace for balance. Savasana should be short or replaced with a seated meditation or pranayama, or perhaps legs-up-the-wall pose.

Kapha pranayama

Bhastrika (bellows breath), *kapalabhati* (skull-shining breath), *bhramari* (bee breath), and external *khumbhaka* (breath retention) are all appropriate pranayama practices for kapha balancing. Victorious breath should be used throughout practice to keep kapha types warm. The *shatkarma* (internal cleansing practices) of *nauli* (stomach churning) and *agni sara* (fire essence practice) are wonderful for kapha to stimulate agni and reduce stagnation.[5]

Pranayama and Asana for the Five Vayus (Subdoshas of Vata)

Figure 20.1 illustrates the vayus' energetic movement and locations.

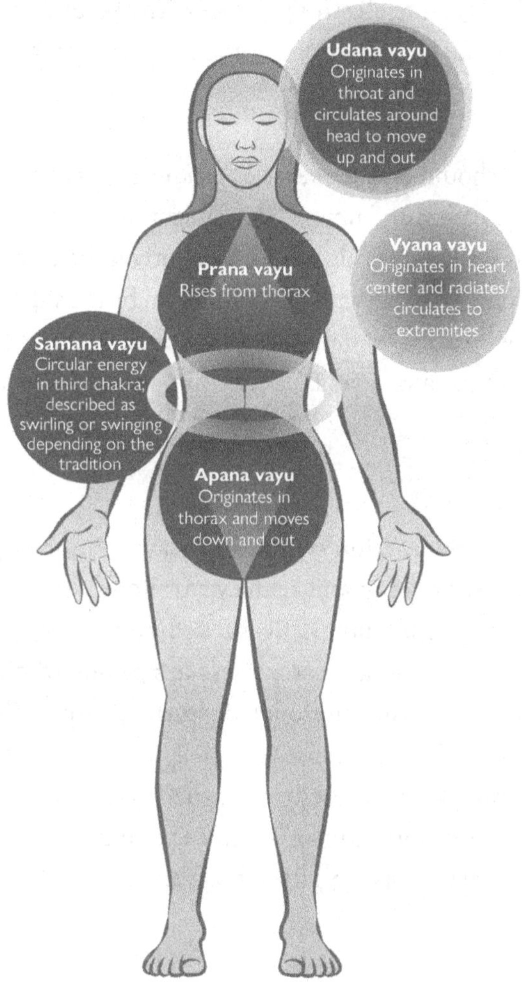

FIGURE 20.1 ENERGETIC MOVEMENT AND LOCATIONS OF THE PRANAVAYUS

Apana vayu

Signs of imbalance in apana vayu include but are not limited to digestive issues like constipation, menstrual issues, infertility issues, inability to feel grounded or sit still, emaciation, exhaustion, anxiety, depression, inability to focus, and forgetfulness.

Pranayama

Breathwork for apana vayu should instill a sense of coming home, groundedness, warmth, and love. Nadi shodhana, ujjayi, dirgha, *chandra bhedhana* (single-nostril breath with inhalation through the left and exhalation through the right), anuloma viloma, and box breathing are all strong choices. The breathwork should be done slowly and completely, not harshly, to create a sense of safety for the nervous system.

Asana

Poses for apana vayu should create a sense of groundedness, stability, strength, and warmth. Asana such as cobra and upward dog are good choices. Standing poses such as warrior I and II as well as chair pose with a drishti on the earth, awareness of the feet, and deep breathing, possibly with the arms down by the sides, may all be helpful as well. When done with arms extended, these standing postures provide a means to regulate both prana and apana vayu. Balances may also be beneficial.

Prana vayu

Prana vayu works in conjunction with apana vayu. Prana vayu allows for the individual to take in fresh energy, and apana vayu allows elimination of that which is spent. Both need to function optimally for well-being.

Signs of imbalance in prana vayu can present in a person who is struggling to get proper sleep or under physical, emotional, or spiritual stress. The imbalance may present as a weakening of the five senses of smell, touch, sight, taste, and hearing. General confusion can also be present, as prana vayu governs the movement of ideas and intelligence. Life force can be lackluster, and those with decreased prana vayu may even have trouble taking a deep breath.

Pranayama

In the breathing process, the inhalation is aligned with prana vayu, and the exhalation with apana vayu.

Prana vayu moves inward and upward. Those with an excess of prana vayu or low apana vayu may appear ungrounded, perhaps walking on tiptoes, and those with low prana vayu or excess apana vayu may appear to sink into the ground and lack the ability to "lift off." Pranayama to create a balance between prana and apana vayu are dirgha, ujjayi, nadi shodhana, anuloma viloma, internal breath retention, and box breathing. Focus on "filling up" with air on the inhalation to increase prana vayu; focus on the exhale to increase apana vayu. Take time to slow down the practice to allow for complete inhalations (or exhalations). Breath retention should be gentle so as not to create grasping or stress in the body.

Performing these breathing exercises with eyes closed and an inward drishti is ideal. As the element of prana vayu is ether, which is subtle and expansive, a focus on the earthy grounding of apana vayu adds balance to the practice.

Asana

A focus on upward movement can be stimulating for prana vayu. Standing postures, especially those including extended arm positions, increase this vayu. Individuals with low prana vayu may benefit from extended mountain, warrior series and the use of kali mudra, with the hands clasped and index fingers extended, overhead. When engaging in these practices, remember to balance with the grounding of apana vayu, feet firmly rooted in the earth. Savasana is another wonderful pose to offer for prana vayu balancing, as it invites an inward focus and settled quality.

Samana vayu

Signs of imbalance of samana vayu include indigestion or other digestive difficulties. Imbalance in this vayu also manifests as mental unrest or inability to be in harmony and can result in a diminished or exaggerated ego. Samana vayu is the gate between the upward-moving prana and downward-moving apana vayus, so an imbalance here can also cause an imbalance in those two vayus. When out of balance, a client may also be making seemingly purposeful unhealthy choices in life physically, psychologically, and spiritually/emotionally.

Pranayama

Surya bhedana, or right-nostril breathing, is appropriate for samana vayu, as it stimulates the digestive fire of agni. This practice is ideally done using *Vishnu mudra* and seated in a calm, cool place.[6] Diaphragmatic breath with three distinct parts (inhaling to first fill the lower third of the torso, then the middle and top thirds), with a focus on slowing the breath and fully expanding the first (lower) third, can also be helpful. External breath retention is also stimulating to samana vayu and can be practiced in moderation to help move the digestive energy.

Asana

Upward bow, wheel, cobra, and upward dog are all useful backbends to stimulate samana vayu. Forward folds like standing forward fold, revolved wide-angle standing forward fold, and seated or standing wide-angle forward fold are all also excellent choices if samana vayu is overactive. Twists can also be healing for overactive samana vayu. Seated twists, supine two-knee twist, and prone twist are possibilities and can be modified as needed. *Mayurasana* (peacock pose) or modified peacock pose is said to stimulate samana vayu by putting pressure on the organs of digestion; this may be contraindicated depending on the individual's health. Also stimulating for digestion and samana vayu is self-abdominal massage while in a pose such as reclining cobbler.[7]

Udana vayu

Signs of imbalance of udana vayu can include indecisiveness, the inability to speak one's mind, a loss of enthusiasm and ambition, and the inability to communicate well. Such an imbalance can also appear as a tightness in the chest and difficulty breathing deeply. A client with decreased udana vayu might describe themselves as having a lazy or slow mind or feeling generally lackluster. Excess udana vayu might present as a newfound sense of arrogance or stubbornness, taking on more than one can handle, or saying more than one should in any given situation.

Pranayama

Because sound is an important principle of udana vayu, bee breath is recommended for breaking up blockages in udana vayu. Using visualization with the breath is another way to stimulate udana vayu. Udana is often aligned with the movement of *kundalini* energy, so visualization of the breath entering through the tailbone from a seated position, traveling up to the crown of the head, and proceeding out as bright, white light would affect movement of udana vayu. Other pranayama for udana vayu, to invoke upward-moving circulatory energy, include skull-shining breath, bellows breath, and internal breath retention.

Asana

Asana that places a focus on the opening of the throat stimulate udana vayu. Upward dog and cobra may be especially beneficial for moving stuck energy in the throat and belly. *Ustrasana* (camel), *matsyasana* (fish), *sasangasana* (rabbit), and shoulderstand all work the throat area and therefore stimulate udana vayu.

Vyana vayu

Imbalance of vyana vayu could look, on the physical level, like poor circulation and possibly malnutrition. Someone with low vyana vayu on a mental level would be alienating themselves, unable to show love and be vulnerable, perhaps unwilling to go out into the world because of fears. They may even appear agoraphobic in extreme cases and be unwilling to try new things. Those with decreased vyana vayu do not want to be the center of attention, as if they want to avoid circulating their own energy (this vayu rules circulation). Bear in mind that those with decreased vyana vayu may seem anxious. Approaching therapeutic protocols with kindness, sensitivity, and love becomes crucial here. Vyana vayu originates in the heart, like prana vayu, and *hridaya* (the heart) is the seat of pure consciousness and unconditional love.

Pranayama

Most important when offering pranayama to support vyana vayu is to consider deep breathing to completely "fill" the body with breath. Offer the visualization of the inhale originating at the heart, radiating out to the fingers, toes, and crown of head and returning to the heart on the exhale. Both internal and external breath retention may also help to stimulate circulation and vyana vayu. Nadi shodhana and anuloma viloma using Vishnu mudra is also wonderful for vyana vayu, as both practices are considered cleansing and detoxifying for the three main *nadis* (energetic channels; see Box 21.1): *ida*, *pingala*, and *sushumna*. The balancing of the nadis allows for energy to flow more freely around the gross and subtle bodies.

Asana

Asana that bring focus to the whole body stimulate vyana vayu, especially when they move from full-body extension of energy to contracted or still states. Beneficial asana can include simple postures such as five-pointed star, warrior II and III, and *ardha chandrasana* half-moon balance, or more complex movements such as sun salutations, done mindfully with pauses between rounds. These practices are exhilarating and create a balance of strength and lightness while building heat and circulation. *Garudasana* (eagle pose) creates a mild tourniquet effect that, when released, stimulates energy flow in the whole body.

Balancing the Koshas

Recall that the *koshas* are the layers, or sheaths, of energies into which the mind manifests (see Chapter 3). Ayurvedically informed practices are particularly useful in addressing koshic imbalances through the principles of like increases like and working with opposites. The most gross sheath, where disease is said to manifest last, is *annamaya kosha*—the food sheath and the body itself.

Annamaya and pranamaya koshas

Employ asana to build physical strength and flexibility in annamaya. Such practices can be tailored to the client's prakruti (nature), vikruti (imbalance), and the kala (time of day, season, and time of life; see Chapter 4). The kriyas of neti, dhauti, nauli, kapalabhati, trataka, and basti (see endnote 5) may be recommended by qualified ayurvedic practitioners.

Practice *dinacharya*, or ayurvedic daily routine, to stabilize the physical body, waking and sleeping, exercising, eating, and doing spiritual work at appropriate times. Practice of *ritucharya*, or ayurvedic seasonal routine, can also be used to stabilize the physical body: Diet, lifestyle, and yogic practices change with the seasons so they balance the doshas that predominate over that time in nature.

Pranayama appropriate for the client's prakruti, vikruti, and kala is helpful for balancing the gross part of pranamaya kosha which, when imbalanced, can lead to many pathologies.

Manomaya, vijnanamaya, and anandamaya koshas

This chapter focuses on asana and pranayama primarily targeted to annamaya and pranamaya, but ayurvedically informed interventions can target each of the intrinsically interrelated koshas.

For example, mantra therapy done in a rhythmic and regular fashion, not erratically, can be used as a daily kriya to affect *manomaya* kosha. Bee breath may pacify manomaya and can be practiced daily, ideally in the morning.

Mantra therapy is perhaps the most beneficial therapy for vijnanamaya and anandamaya kosha ayurvedically. Simple, sattvic, and expansive mantras such as Om are recommended. Find a mantra acceptable to the client's faith tradition (see Chapter 17).

Balancing the Subtle Essences

Recall from Chapter 4 that the subtle essences of *prana*, *tejas*, and *ojas* are similar to the tridosha in that they are composed of the same five elements and align with the balance of vata, pitta, and kapha, respectively, in a person's prakruti, but they reflect the subtler of the elemental pair they represent. They are the refined form of the dosha. As with ayurvedic approaches to balancing the doshas, like increases like, and treatment can be with opposites. The subtle essences may be imbalanced along with, or independent of, any imbalances in the dosha with which they align.[8]

Prana

An increase in prana can lead to a general sense of restlessness and erratic mood. It can also lead to overzealous behavior and the inability to focus on any one thing at a time. A decrease in prana usually presents as a sense of the client being closed off. Those who were open before may lack creativity or the inability to be close in relationships, or they may be confused and isolated. Prana governs the body's cardiopulmonary systems, and thus severe imbalances can lead to respiratory and heart conditions.

To balance prana using pranayama is ideal; consider the idea of bringing vital essence into the body. Pranayama while in seated postures such as *padmasana* (lotus), easy pose, or *swastikasana* (auspicious pose), or seated in a chair as a modification, is suggested. Yoga poses that open the lungs and invite a sense of receptivity, such as backbends and lateral stretches, will aid in promoting pranic balance.

Tejas

High tejas will present as anger, irritability, inability to control aggression, anxiety, stress, emaciation, overall mental/physical and emotional/spiritual tension, and insatiability. When tejas is decreased, a person may have an "identity crisis," feel disenfranchised, lose their sense of purpose, be spiritually bereft, and feel overall physically, mentally, and emotionally lackluster. Imbalanced tejas can lead to mental disease, such as depression and anxiety disorders, but because tejas is the source of cellular intelligence in the body, it can also lead to chronic illnesses, such as autoimmune conditions, in which the body responds inappropriately.

Asana and pranayama that increase agni balance tejas. Energetically activating the digestive organs and samana vayu with twists, backbends, sun salutations, and poses that use the arms are all key to balancing tejas. Use of the arms also elevates prana vayu, which aids in activation of samana vayu by bringing energy to the upper body. The overall more robust circulation also supports the digestive organs.

Pranayama such as skull-shining breath, bellows breath, right-nostril breathing, and retentions all increase fire. Agni sara kriya and nauli are both powerful aids to increase tejas. Cooling practices synonymous with those listed above to pacify pitta dosha decrease tejas.

Ojas

When someone has balanced ojas, they are full of life, appear sattvic and healthy, and have good immune strength, as well as mental, emotional, and spiritual strength. They have a sense of contentment and stability and an overall glow. Diminished ojas results in low immunity, infertility, a general sense of depletion, lackluster energy, weakness, and emaciation. More serious invasive conditions can prey on depleted ojas, including cancers and infections such as meningitis.

Although "too much" ojas is not possible, *ama* can build up from too much of a good thing (e.g., rest, rich foods). Ama is considered undigested matter that is circulating in the body as toxins. Someone with ama in their body will appear heavy, possibly both physically and psychoemotionally, and unwell.

Practicing yoga appropriate for one's prakruti and meditating daily increases ojas. Maintaining a sense of love and joy throughout a practice will also help. Taking adequate rest at the end of a yoga session and making sure one is rested prior to practice also support ojas. Yoga therapy for building ojas should leave the client feeling energized and full, never depleted, and always as if they still have something in their energy banks for later. Practicing yoga at the same time daily and doing *metta* (loving-kindness) meditation both promote healthy ojas.

Summary

This chapter provides yoga therapists with a way to consider the skills derived from ayurvedic assessment to benefit clients. The review of prakruti, or original nature, and asana and pranayama recommendations for various prakruti and vikruti from an ayurvedic practitioner, prompt thinking through the elemental considerations that might promote balance.

Sattva, rajas, and tamas are the three ever-present gunas of nature, creating balance in concert with one another (see Chapter 4). Yoga therapists promote optimal balance among sattva, rajas (activity, movement, energy, heat, creation, desire, and craving), and tamas (inertia, darkness, heaviness, dullness, and obstruction). The mind constantly utilizes all three gunas, and many people tend toward one of the three more than the others. Through yoga and lifestyle, one should aim to generally increase sattva and decrease rajas and tamas if they appear unbalanced or outside the bounds of their normal state of existence in the mind.

Ayurveda recognizes many different concepts in individuals, from the tridoshic composition of vata, pitta, and kapha that is central to an individual's nature and present state (prakruti and vikruti), to the vayus or subdoshas of vata, the koshic "sheaths," and the subtle essences of prana, tejas, and ojas—the doshas refined.

Each of these constructs promotes health when balanced. Ayurvedic practitioners recognize that with any imbalances, like increases like and opposites may be helpfully employed.

The chapter focuses on annamaya and pranamaya kosha to enable beginning yoga therapists to more readily grasp how to do this work in what are thought of as the "denser" realms. It is recommended that clients who wish to pursue an ayurvedic approach to yoga therapy in the subtler realms of manomaya, vijnanamaya, and anandamaya kosha begin their journeys with a visit to an ayurvedic practitioner. When offered through an ayurvedic lens, yoga therapy asana and pranayama techniques may play an ideal role to help to restore balance in annamaya kosha.

Additional Resources

Finlayson, D. (2018). The role of ayurvedic assessment in yoga therapy. *Yoga Therapy Today*, Summer, 40–43.

See also the resources listed in Chapter 4.

Endnotes

1 Information on ways to consider appropriate care strategies can be found in Section II of this book. For structural contraindications, review Chapter 8 (and Chapter 18). For physiological contraindications, review Chapter 7, including Boxes 7.1–7.7. For mental health considerations, review Chapters 11 and 12.

2 Ayurveda, like yoga, has been an oral tradition. The colonization of India interrupted the natural development of this traditional medicine with the introduction of conventional Western medicine and the relegation of ayurveda to second-class status; see Berger, R. (2013). *Ayurveda made modern: Political histories of indigenous medicine in North India, 1900–1955* (Cambridge Imperial and Post-Colonial Studies Series). Palgrave Macmillan. These circumstances have led to a dearth of peer-reviewed academic research to support ayurvedic protocols other than pharmaceutical-type interventions. Additionally, as noted in Chapter 4, extant source texts are typically inaccessible and often only roughly translated.

This chapter offers for readers' critical consideration and exploration recommendations that have been handed from a teacher to a student. Through the discussion of the tools of yoga and the way of seeing a client through the ten pairs of opposites, it is hoped that beginning yoga therapists will be able to think for themselves "elementally." Using these methods of thought and observation can then enhance delivery of asana and pranayama interventions in a way that honors this tradition.

Additional study is recommended for those interested in more deeply incorporating ayurvedic principles into yoga therapy practice.

3 See, e.g., Haas, N. (2012). *Health and consciousness through ayurveda and yoga*. Mata Amritanandamayi Research Center.

4 Any posture or sequence that involves an inversion or places the head below the heart warrants caution for clients with eye- or head-pressure issues or glaucoma or with uncontrolled hypertension (high blood pressure). Consult the client's other healthcare providers for guidance, describing the specific proposed exercise(s) in simple language. See also Box 7.3.

5 Be aware that these types of deep pranayama practices are contraindicated for anyone pregnant, dealing with abdominal discomfort, suffering from an abdominal injury or hernia, or living with inflammatory bowel disorders that could be disrupted by these *kriyas*.

The *Hatha Yoga Pradipika* describes six cleansing techniques, the *shatkriya* or *shatkarma* (six actions) and variations, that prepare the system for further practice: *neti* (nasal lavage), *dhauti* (internal cleansing; agni sara is one type), *nauli* (stomach churning), *kapalabhati* (skull-shining breath), *trataka* (concentration or fixed gazing), and *basti* (enema). See Muktibodhananda, S. (2012). *Hatha yoga pradipika* 2.21–38. Yoga Publications Trust.

6 Vishnu mudra is traditionally performed with the right hand. The index and middle fingers curl toward the palm, leaving the ring and little fingers as straight as possible; for alternate-nostril breathing practices the thumb gently presses the right nostril closed, and the ring finger gently closes the left. Chapter 21 offers additional vayu-balancing mudra practices.

7 The client applies pressure in a circular motion, starting at the lower right of the abdomen below the navel and moving up the right side, across just under the rib cage, and down the left side. This can be done with blocks or pillows supporting the knees, or seated in a chair, so the client is not straining while trying to move samana vayu.

8 Frawley, D. (2012). *Soma in yoga and ayurveda: The power of rejuvenation and immortality* (pp. 96–98). Lotus Press.

21

Mudra and Bandha

MARSHA THERESE DANZIG

Every day, whether consciously or unconsciously, everyone uses their hands to create meaningful gestures. From the open-palmed wave at a neighbor to the OK sign in response to an inquiry, people bring their hands together in particular arrangements that powerfully convey messages. Walking around tight-fisted for an extended period would create reverberations in physical posture, respiration, and demeanor. Brought into both hands and held at the navel, the same shape can bring awareness to sensations in the body and a focus on anger being discharged; *mushti mudra* is a gesture intended to support the release of intense emotions.[1]

A mudra is just that, a gesture—one with deep roots in yogic tradition and deep meaning on the physical, mental, emotional, and spiritual levels. A gesture can be considered a small or large offering of a part of oneself to someone or something else for a particular result. According to scholar Georg Feuerstein, one root of the word mudra is *mudd*, or joyous delight (in the Divine) that enables the mind to be absorbed into bliss.[2]

The History of Mudra

Mudras are believed to have their roots in the Indus civilization, during the Vedic era, dating back to more than 2,000 years BCE. Mudras were used ritualistically, during dance, meditation, and in artistic expression.[3] Mudras form a major iconography within Hindu images both ancient and contemporary, and remain a part of everyday life in India. For example, greeting someone by bowing and saying *namaste*, with the hands in a prayer position at the heart (*anjali mudra*), is a common sign of respect.

Natyashastra (theater or dance of the *shastras*, or texts), a Hindu text from the 1st or 2nd century BCE, maps out how mudras are to be used to signify specific spiritual principles within traditional dances. Mudras are the key component of these dances, from which stories emerge. There are 28 to 30 *asamyukta* (single-handed mudras) and 24 *samukta* (two-handed mudras) classically used in *natyashastra*.[4]

Buddhism, Hatha Yoga, tantric rituals, and Indian martial arts all have used mudra as part of their practices for centuries. Mudras are also found in Christian iconography. The *hamsa*, or hand of God (believed to be from ancient Egypt), is used by Christians, Muslims, and Jews and predates all three religions.

A mudra is also referred to as a seal, as the fingers come together in specific patterns of closure. The combination of fingers produces various outcomes for the practitioner. As in the rest of the physical body, consciousness imbues the fingertips, fingers, palms, backs of the hands, and wrists. With more than 100,000 nerve receptors in the hands and 3,000 nerve receptors in each fingertip alone,[5] the hand is especially sensitive, creating the equivalent of an electric circuit that sends currents to the brain and body when placed into a mudra. The cortical homunculi are maps of the sensory-motor brain that mirror the parts of the body. The hands make up nearly one third of the sensory cortex and even more of the motor cortex and are themselves a microcosm of the brain and body. The hands convey a great deal of information to the brain.

In addition to hand mudras, certain full-body mudras, *bandhas* ("locks" in the chin area, abdomen, and groin; see Box 21.1), and tongue and chin placements serve as seals.[6] Historically, seals represented a mark or oath. A seal on a document indicated not only ownership but also importance. In the same way, a mudra is like an internal oath to a spiritual principle that has a higher, more important purpose, whether it represents a deity or a feeling being expressed. Body mudras are meant to balance all five elements, thereby ridding the body of disease. The *Goraksha Paddhati*, a Hatha Yoga text from around the 12th century CE, speaks of the body mudras as paths to liberation that awaken *kundalini*, or dormant energy potential.[7]

Another aspect of mudra is *marmas*, which are similar to acupuncture points in the body. They bring the *mahad* (*mahat*), or primordial innate intelligence, into form and consciousness as sensitive points in the body where *prana*, or life force, is most concentrated or blocked.[8] Practicing certain mudras is thought to stimulate marma points to move energy through the body.

BOX 21.1 WORKING WITH GRANTHI AND BANDHA

DIANE FINLAYSON AND LAURIE HYLAND ROBERTSON

In the same way the circulatory system allows blood to flow through *annamaya kosha*, *pranamaya* is thought to make use of a similar subtle circulatory system to move life force through the subtle body. This energetic system is defined in philosophical form through the chakra system of Tantra, and it aligns with yoga, ayurveda, and Jainism. The circulation of pranamaya has cross-cultural correlations with many of the world's mystical traditions, including Judaism/Qabbalah, Chinese medicine, and Egypt's Kemetic understanding of the worlds without and within.

In Tantra, the *nadis* function as the veins and arteries of the life force, and the chakras are "wheels of energy" on the main energetic artery, *sushumna*. Beginning in the 20th century with the inception of contemporary psychotherapy and advances in the understanding of human development, the chakras have also taken on significance in human developmental stages.[9] (See Chapter 2 and Box 7.1 for additional notes on the chakras.)

Activation of the *bandhas*, energetic locks similar to dams in a waterway system, assists with titrating the movement of life force (*prana*) and unblocking the *granthis*, energetic knots that prevent the free flow of prana through sushumna nadi. Working with the pranamaya sheath offers opportunities to create free flow of energy in the human system through pranayama, mudra, and mantra, and aids clients in integrating lessons for the *manomaya* sheath based on the condition of the granthis.

Creating a manageable flow of energy in sushumna prepares the energetic system for liberation through the rise of essential life force from *muladhara* (the root), up sushumna, and through *sahasrara* (the crown chakra). Appropriate use of the bandhas may be helpful in preventing psychic damage during awakening, or liberation, experiences.[10]

Granthi

The *granthis* are explained in the *Hatha Yoga Pradipika*.[11] These knots prevent the free flow of prana, so loosening them is important for various stages of human development.

Brahma granthi is associated with the first two chakras (*muladhara* and *svadisthana*) and their survival and instinctive functions. This granthi, which may be addressed by working with *mula bandha*, hinders growth by keeping an individual attached to physical comforts, including wealth.

Because ***Vishnu granthi*** relates to the *manipura* and *anahata* chakras, this blockage affects physical, mental, and emotional functioning:

> Manipura sustains *pranamaya kosha*, the energy body, governing the digestion and metabolism of food. Anahata sustains *manomaya kosha*, the mental body, and they both affect *annamaya kosha*, the physical body. Once Vishnu granthi

is transcended, one is no longer bound by physical, mental and emotional attachments. Relationships and energy become more universal, rather than being limited by personal preferences or aversions.[12]

Working with *uddiyana bandha* is said to aid Vishnu granthi.[13]

Rudra granthi, associated with the *vishuddha* and *ajna* chakras, is involved with egoic identification. Removing this blockage, via *jalandhara bandha*, results in dissolution of individual identity and the eventual return to original consciousness.

Bandha

According to Swami Satyananda, "The *Hatha Yoga Pradipika* deals with bandhas and mudras together and the ancient tantric texts also make no distinction between the two."[14] The bandhas can be engaged and exercised in ways that allow the individual to overcome the drawbacks of the granthis. In contemporary practice, bandhas are extensively incorporated in mudra as well as pranayama and asana techniques.

As noted elsewhere in this text, directly correlating yogic concepts with Western scientific knowledge is not always possible (or appropriate). However, it may be useful to consider the three main bandhas referred to in the *Hatha Yoga Pradipika* in light of three key anatomical diaphragms. *Jalandhara*, the throat lock, corresponds to the "diaphragm" of the thoracic outlet.[15] *Uddiyana bandha* is in the area of the respiratory diaphragm,[16] and *mula bandha* may be correlated with the muscles of the pelvic floor.[17] Attention to the use of the bandhas provides a means of containment and correct use of prana. Application of the bandhas in a manner consistent with the needs of a client can promote beneficial flow of energy throughout pranamaya.

Relationship to pranavayus and applications of bandha

One yoga therapy assessment tool is the reading and understanding of the five winds of *vata* from ayurveda (the *pranavayus*; see Chapter 4). For instance, a client with overabundant prana vayu may be guided in the use of jalandhara bandha, with or without mudra and mantra. One with excess *apana vayu* may benefit from the use of mula bandha to help keep the life force in the system. The use of uddiyana bandha may be beneficial for those with digestive issues. Use of all the bandhas in conjunction, *maha bandha*, promotes the use of energy for spiritual transformation and provides the means of generating the personal energy required to fulfill the client's *dharma*.[18]

When working with a client it is important to cultivate awareness of the physical tension held around each bandha, and to note that gross muscular engagement is not synonymous with bandha engagement. That is, lifting the pelvic floor muscles gently up and in, for example, is a beginning for accessing the energetic containment of mula bandha but not the complete practice. Additionally, cultivation of the ability to deliberately engage and disengage the musculature around each bandha is important, as is the assiduous avoidance of strain. Cuing clients to build such awareness offers the possibility for supple strength to support range of motion alongside the transformational possibility of manipulating one's own energies.

Yogic Function

Mudras are mind-body tools for addressing experiences such as fear, anger, and pain as well as peace, balance, and insight. The subtleties of the sensory nerves in the hands have a direct correspondence to the *vayus* (flows of prana through the body) and the *chakras*[19] (subtle energy centers in the body; see Box 21.1). Correctly combining the fingers in various positions is thought to have a precise impact on the systems of the body.[20] The habitual *vrittis*, or fluctuations of the mind described in the *Yoga Sutras*, can also be addressed by continuous practice of specific mudras.

Each mudra has a unique function, often relating to an emotion, a health concern, a prayer, or the invocation of a deity who represents a certain quality the practitioner is seeking. The texts and traditions from which mudras come sometimes refer to them as magical cures. For example, the *Hatha Yoga Pradipika*'s description of *nabho mudra* (mudra of the sky), where the tongue presses into the roof of the mouth while the practitioner focuses on the inner eye, is said to cure all diseases.[21]

For hand mudras, each finger corresponds to one of the five basic elements. In the tradition of Vedic astrology[22] (*jyotish*), which includes palmistry, the thumb is fire (*agni*), the index finger is air (*vayu*), the middle finger is ether (*akash*), the ring finger is earth (*prithvi*), and the little finger is water (*jala*). In the tradition of ayurveda, according to Vasant Lad,[23] the thumb is ether, the index finger is air, the middle finger is fire, the ring finger is water, and the little finger is earth. Bringing physical, mental, and energetic attention to the various combinations of these fingers/elements is meant to address imbalances of the body, mind, and spirit. Each finger also corresponds to one of the five vayus. (See Chapter 4 for more information on the *pranavayus*, the five subdoshas of vata.)

Consider *gyan/jnana mudra*, or symbol of Om, which brings the thumb and forefinger tips together in an O shape. Too much vayu (forefinger) and we can become full of hot air (wind). Too much fire (thumb) and we can become zealots with no real sense of direction. Combining these two elements of fire and air creates the symbol of Om, or harmony and balance. Symbolically, the thumb represents Brahman, or highest consciousness. The ring finger is referred to as the individual self. The three extended fingers represent the *gunas*, or attributes of nature (see Chapter 3): The middle finger is *sattva*, or harmony; the ring finger is *rajas*, or action; and the little finger is *tamas*, or inaction. Bringing the index finger and thumb together is meant to create a loop of energy that pulls one inward. Although the origin of mudra in yogic tradition remains a mystery, gyan mudra is mentioned in the *Siva Purana*,[24] a Hindu text from possibly the 1st or 2nd century CE.

Mudra Practice

There are five main types of mudra:

- ***hasta mudras*** (hand mudras)
- ***bandhas*** (internal body locks)
- ***kaya mudras*** (full-body mudras)
- ***mana mudras*** (head, tongue, and mouth mudras)
- ***adhara mudras*** (groin/perineal mudras)[25]

The majority of mudras are hand mudras, with other more esoteric techniques such as perineal mudras being used as needed. Hand mudras can be either easy or challenging, depending on the placement of fingers.

The practice of mudra starts with intention and identification of the mudra that would best speak to the present need. Slow breath, conscious focus, and a meditative mindset are additional keys to mudra practice. Most hand mudras are gentle, with fingertips touching lightly. Hand mudras are stand-alone practices, but they can be included in yoga *asana*, meditation, or mantra practice.

Mudras are typically performed in *sukhasana* (easy seat), *vajrasana* (kneeling), *padmasana* (lotus), or another relaxed seated pose and held for 5 seconds to 15 minutes or longer; however, the operation of the habitual vrittis means that longer holds in some cases may aggravate a condition rather than resolve it. Pushing to accomplish a long hold can indicate a mind in a state of *vikalpa*, or wishful thinking.

The benefits of mudras have been gleaned over centuries of practice and tradition.[26] The rich science of yoga has given context and meaning to mudras based on the experience of the yogis who practiced and documented their benefits rigorously.[27] Little Western research has been done on mudra, but complementary studies on acupressure,[28] acupuncture, and marma[29] points support their potential mechanisms. Anecdotally, many mudra practitioners note positive changes in demeanor, pain level, stress, and aggravated emotions.

Common mudras, including a representative practice to affect each of the five vayus, are illustrated in Table 21.1.

Table 21.1 Common hand mudras

Mudra		Practice Steps	Purpose	Example Client Need
Prana	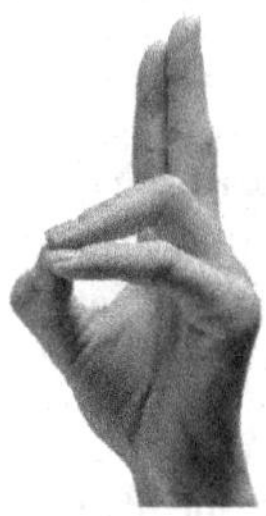	Press the thumb tip to the tips of the ring and little fingers; extend the index and middle fingers	Increase life force; direct prana to most needed areas in the body, mind, or spirit; associated with the heart and connection; air element	Increased energy
Apana	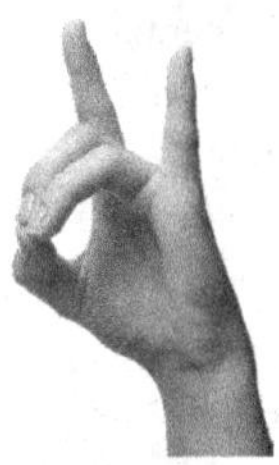	Press the thumb tip to the tips of the ring and middle fingers; extend the little and index fingers	Support healthy digestion, elimination, and detoxification; associated with releasing; earth element	Release of worry
Vyana	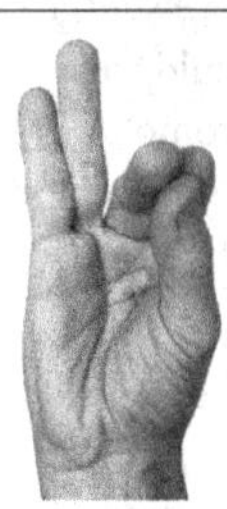	Press the thumb tip to the index and middle fingertips; extend the ring and little fingers	Support the heart and lungs; balance blood pressure; associated with pelvic bowl; water element	Blood pressure regulation
Samana	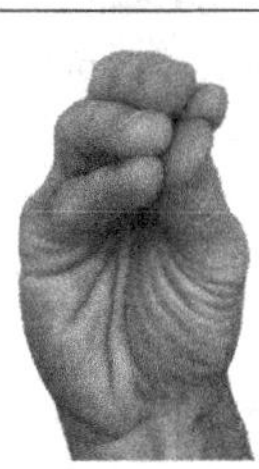	Press all four fingers to the thumb tip	Support healthy digestion and absorption; associated with the respiratory diaphragm; fire element	Metabolism stabilization

Mudra		**Practice Steps**	**Purpose**	**Example Client Need**
Udana	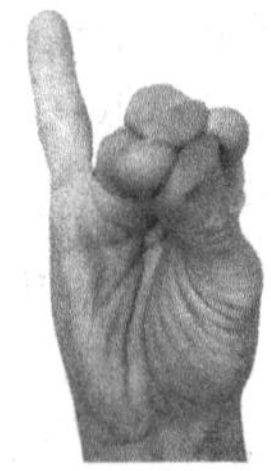	Press the index, middle, and ring fingers to the tip of the thumb; extend the little finger	Balance the thyroid and parathyroid glands; support the respiratory system and throat; associated with speech; ether element	More clearly speaking one's mind
Varuna	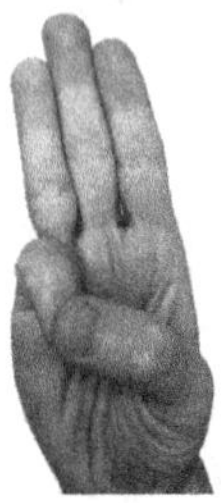	Fold the little finger under the top of the thumb	Promote an attitude of ease; balance the water element; represents Varuna, god of water	Release of feelings of tension
Prithvi	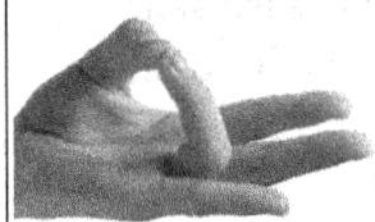	Place the thumb and ring finger together while extending the other fingers	Promote a feeling of being settled; relieve anxiety; represents Mother Earth in Hindu	Release of upset and anxiety
Dhyana	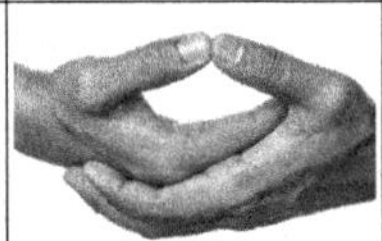	With the palms turned up, place the right palm on top of the left with the thumb tips touching; rest the hands at the navel area	Enhance meditation; increase mental balance; calm overreactivity	Decreased overreactivity
Uttarabodhi	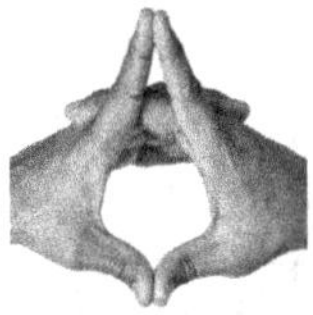	Interlock the fingers; extend the thumb and index fingers apart, creating space between all the fingers	Boost self-confidence; soothe worry; build trust in life; promote release into limitless potential	Release of constriction caused by thoughts and beliefs
Padma	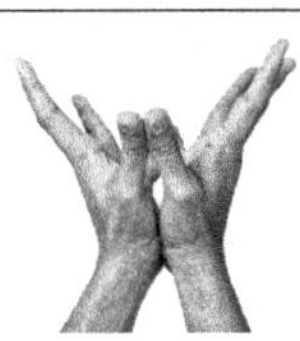	Press the heels of the hands and the tips of the thumbs and little fingers together; spread the other fingers open	Open the heart; release mistrust; promote accepting inner beauty and opening to the spirit of bliss; associated with Lakshmi	Reconnection to bliss

Besides these well-known hand mudras, the traditional texts mention additional mudras. According to the *Hatha Yoga Pradipika*, these are resourced from Shiva himself and designed to destroy old age and death. Originally meant to be kept secret and passed on from guru to student, they are now available to all with the caveat that they were likely viewed as extremely potent and should therefore not be used casually or without respect. When teaching these specific mudras to yoga clients, it is recommended that yoga therapists honor their power and do not teach them lightly.

Unlike the gross effects of asana, many yoga therapy clients may be unable to sense the subtle energy involved in mudra and therefore have more difficulty perceiving the effects of the practice. Skillful yoga therapists will meet clients where they are in terms of cultural understanding, framing mudra—or indeed any practice—in a way that resonates with the client's mindset and current needs. The yoga therapist might discuss the various gestures used daily by people to communicate in specific cultures: For instance, the rich, emotion-filled lexicon of American Sign Language, waving at a neighbor, and gesticulating in anger at another driver all evoke particular energies.

Also, as in any practice, yoga therapists should be prepared to modify mudra in accordance with individual capacity. Mudras can be inaccessible for those with disabilities that affect the hands in particular, such as rheumatoid arthritis, although in some cases attention to continued mobility may be helpful for maintaining remaining range of motion. Practices can include guided imagery and other components to achieve the intended energetic effects. For example, for a client unable to fully "seal" a mudra by touching fingertip to fingertip, the yoga therapist might encourage gentle movement of the hands to the edge of resistance while the client envisions the fully sealed mudra, thus bringing energy and awareness to these areas of the body. Extended mudras like *kali mudra* raised overhead in warrior I may be inaccessible to those with arthritis in any part of the upper body from fingers to neck, so the yoga therapist may recommend a simpler shape like anjali mudra while the client envisions joining their hands overhead.

Bandha

The bandhas are internal body locks that redirect the flow of vayus in the body-mind.[30] Just as locks are used by farmers to change the flow of water for irrigation, the bandhas "irrigate" the body's systems and change the flow of prana for various purposes.

Bandhas are said to maintain and lift the inner organs and support the outer body, including bones and muscles. They are a way of sealing in energy, keeping the mind from de-identifying with the Self. These internal mudras are intended to conserve energy so it can be used efficiently. Bandhas also work with the chakras and glands. Activating the *uddiyana bandha*, or navel lock, for example, is said to support the second and third chakras as well as the gonads, adrenals, and pancreas. Because body mudras are so potent, they are best taught by someone well-qualified, ideally in a more individualized therapeutic yoga setting where the client can be safely monitored. See Box 21.1 for more information.

The three principal bandhas

- ***Mula bandha*** (root lock): The pubic bone is drawn toward the tailbone as the perineum lifts up and in and the breath is kept steady. Mula bandha stabilizes the pelvis, provides an inner lift for the center of the body, may help to address incontinence, and redirects apana vayu upward to awaken kundalini or higher consciousness.
- ***Uddiyana bandha*** (navel lock): The navel is drawn in toward the spine, then the lock is gently internally lifted up toward the bottom of the heart. Uddiyana bandha reverses apana vayu to interact with prana and samana vayu at the navel, creating fire in the belly and continuing to redirect the flow of kundalini up the *sushumna*, or energetic spine.
- ***Jalandhara bandha*** (chin lock): The top center of the heart is drawn up toward the chin as the shoulders drop. This bandha pushes the prana vayu at the heart down into the navel, again to activate the core and stimulate kundalini.

Body Mudra

Body mudras look similar to asana, but their purpose is quite different. In asana, the body is placed into positions to still the mind, physically releasing blocks and tensions to prepare for meditation. The body mudras, on the other hand, are concentrated on the management of prana, with a deep inner focus on activating kundalini energy. *Janu sirsasana* (head-to-knee pose) and *maha mudra* are perfect examples. Janu sirsasana lengthens and flexes the spine, flexes both hips and externally rotates the hip of the flexed knee, lengthens the hamstrings, and quiets the mind. Maha mudra has the same shape as janu sirsasana but keeps the spine extended via the inner lift of the three bandhas and includes a focus on activating kundalini over time.

Examples of body mudra and practice methods are shown in Figure 21.1, and head mudra are shown in Figure 21.2 (perineal mudra is used less often in Western yoga therapy settings).

Draw the left foot into the groin as the right leg is extended, foot flexed. Reach toward the left foot. Apply all three bandhas as the breath remains steady. Switch legs.

This practice is used to redirect sexual energy toward heightened spiritual awareness.

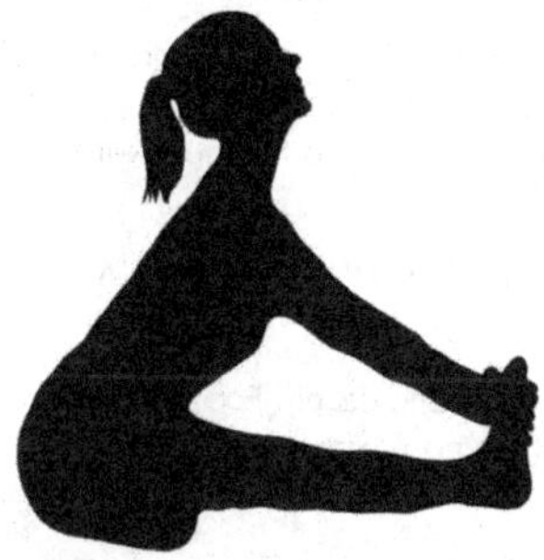

FIGURE 21.1A *MAHA MUDRA* (GREAT SEAL)

Sit with one hip at a wall. Twist onto the back, letting the back of the legs rest on the wall above the hips.

This mudra is meant to relax the pelvis and legs, reduce swelling in the limbs, and lessen lower back pain.

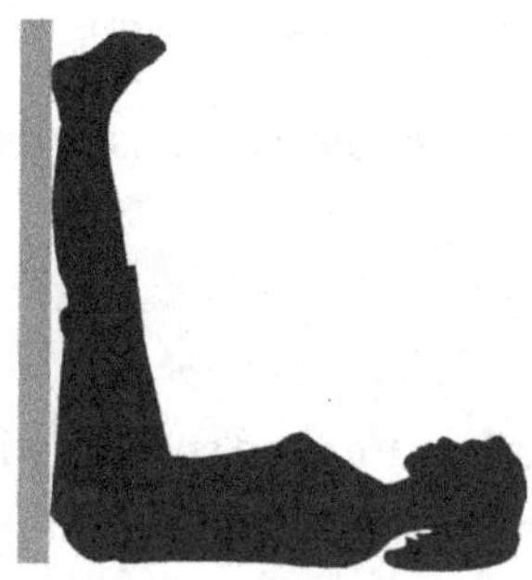

FIGURE 21.1B *VIPARITA KARANI MUDRA* (INVERTED-LEG POSE)

Sit with the hands firmly pressing on the floor or knees. Practice a few rounds of *bhastrika* breath to clear the body and mind, then draw the navel deeply back and up, churning the belly as the breath is suspended. Exhale and release when needed. Perform two to three times.

The purpose of this mudra is to awaken and release latent energy, or kundalini, for greater health and spiritual consciousness.

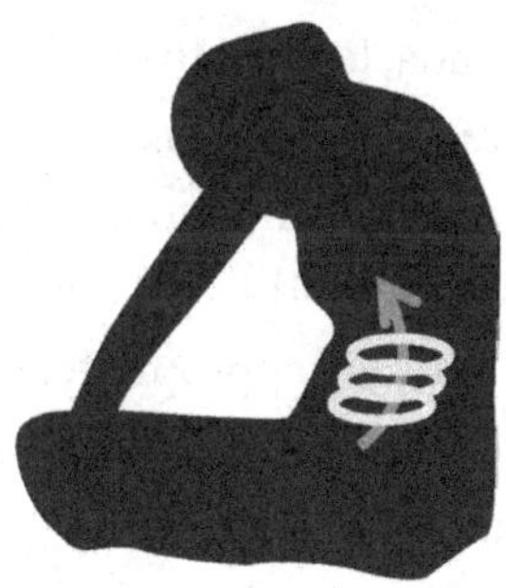

FIGURE 21.1C *SHAKTI CHALANA MUDRA* (SHAKTI-AWAKENING MOVEMENT)

Relax the eyes and breathe deeply. Focus the eyes on the third-eye center between the eyebrows. Start with a small amount of time (e.g., 5 seconds), increasing as possible.

This mudra is said to stimulate the pineal gland, calm the mind, and increase the ability to meditate. It is not recommended for those with eye strain.

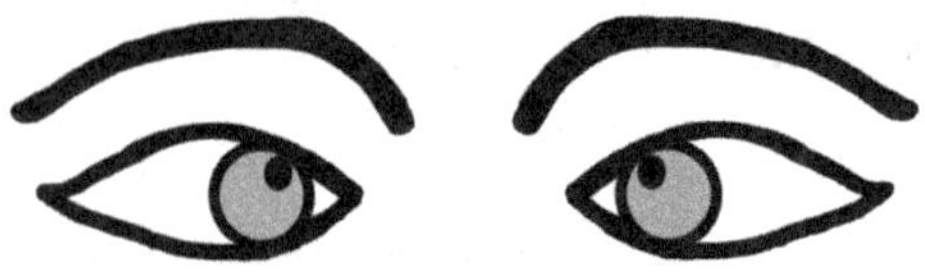

FIGURE 21.2A *SHAMBHAVI MUDRA* (EYEBROW-CENTER GAZING)

Relax the eyes and breathe deeply. Focus the eyes on the tip of the nose. Start with a small amount of time (e.g., 5 seconds), then increase as possible.

This mudra is said to increase concentration. It is not recommended for those with depression, as it is a deeply introspective practice that can therefore promote rumination.

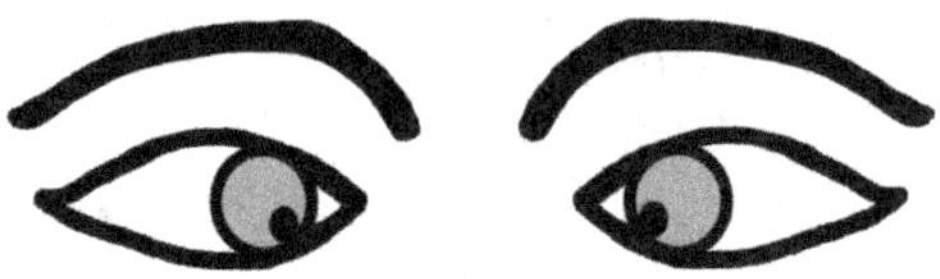

FIGURE 21.2B *NASIKAGRA MUDRA* (NOSE-TIP GAZING)

Summary

Although mudras are used sparingly in Western yoga practice, they are extremely useful within a yoga therapy session. Mudras are often possible when asana and other practices may be inaccessible, although mudra themselves may be difficult because of conditions such as arthritis or amputation. They can be held for longer periods than asana, leading to deep states of inner awareness and therefore healing. Mudras may reach people in subtle ways that bypass the overthinking or fearful mind. The practices can help clients tap into their spirituality and expand their consciousness when other practices, such as mantra or meditation, may not be palatable or culturally appropriate.

Many mudras, such as prithvi mudra, are intended to address emotional struggles, making them ideal for helping clients to increase awareness around anxiety, depression, or grief, or before a concerning medical procedure. They seem to have a quick effect on the body, breath, mind, and emotions, which can be helpful when a client is struggling to stay present. Evidence suggests that mudra may be effective for people with Alzheimer's disease[31] and in heart attack prevention.[32] Mudras may also be useful for people with posttraumatic stress disorder (PTSD): Some research shows that somatosensory processing can be inhibited in PTSD,[33] and mudra may provide a gentle way to restore somatosensory function.

Mudra is a self-empowering tool for yoga therapists to offer to clients for inspiration toward their own well-being. As suggested by research in other fields, consistent practice, especially at the same time each day, may produce the best results.[34] The most productive way for yoga therapists to support clients with mudra is, arguably, to observe their effects during their own personal practices. Because people seek yoga therapy for a variety of reasons, from physical pain to anxiety, mudra specific to these needs can be part of an individualized care plan. Most mudra practices can be done anywhere, at any time. Mudras are an easy way to make the healing art of yoga accessible to all.

Additional Resources

Dev, K. (2012). *Mudras for healing (Mudra vigyan: A way of life)*. Aacharya Shri Enterprises.

Feuerstein, G. (2013). *The yoga tradition: Its history, literature, philosophy, and practice*. Hohm Press.

Hirschi, G., Grimm, C. M., & Ito, J. (2016). *Mudras: Yoga in your hands*. Weiser Books.

Mallinson, J. (2004). *The Gheranda Samhita: The original Sanskrit*. YogaVidya.com.

Mesko, S. (2013). *Healing mudras: Yoga for your hands*. Mudra Hands Publishing.

Muktibodhananda, S. (2012). *Hatha yoga pradipika* (3.1–102). Yoga Publications Trust.

Saraswati, N. S. (2014). *Mudra vigyan: Philosophy and practice of yogic gestures*. Yoga Publications Trust.

Saraswati, S. (2015). *Asana pranayama mudra bandha*. Yoga Publications Trust.

Endnotes

1 Hirschi, G., Grimm, C. M., & Ito, J. (2016). *Mudras: Yoga in your hands*. Weiser Books.

2 Feuerstein, G. (2013). *The yoga tradition: Its history, literature, philosophy, and practice*. Hohm Press.

3 Feuerstein, *The yoga tradition*.

4 Muni, B., & Ghosh, M. (2016). *Nāṭyaśāstram: A treatise on ancient Indian dramaturgy and histrionics*. Chaukhamba Surbharati Prakashan.

5 Hancock, E. (1995). A handy guide to touch. *Johns Hopkins Magazine*, April. https://pages.jh.edu/jhumag/495web/touch.html

6 According to the *Hatha Yoga Pradipika* (written between the 6th and 15th centuries CE), *Gheranda Samhita* (written in the 19th century CE), and *Shiva Samhita* (written between the 17th and 18th centuries CE). See Chapter 2.

7 Feuerstein, *The yoga tradition*.

8 Lad, V., & Durve, A. (2016). *Marma points of ayurveda: The energy pathways for healing body, mind & consciousness with a comparison to traditional Chinese medicine*. Ayurvedic Press.

9 Washburn, M. (1995). *The ego and the dynamic ground: A transpersonal theory of human development* (p. 199). State University of New York Press.

10 Srinivasan, T. M. (1991). Pranayama and brain correlates. *Ancient Science of Life*, *11*(1–2), 2–6.

11 Svatmarama. (2012). *The hatha yoga pradipika* (B. D. Akers, Trans.). YogaVidya.com.

12 Saraswati, S. ([2009] 2015). *Asana pranayama mudra bandha* (4th ed., p. 472). Yoga Publications Trust.

13 Bhardwaj, A. (2019). *Celebrating life with yoga*. D. K. Printworld.

14 Saraswati, *Asana pranayama mudra bandha* (p. 471).

15 Clients may be able to locate these muscles by gently practicing posterior cervical translation, an exercise that strengthens the deep cervical flexors by drawing the chin toward the chest while keeping the crown of the head level.

16 *Uddiyana bandha* literally translates as "flying-up" lock, referring to the engagement of rectus abdominus, analogous to "drawing the navel toward the spine." When working with the bandhas, especially uddiyana, it may be useful to consider the image of the "tension of an egg yolk" for cuing abdominal containment to create resilience without rigidity.

17 Clients may be cued to locate these muscles by practicing stopping the flow of urine, although habitually doing so may result in incomplete bladder emptying and is not recommended. As yoga therapists it is important to guide clients correctly.

Mula bandha is located in slightly different areas for men and women. For men, the area of contraction is between anus and testes, whereas for women the muscles engaged are those behind the cervix, where the uterus projects into the vagina (Saraswati, *Asana pranayama mudra bandha* [p. 478]). It is often difficult for the client to access these areas, and working with *ashwini* and *shajoli/vajroli mudra* may be used to develop the awareness and sensitivity required to work successfully with mula bandha.

18 Some teachers, including those of the Satyananda lineage, recommend that the individual bandhas be learned prior to using them together in maha bandha.

19 Radha, S. S. (1996). *Kundalini yoga for the West: A foundation for character building, courage and awareness.* Timeless Books.

20 Formal research on the effects of mudra is sparse but emerging. See, e.g., Kumar, K. S., Srinivasan, T. M., Ilavarasu, J., Mondal, B., & Nagendra, H. R. (2018). Classification of electrophotonic images of yogic practice of mudra through neural networks. *International Journal of Yoga, 11*(2), 152–156.

21 Muktibodhananda, S. (2012). *Hatha yoga pradipika.* Yoga Publications Trust.

22 Dev, K. (2012). *Mudras for healing (Mudra vigyan: A way of life).* Aacharya Shri Enterprises.

23 Lad, V. (2009). *Ayurveda: The science of self healing.* Lotus Press.

24 Shastri, J. (2005). *The siva purana.* Motilal Banarsidass.

25 Saraswati, S. (2013). *Asana pranayama mudra bandha.* Yoga Publications Trust.

26 Dev, *Mudras for healing.*

27 Kumar et al., Classification of electrophotonic images.

28 Mehta, P., Dhapte, V., Kadam, S., & Dhapte, V. (2017). Contemporary acupressure therapy: Adroit cure for painless recovery of therapeutic ailments. *Journal of Traditional and Complementary Medicine, 7*(2), 251–263.

29 Schrott, E. G., Raju, J. R., & Schrott, S. (2016). *Marma therapy.* Singing Dragon.

30 Avalon, A. (1974). *The serpent power: The secrets of tantric and shaktic yoga.* Dover Publications.

31 Khalsa, D. S. (2015). Stress, meditation, and Alzheimer's disease prevention: Where the evidence stands. *Journal of Alzheimer's Disease, 48*(1), 1–12.

32 Tripathi, D., Kalantri, Y., Kumar, H., Chitnis, V., et al. (2017). Effect of yoga hand mudra on cardiac and neurological parameters in preventing heart attack. *Research Journal of Recent Sciences, 6*(2), 16–20.

33 Badura-Brack, A. S., Becker, K. M., McDermott, T. J., Ryan, T. J., et al. (2015). Decreased somatosensory activity to non-threatening touch in combat veterans with posttraumatic stress disorder. *Psychiatry Research: Neuroimaging, 233*(2), 194–200.

34 Arlinghaus, K. R., & Johnston, C. A. (2018). The importance of creating habits and routine. *American Journal of Lifestyle Medicine, 13*(2), 142–144.

22

Yoga Nidra Healing

UMA DINSMORE-TULI

Nidra is the Sanskrit word for sleep. Yoga nidra literally means the yoga of sleep, or the sleep of yoga. In practical terms, yoga nidra is a form of yoga requiring no physical movement whatsoever: Anyone who can breathe, and anyone who has ever, even once in their lives, fallen asleep, can practice yoga nidra. It is essentially a horizontal meditation on the act of falling asleep, although it can also be practiced seated, standing, or indeed, with experience, in any situation. For beginning yoga students, yoga nidra will likely be more accessible than a seated meditation practice, but for experienced practitioners it can be an exquisite entry into the meditative heart of yoga. Its key characteristic is effortlessness and surrender because there is nothing to do but listen and rest. Yoga nidra is a state of consciousness, a way of being rather than a technique to master. This sleep that is not sleep invites one into the liminal boundaries of consciousness between one state and another, between ordinary consciousness and the underlying, superconscious state of *turiya*, states of being, not doing.[1]

Although every tradition of yoga nidra has its own unique form, many are based on a similar underlying structure, usually in this order:

1. **Preparation:** Gathering together and doing everything needed for a beneficial practice can include restorative propping and review of any issues being addressed.

2. **Settling:** This demarcation between the everyday state of consciousness and the state of yoga nidra may involve reference to elemental resonances (see Chapters 3 and 4).

3. ***Sankalpa*:** One's resolution or resolve may be focused in the space of the spiritual heart, which is identified as the location of the yoga nidra state

of consciousness. The sankalpa may be preceded by an intention for the practice or the creation of a safe space.

4. **Rotation of consciousness (body scan):** Many different itineraries through the body can be used, each with its own rationale.[2]

5. **Pairs of opposites:** This element of practice can take many forms, from the straightforward (e.g., heavy and light) to those used for specific aspects of psychological exploration or growth (e.g., confidence and confusion).

6. **Breathing and awareness of points of contact:** Bringing conscious attention to the breath may include counting breaths. Noticing connections between the body and the surface on which it rests can either deepen the connection to the experience of yoga nidra or serve as a reassuring reminder of the physicality of the body and the ground.

7. **Visualizations in *chidakasha*:** The purpose and nature of visualizations in the mind space depend on the intention of the yoga therapist and/or client. Some introduce images of journeys or archetypal images, and others invite people to notice whatever arises naturally.[3]

8. **Sankalpa:** The sankalpa may be repeated to deepen the effect and connection.

9. **Externalization and return to everyday state:** This phase of yoga nidra often includes a return to intention/safe place or an invitation to carry the benefits of practice into everyday life.

10. **Finish:** The process of exiting the state of yoga nidra is often just as long as the process of entering into it. Because people may be in quite an impressionable and relaxed frame of mind traditional forms usually close the practice by sharing chants, prayers, or uplifting readings. In a secular context, the need for proper closure can be met through sharing carefully chosen poetry, song, or sounds.

Yoga nidra is a journey that starts and ends in the physical body and an everyday state of consciousness. Clear starting and ending points contribute to making yoga nidra a safe vessel in which to explore other aspects of the body-mind and other states of consciousness. (See also the ideas for creating safe containers of practice in Chapter 14, and note that, e.g., not all forms of yoga nidra are trauma-informed. Some practices could be triggering, or even unsettling for those with anxiety.)

Nidra Shakti

Nidra Shakti, the "power of sleep," is the active ingredient of all yoga nidra, regardless of form, school, or lineage. Nidra Shakti can be understood to be a form of the goddess Kali, who is time herself and one of the many faces of Shakti, the power of life. Nidra Shakti is praised in these terms in a 5th-century Indian devotional hymn "Devi Mahatmaya": "To the Divine Goddess who resides in all existence in the form of Sleep, we bow to Her; we bow to Her, continually we bow, we bow" (5.23).[4] (For more detailed explorations of the nature of Shakti in yoga therapy, see Chapter 15.)

Perceiving the presence of Nidra Shakti within yoga nidra offers an understanding of the *adaptogenic* nature of yoga nidra experiences, that is, the intelligent power of Nidra Shakti ensures that what is needed is received. For example, tired people can sleep, sick people can heal, humans looking for inspiration can receive solutions to problems—and spiritual seekers can experience yoga nidra as a deeply meditative journey. Yoga nidra has the potential to meet clients where they are, and so respond to the particular needs of each person, in each dimension of their being, just as necessary.

Postlineage Yoga Nidra

Postlineage yoga is a term created by yoga teacher and researcher Theodora Wildcroft.[5] It does not mean antilineage or no lineage, but instead refers to an approach to yoga that places practitioner, teacher, or yoga therapist in a place of freedom, without the obligation to adhere to the teachings of a single source. Effective therapeutic applications of yoga nidra are by definition postlineage—drawing on a multiplicity of approaches inspires the possibility to be fully responsive to client needs. To understand what this means in practical terms for the use of yoga nidra in yoga therapy, it is necessary to have a sense of the major different lineages currently offering yoga nidra teachings and trainings.

In Europe, the most widespread approach to yoga nidra is Satyananda Yoga Nidra, the method devised by Swami Satyananda Saraswati in the 1960s. This method was among the inspirations for Richard Miller's development of iRest Yoga Nidra, one of the most popular forms in the United States. Both of these methods have a similar framework to the I AM method of yoga nidra presented by Amrit Desai, whereas the Himalayan Institute's approach to yoga nidra, as taught by Swami Rama, offers a longer practice that differs structurally from the previous three methods but arguably leads to similar states of being (see Table 22.1 for more detail).

Table 22.1 Major contemporary yoga nidra lineages

Lineage/School/Teacher	Milestones in Development
Swami Satyananda, from 1952 to 1984	1952–1984 Swami Satyananda Saraswati teaches and lectures on yoga nidra worldwide, training students in the techniques he developed 1974 *Yoga Nidra* ("blue book")
Bihar School of Yoga, from 1964	1971 Swami Pragyamurti starts teaching Satyananda yoga nidra in the UK 1979 Satyananda *Yoga Nidra* recordings by Swami Pragyamurti 1993 Swami Niranjanananda (Satyananda's successor) describes three preliminary levels of Satyananda yoga nidra in *Yoga Darshan*
Scandinavian School of Yoga and Meditation, from 1970	1978 Swami Satyananda's European disciple Swami Janakananda (Denmark) makes yoga nidra recordings that include innovative soundscapes and music and trains yoga teachers to deliver the practice
Richard Miller, from 1970	1970 Richard Miller first experiences yoga nidra in an Integral Yoga class and continues to practice the technique, developing a theory and practice of yoga nidra informed by non-dual psychotherapy and Western psychology 1987 Formation of the Integrative Restoration (iRest) Institute 2005 Publication of *Yoga Nidra: A Meditative Practice for Deep Relaxation and Healing* 2015 *The iRest Program for Healing PTSD: A Proven-Effective Approach to Using Yoga Nidra Meditation and Deep Relaxation Techniques to Overcome Trauma*
Swami Rama, from 1971	1971 Swami Rama demonstrates yogic meditative techniques including yoga nidra at the Meninger Institute 1971 Formation of the Himalayan Institute, which has an intention to preserve and share the teachings of Swami Rama 1988 Publication of *Path of Fire and Light* (Vol. 2), describing two of five methods of yoga nidra 2011 Veda Bharati (Swami Rama's disciple) hosts conference where he identifies four levels of practice and sponsors an international conference on yoga nidra to promote discussion between practitioners and researchers
Modern academic developments, from 1975	1975 Herbert Benson, US pioneer in mind-body medicine, publishes *The Relaxation Response*, describing many of the practical strategies also present in yoga nidra 2005 Mark Singleton, a UK yoga researcher, publishes *Salvation Through Relaxation: Proprioceptive Therapy and Its Relation to Yoga*, identifying the impact of Western proprioceptive therapies on development of yoga nidra 2003 N. C. Panda, an Indian academic, publishes *Yoga Nidra, Yogic Trance: Theory, Practice and Applications*, identifying yoga nidra as an autosuggestive, self-hypnotic phenomenon

Rod Stryker, from 1999	1977 Rod Stryker starts studying yoga 1999 Rod Stryker meets his current teacher, Pandit Rajmani Tigunait, spiritual head of the Himalayan Institute, and releases his first yoga nidra audio recordings 2013 Publication of *The Four Desires: Creating a Life of Purpose, Happiness, Prosperity, and Freedom*, about *sankalpa* as a means of goal setting and recognition of *dharma* Currently one of the senior teachers at the Himalayan Institute
Yoga Nidra Network, from 2010	2010 Sitaram Partnership (Uma Dinsmore-Tuli and Nirlipta Tuli) launches the first comparative yoga nidra teacher training course in the UK, under the auspices of Yogacampus as a module of the Yoga Campus Diploma in Yoga Therapy 2011 Foundation of the Yoga Nidra Network to promote comparative studies and hybrid creative and therapeutic uses of yoga nidra 2014 Total Yoga Nidra Foundation Course (now known as the Immersion Course) launched

Note that the table does not include Amrit Desai's I AM method of yoga nidra.
Adapted with permission from Dinsmore-Tuli, U., & Tuli, N. C. N. (2011–2020). *Total Yoga Nidra online foundation workbook*. Sitaram and Sons.

Acknowledging that each of these different schools offers some beneficial approaches to yoga nidra, and that they are all distinct but related, leads to a better understanding of the applicability of a postlineage approach in which the yoga therapist is free to utilize from each school the most relevant and appropriate aspects to meet a client's needs. Many training providers equip facilitators with a single standard script for use in all situations and discourage departure from that scripted presentation or set of enquiries. The yoga nidra form discussed in the remainder of this chapter, Total Yoga Nidra, is one characterized by responsiveness, as it employs co-creative strategies together with elements from the previously mentioned schools.

It is important to recognize that this postlineage approach is entirely independent of any gurus or spiritual guides. When making choices about yoga nidra methods—or trainings—it is worth considering the abuses of power hidden within many of these training organizations and asking, "Does this level of power imbalance matter to me and the clients I serve? What kind of yoga therapy does this method permit?"[6]

Conditions for success

Five characteristics of postlineage yoga nidra are of particular relevance to yoga therapists. To provide appropriate yoga nidra for yoga therapy clients, it is advisable that

- the facilitator is capable of adapting the practice to the individual
- the practice is responsive to time and place
- the facilitator is trauma-informed and attentive to the needs of the moment
- the facilitator is in service to the client
- the facilitator is capable of drawing on multiple forms and methods as needed, limited neither by adherence to a single form/script nor by ignorance of any other options

Although standardized one-size-fits-all practices of yoga nidra may be therapeutic, its adaptogenic power may be most potent when the facilitator is free to respond to the client, delivering practices directly relevant to present needs rather than following a particular script. The five conditions of postlineage yoga nidra empower co-creative healing, wherein the yoga therapist offers the client a uniquely tailored experience.[7]

Responsive, client-centered yoga nidra

The essential element of trust enables the client to relax within the felt sense that the yoga therapist is fully present, responsive, and attentive to the co-creation of an appropriate yoga nidra. To achieve this, yoga therapists themselves need to be free from any fears of departing from a set script, or fears that they lack resources to meet any need that may arise. In effect, this means the yoga therapist needs to be sufficiently competent and confident in more than one method of yoga nidra. In this context, to be postlineage is to be free to trust the integrity of personal and professional experience as a reliable intuitive guide to what may be helpful for the client. It is to welcome with humility the authority of the wisdom of Nidra Shakti by creating conditions that allow for this intuitive and potent force to move freely between client and facilitator.

Before offering any yoga nidra practice, humility also requires that the therapist ask, "How long have you got for this?" If the client replies, "Well, I think I might find 13 minutes," there is no point in creating a technically brilliant 30-minute practice.

Because yoga nidra is a practice that powerfully reconnects one to intuitive wisdom, it is vital that any yoga therapist wishing to share yoga nidra explore its practices and use them themselves. Daily experience enables yoga therapists to confidently trust the heart of their intuitive inner wisdom when co-creating yoga nidra practices with clients. An instinctive, spontaneous approach does not obviate the need for sound clinical reasoning, nor preclude its use. Intuition and discernment based on a working knowledge of classical structural elements can work together to effect individually meaningful change in a client without strictly following a protocol.

Affirming at the beginning and end of the practice, "With great respect and love, I honor my heart, my inner teacher,"[8] invites client and therapist to occupy a shared field of intuitive connection and trust. The power of reconnecting to the heart's wisdom through this affirmation transforms the understanding of yoga therapeutic alliances, enabling the beginning yoga therapist to recognize postlineage, co-creative therapeutic yoga nidra as a reliable way for clients to access their own intuitive wisdom—potent medicine indeed.

Clinical Use of Yoga Nidra: Case Application

The scope for the therapeutic application of yoga nidra, particularly when approached with the principles of a postlineage approach, is vast. There are many ways to use yoga nidra within yoga therapy, and the following case history explores just one application: preparation for and recovery from surgery in the context of perimenopause. The issues addressed include uterine fibroids, a midlife reevaluation of femininity, and the experience of deep uncertainty during preparation for possible hysterectomy. Many of the issues here are relevant for all clients encountering similar combinations of stressors presurgery amidst life-stage challenges.

"Cassie," a 45-year-old psychotherapist, had experienced extreme menstrual pain since menarche.[9] She developed uterine fibroids in her 30s and had been on hormonal birth control for decades. Cassie had recently undergone a series of invasive tests to ascertain whether the fibroids in her womb could be removed, or whether she would need a hysterectomy. The tests showed no certain outcomes, so Cassie was preparing for surgery to remove the fibroids with the option for a full hysterectomy if necessary. She was in a place of deep uncertainty and fear.

Cassie had practiced Iyengar Yoga for 20 years but had never experienced yoga nidra until she attended a women's yoga circle. When she subsequently arrived for her first yoga therapy session, she reported feeling confused and anxious: "[I'm] not sure if I will need a hysterectomy or not, so I'm looking for yoga therapy to recover after surgery, to help me feel whole and connected, with or without my womb."

Although Cassie was seeking yoga therapy for postsurgical recovery, it also became crucial to her navigation of the uncertainty of the outcome of the surgery. Many with gynecological problems are prepared for investigative surgery on this basis, signing permission for a full hysterectomy in the event that surgeons deem it necessary. This places people in intense uncertainty.

Cassie explained that a major issue troubling her preparation for surgery was that she had never felt any positive connection to her experiences as a woman. She spoke of deep physical suffering, regret, and anger. She described sadness that it was only now, in perimenopause, as she faced the prospect of losing her womb, that she felt moved to connect with her femininity and the rhythms of her menstrual cycle.

Cassie was a single mother, her daughter edging toward puberty. As she spoke about her own femininity, it became clear that her relationship with her daughter's imminent menarche was an important aspect of Cassie's capacity to reconnect and make peace with the prospect of losing her own womb:

> My daughter's coming up for her first period. It's shaken me up. I'm re-visiting my own deep resistance to womanhood. I don't want her to suffer like me. I've tried to bring a positive feminine presence to my daughter's life. I've been open about menstruation, and encouraged her to go to local "sister circles": the great young women who run these groups help girls embrace their moon times. A different world from my first period, [which was] such a source of shame and pain for me.

Cassie explained that, sadly for her and her daughter, "when the headmaster of my daughter's school discovered she was attending the girls' circles, he told me this was incompatible with education at his school. He told me if my daughter continued to attend these circles, he would expel her." Cassie was distressed enough by this experience to speak about it in a women's yoga therapy circle she attended after the initial individual yoga therapy session: "I think he's very wrong, but I have no choice. I know the girls' circles built my daughter's self-respect and confidence. But I don't want her to be expelled, so I have had to stop her going to the girls' circles."

Cassie was distressed about the decision she had to make. The dynamic of the school's opposition to her daughter's menstrual meetings directly affected Cassie's own health. Her conflict around her daughter's school mirrored a deeper conflict within herself. She regretted that, just as she had begun to reconnect with neglected and painful parts of herself (her womb life and cycles of feminine power), she had also agreed to the possibility of having her womb removed and entering into surgical menopause. At the same time Cassie was seeking to embrace her femininity and heal her relationship with her womb, and with perimenopause, she felt she had no choice but to honor the medical approach to preserve her health, including the possibility of hysterectomy during investigative surgery. She was holding the two opposites together, just as she managed the dynamic with her daughter's school.

Co-creating yoga nidra practices for yoga therapy clients

Cassie's experience is a vivid example of the intimate and powerful relationship between personal health and social context. Yoga therapy is well-placed to address this interface. In particular, because yoga nidra welcomes dynamic tension between pairs of opposites, it is often a helpful practice for those struggling to be well, or to prepare for surgery, during periods of uncertainty.

When asked how much time she had, at what time of day, Cassie replied that she thought she could manage 15 minutes before breakfast. In practical terms, co-creating a yoga nidra with a client for therapeutic purposes has some similarities to tailoring. Imagine visiting a tailor to order a bespoke coat for a special occasion, selecting the color and material, its weave or pattern, and consulting with the tailor on how to adapt classic styles to create the ideal coat. The tailor would cut that coat according to the grain, weight, and width of the chosen cloth to fit the customer's current shape and form. This is the equivalent of agreeing on basic parameters of length and general theme of co-creative yoga nidra—in Cassie's case, for example, a 15-minute practice for morning use, with an intention to invite reconnection to feminine cyclical rhythms to nourish well-being in preparation for surgery.

Back in the tailor's workshop, after the initial choices of cloth and cut, the customer would rely on the tailor's skill, judgment, vision, and expertise to stitch a unique and well-fitting coat to meet their needs. To make a client's practice requires skills and experience of multiple yoga nidra structures, together with an intuitive sense of what feels right for the client (based on what they have shared), to integrate their specific words and requests into the nidra, rather like the tailor working personal preferences together with well-known classic styles to create something unique, well-fitting, and suited to the occasion. Because clients often present with a number of issues simultaneously, for example requesting not only a practice to prepare for surgery but one to reconnect to cyclical rhythms, or to "recover forgotten parts of myself," a yoga therapist needs to be prepared to make a number of choices, cutting the coat of the client's yoga nidra practice from the cloth of whatever agreed theme is the most nourishing.

The classic yoga nidra framework of a ten-part structure, as described at the beginning of this chapter, is fairly standard in most schools of yoga nidra. Within this structure it is possible to integrate a body scan along a range of itineraries. Cassie, for example, practiced following the itinerary of the Himalayan Institute's 61 points because she had enjoyed this in her women's yoga circle. Because Cassie had declared that she was "not a visualizer," she was given the invitation to "*feel* morning light warming the land of [her] body" instead of "seeing" the points. She had also requested the integration of an embodied experience of cyclical wisdom, so the nidra created for her included a four-part seasonal breath in the settling and breath awareness sections to encourage a connection with the inner seasons through every breath. The in-breath was springtime and the out-breath was autumn, with the fullness of the inhalation welcomed as summertime and the pause after exhalation as winter; each component of the four-part breath corresponded with a season, breathing around the cycle of the year. This gave Cassie time and space to rest and welcome all that arose as the rhythm of the seasonal breath moved through the world of her body. Every word or phrase used was either Cassie's own or one shared around cyclical reconnection, especially the "seasons of the menstrual cycle" that Cassie had explored in the women's yoga circle.

A yoga therapist needs to be fully attentive and responsive to the client throughout the whole practice. This is only possible if they are sufficiently familiar with the structure of yoga nidra so that it is no longer a conscious effort to recall it. In this way, it becomes possible to focus instead entirely on the client, working away from one's notes or script to intuitively feel into what to say.

It is important to emphasize that all yoga nidras co-created for yoga therapy sessions need to be securely boundaried by the agreed-on time limit and the classic structure. As the yoga therapist delivers the yoga nidra experience, they must keep an eye on the client for signs of how that experience is progressing. Based on the observation of the client (change in breathing patterns, gut activity/gurgling, fluttering eyelids or eye movement), the yoga therapist must be ready to improvise with wording, pauses, and tone to guide the session in a way that keeps the client floating between deep rest and dreamless sleep. Each co-creative therapeutic yoga nidra is a practice that never before existed in precisely the form that is being uniquely tailored to the client's requirements at this phase in their life, providing them with a well-fitting coat of nourishment and cyclical reconnection.

It is helpful to record yoga nidra practices delivered in a session on the client's device to enable them to listen to it each day. In the case of Cassie, daily listening helped her to "sense how I might feel if I wake up with no womb. I feel more able to welcome whatever that might mean for me, including moving directly into menopause."

As Cassie was scheduled for surgery the following day and would be spending a couple of days in the hospital, followed by postoperative healing, the second individual yoga therapy session was an opportunity to co-create a second yoga nidra practice. This was similar to the first (familiarity and repetition can be healing and reassuring) but for 30 instead of 15 minutes, giving Cassie options for shorter or longer practices. The new practice integrated four moon phases, synchronized with breath in settling and in the pairs of opposites section, inviting Cassie to experience inhalation as waxing moon and exhalation as waning moon; it also offered the 61-point rotation as a way to feel quiet moonlight illuminating the night sky of the body.

Cassie called after surgery to report that she had a full hysterectomy:

> As I rested in yoga nidra, before and after the surgery, I could feel myself getting back into connection with the rhythms of my life. I was disconnected for so long. Those nidras helped me to pause, listen into myself, and welcome who I am.

As can be seen with clients in a range of circumstances, Cassie valued the reconnective power of yoga nidra to support her as a whole, vital being. The practice helped her to place the experience of womb loss in context of the wider cycles of her life.

If Cassie's sessions had simply focused on the possibility of hysterectomy, they might have been helpful for her physical recovery or for managing anxiety.[10] However, such an approach would have isolated this experience from the rest of her troubled relationship with her femininity. This would have bypassed some of the deeper issues, and possibly sabotaged postsurgical healing, because it would have disrespected Shakti by disenfranchising Cassie from the chance to engage consciously with the siddhi of menopause (see Chapter 15) and its resonance with her daughter's imminent menarche. These factors were all part of the clinical picture, and all, subliminally but powerfully, were included within the seasonal and lunar language of the co-created yoga nidra practices. Integrating yoga nidra within yoga therapy can help a client to maintain a sense of the whole picture through one effortless practice of accepting what is.

Cassie continued to practice yoga nidra several times daily immediately after surgery, from which she made an excellent recovery. She is now fully restored to vitality and wellness, embracing her postmenopausal energy through a cyclical connection with lunar rhythms, with the rhythms of her daughter's menstruations, and with a heightened awareness and respect for the movements of Shakti in her life. The experience enabled Cassie to rediscover her connection to cyclical wisdom and to trust in her capacity to thrive as a conscious and empowered postmenopausal woman: "I feel whole again (without a womb!). Totally able to welcome my femininity in this phase of my life and to be in the rhythm of living well."

Summary

Yoga nidra represents an awakening process, but *rest* is paradoxically required to awaken consciousness and connection to these rhythmic cycles. The sleep of awakening that is yoga nidra prompts a sense of reconnection through which a sense of planetary responsibility can be awakened: A recognition can arise that the rhythmic cycles nourishing one's own health are the very same cycles nourishing the whole of life.

As a species, we cannot hope to restore rhythms and cycles with*out*, in the wider world, unless and until respect for these cycles *within* the world of the body has been restored. This embodied sense of reconnection brings one's awareness back home, into right relation with all life on the planet. Co-creative yoga nidra is a potent medicine to help humans to listen in, rest well, and step back into rhythm with the worlds of their own bodies and the world they inhabit—personal reconnection for planetary healing.

Additional Resources

The recording made for Cassie is her private poetry, but other nidras recorded in other environments with similar intentions are available from the author's Yoga Nidra Network. See, e.g., "Rhythmically attuned to the dance of the moon" (www.yoganidranetwork.org/mp3/rhythmically-attuned-dance-moon) and Dinsmore-Tuli, U. (2018). *Yoni nidra* [Album]. Sitaram and Sons.

Birch, J., & Hargreaves, J. (2015, Jan. 6). Yoganidrā: An understanding of the history and context. *The Luminescent*. www.theluminescent.org/2015/01/yoganidra.html

Boyes, D. (1973). *The yoga of awakened sleep* [in French]. Epi Editeurs.

Brody, K. (2017). *The daring to rest yoga nidra meditation program: A 40-day journey to break the cycle of fatigue and restore vitality, purpose, and power* [Album]. Sounds True.

Desai, K. (2017). *Yoga nidra: The art of transformational sleep—Restore your health, reshape your life and change your destiny*. Lotus Press.

Dinsmore-Tuli, U. (2020). *Yoni shakti: A woman's guide to power and freedom through yoga and tantra*. YogaWords.

Dinsmore-Tuli, U., & Tuli, N. (2014). Total Yoga Nidra and Swami Satyananda: Where we stand now—A statement from the Yoga Nidra Network. www.yoganidranetwork.org/article/total-yoga-nidra-and-swami-satyananda-where-we-stand-now

Miller, R. (2005). *Yoga nidra: A meditative practice for deep relaxation and healing*. Sounds True.

Parker, S., Bharati, S. V., & Fernandez, M. (2013). Defining yoga-nidra: Traditional accounts, physiological research, and future directions. *International Journal of Yoga Therapy*, *23*(1), 11–16.

Saraswati, S. (1984). *Yoga nidra*. Yoga Publications Trust.

Stiles, M. (2000). *Structural yoga therapy: Adapting to the individual*. Red Wheel/Weiser.

Endnotes

1 Dinsmore-Tuli, U. (2021). *Nidra shakti: A decolonising encyclopaedia of yoga nidra*. Sitaram and Sons.

2 E.g., following the layout and proportional representation of the brain's sensory and motor cortices, or in accordance with yogic anatomy (*panchamaya kosha*) or ayurvedic *marma* points. Rotation of consciousness is rooted in the practice of *nyasa*. Medieval Hatha Yoga manuals mention yoga nidra as a philosophical concept, a state of awareness rather than a multistep technique. The descriptions of nyasa in these manuals are similar to the movement of consciousness around the body in contemporary yoga nidra techniques.

3 The prescriptive images may be related to traditional foci for spiritual growth and development, e.g., meditating upon the image of one's own corpse or inviting images of spiritual teachers for the purposes of deepening a connection to these figures.

4 Coburn, T. B. (1991). *Encountering the goddess: A translation of the Devī-Māhātmya and a study of its interpretation*. State University of New York Press.

5 Wildcroft, T. R. (2018). Patterns of authority and practice relationships in "post-lineage yoga" [Doctoral dissertation, Open University]. http://oro.open.ac.uk/59125/1/thesis_TRW19.pdf

6 Independence is a significant choice to make when the leaders of three out of the five main schools of yoga nidra (Swami Rama, Swami Satyananda, and Amrit Desai) were either convicted of sexual and financial abuses (Rama and Desai) or have been found to be ultimately responsible for abuses committed within the organizations that promulgate their methods of yoga nidra (Swami Satyananda).
Australian Royal Commission of Investigation into Institutional Responses to Child Sexual Abuse. (2014). Case study 21: Satyananda Yoga Ashram. www.childabuseroyalcommission.gov.au/case-studies/case-study-21-satyananda-yoga-ashram
Dushkin v. Desai. (1998, Aug. 27). Memorandum regarding defendant's motion to dismiss. http://ma.findacase.com/research/wfrmDocViewer.aspx/xq/fac.19980827_0000200.DMA.htm/qx
Falk, G. D. (2009). *Stripping the gurus*. Million Monkeys Press.
Pankhania, J., & Hargreaves, J. (2017, Dec. 22). A culture of silence: Satyananda Yoga. *The Luminescent*. www.theluminescent.org/2017/12/a-culture-of-silence-satyananda-yoga.html
Patel v. Himalayan International Institute of Yoga Science and Philosophy of the USA. (1997, Sept. 4). Memorandum of judgment made by Chief Judge Vanaskie. http://web.archive.org/web/20100527120709/http://www.pamd.uscourts.gov/opinions/vanaskie/94v1118.pdf
Webster, K. (1990, Dec.). The case against Swami Rama of the Himalayas. *Yoga Journal Magazine*. www.scribd.com/document/515557/The-Case-Against-Swami-Rama-of-the-Himalayas

7 Note that a growing body of evidence, generally from studies of more standardized approaches, suggests yoga nidra's capacity to change health outcomes. See, e.g., Kim, S. D. (2017). Psychological effects of yoga nidra in women with menstrual disorders: A systematic review of randomized controlled trials. *Complementary Therapies in Clinical Practice*, *28*, 4–8.

8 Attributed to Swami Muktananda.

9 Client material is shared with permission.

10 Kamakhya, K. (2008). A study on the impact on stress and anxiety through yoga nidra. *Indian Journal of Traditional Knowledge*, *7*(3), 401–444.

23

The Use of Meditation in Yoga Therapy

KEISHIN KIMURA (translated by Madoka Chase Onizuka)

Meditation facilitates the transformation necessary for Self-realization, and understanding the role of meditation as a spiritual practice informs the use of meditation in yoga therapy. Yogic scriptures and sages say that mistaken identity (conjunction between Seer and seen, or conflating *prakriti* and *purusha*) is the cause of suffering.[1]

In Yoga Sutra 2.5, Patanjali explains that ignorance (*avidya*) causing mistaken identity is "the conviction of permanence, purity, happiness and self in what are really impermanent, impure, painful and not self."[2] In yoga therapy terms, these are cognitive errors made by the *buddhi*, the faculty of the four functions of the mind that encompasses higher mind and discernment. This suffering causes distress that disrupts the various *koshas* (layers of being) and can be considered to be at the root of the lifestyle disorders prevalent around the world today.[3]

Meditation educates the buddhi, dispelling ignorance, and thus lessens the disturbances to the koshas and leads to improved overall health. Contemporary research literature often defines meditation as *mindfulness*, *meditation*, or *mindfulness meditation*. Buddhist-anchored forms of mindfulness, loving-kindness meditation, and more recently iRest protocols are the most commonly researched types. For the purpose of yoga therapy, this chapter divides meditation into two categories: First is Vedic meditation as explained in the Upanishads. The other category treats all eight components of Patanjali's yoga as meditation.

Vedic Meditation

Vedic meditation is a four-step practice that directly addresses the buddhi's cognitive errors, the sources of suffering. The buddhi is the intellect, the psychological organ responsible for discernment and decision-making (see Chapter 11). In the *Bhagavad Gita* and *Katha Upanishad*, the buddhi is likened to the driver of a horse-drawn chariot. The body of the chariot is the physical body, in which sits a silent passenger, the Self. The driver of the chariot is the buddhi, and it holds the reins (*manas*, the sensory-motor mind) to guide ten horses. These ten horses represent the organs of action and perception (*karma* and *jnana indriyas*, respectively).[4]

Manas transmits information between the horses and the buddhi. If the buddhi is skillful, it can exercise wise control of the horses, of the information arising from actions and perceptions, and the chariot and its passenger ride smoothly along the road of life. If not well-trained, however, the buddhi cannot control the organs of perception and action and the horses run amok, blindly chasing pleasure and seeking to avoid pain.

Vedic meditation educates the buddhi to become aware of its own ignorance—the cognitive errors that mistake impermanence for permanence, impurity for purity, pain for pleasure, and not-self for Self. Its use in yoga therapy offers clients the experience of self-transformation and wisdom to address and overcome life's challenges.

The *Brihadaranyaka Upanishad* (4.5) introduces Vedic meditation in a conversation between the sage Yajnavalkya and his wife, Maitreyi. When he decides to leave to pursue an ascetic life, Yajnavalkya promises to give Maitreyi enough money to live out her days. She objects, arguing that money will not give her the liberation she seeks. In response, Yajnavalkya teaches her the four steps of Vedic meditation to awaken to the true Self: "The Self, my dear Maitreyi, should be realized—should be heard of, reflected on, and meditated upon. When the Self, my dear, is realized by being heard of, reflected on, and meditated upon, all this is known" (4.5.6).[5]

As Yajnavalkya explains, Vedic meditation comprises the four steps of hearing about (*shravana*), reflecting on (*manana*), meditating on (*nidhidhyasana*), and profound knowledge (*jnana*). It is important to remember that, traditionally, the object of Vedic meditation is realization of Self (i.e., ultimate health). The four steps are detailed below.

The steps of Vedic meditation

Step 1: Shravana

In shravana, students traditionally either read yogic scriptures or listen to a guru's discourse. In contemporary yoga therapy settings, the yoga therapist and client agree on a theme for reflection, and the yoga therapist's explanation of the theme exposes the client to new perspectives. The therapist proposes a simple theme that is most appropriate for the client's needs, in line with the therapeutic goals they have co-created.

When first beginning Vedic meditation, it is generally advised to start with simple, positive, non-judgmental themes, especially if the client exhibits depression or self-critical tendencies. Themes that challenge deeply ingrained beliefs may trigger many emotions or traumatic memories. Respecting the client's pace will help the yoga therapist to ensure that the client has the tools to handle their emotions before embarking on challenging inquiry.

In selecting a theme, it is also important to remember that meditation transforms a client's behavior, bringing them closer to yoga's definition of ultimate health—liberation from attachment with knowledge of the difference between Seer and seen. It is recommended, therefore, that Vedic meditation be instructed in a way that enables clients to relive experiences of high-quality behavioral transformation that they have already (and likely unknowingly) accomplished. If someone has challenges with being truthful, for example, silent reflections on a time they were truthful—and the resulting positive outcomes—would reinforce their understanding of the benefits of *satya*. A theme for someone who tends to be negative or blame others could relate to recent occasions when they felt gratitude. Someone who tends to think they are incompetent could be invited to recall three things they successfully accomplished.

Understanding how yoga defines health and the obstacles (*kleshas*) to attaining it enables the therapist to skillfully choose themes that help the client to dispel their own ignorance. *Kaivalya* is equated with perfect health (or freedom),[6] so the characteristics of one who has attained kaivalya are useful standards by which to measure health in yoga therapy.[7]

One example of a characteristic of perfect health is freedom from attachment. The concepts in these two verses of the *Bhagavad Gita* could be used to reflect on how the obstacle of attachment plays out in life (2.62–63):

> When you keep thinking about sense objects, attachment comes. Attachment breeds desire, the lust of possession that burns to anger.
>
> Anger clouds the judgment; you can no longer learn from past mistakes. Lost is

the power to choose between what is wise and what is unwise, and your life is utter waste.[8]

Finally, it is important that the client is in agreement with the theme before embarking on the next step.

Step 2: Manana

After the dialogue of shravana comes the second step: manana, the silent self-reflection on thoughts that is a precursor to the immersive experience of meditation. This step can reveal the cognitive errors causing attachment and stress. Discussion between yoga therapist and client after manana further educates the buddhi.

During manana, yoga therapist and client sit together, reflecting on the same theme; depending on the client's condition and capacity for concentration, manana might last from ten seconds to several minutes.[9] Manana may be longer in spiritual practices, but in yoga therapy sessions with limited time, a few minutes of manana provides sufficient content for discussion and preparation for the next step, nidhidhyasana, which prompts clients to bring their insights off the cushion and into daily life. After the silent contemplation of manana, the therapist may share a simple and short explanation of their own experience. After the client shares, the therapist can ask open-ended questions to help deepen the client's insight and reinforce any positive changes. Useful prompts may include

- Tell me more about that.
- What does that mean to you?
- In what other ways…?
- How would you…?

As a general example continuing on the theme of attachment, someone with self-esteem issues and perfectionist tendencies could reflect on thoughts and feelings that arise when attachment to perfection is strong. Another approach could be to recall a time when the person acted without the attachment to perfection. In either case, when the buddhi notices that such attachment leads to anger and judgment rather than happiness (cognitive error of pain for pleasure), letting go of this mental pattern may be easier.

Steps 3 and 4: Nidhidhyasana and jnana

After discussing the results of manana, the yoga therapist guides the client into nidhidhyasana, a transformational part of the plan of care. The therapist reinforces positive insights from manana and encourages the client to continue observation of these thought patterns while going about everyday life outside sessions. This step may additionally involve trying a new behavior pattern or simply noticing whether an insight that arose during manana remains accurate in daily life. During nidhidhyasana, new questions may emerge, and these can be discussed at the next yoga therapy session. Eventually, the insight is mastered and becomes the deep knowledge represented by jnana.

These stages of Vedic meditation enable yoga therapy clients to purify the many memories of attachment stored in *citta*, the "storehouse of memories" located in the physical sheath, *anandamaya kosha*.[10] As the buddhi becomes more skilled, it interprets both past memories and present events in more *sattvic*, balanced ways. With this purification, the buddhi makes fewer cognitive errors, leading to a smoother ride for the chariot, passenger, and horses.

The Eight Limbs as Meditation

According to Patanjali, yoga is by definition about the mind: *Yogas chitta vritti nirodah*, or "Yoga is restraining the mind-stuff (Chitta) from taking various forms (Vrittis),"[11] or "restriction of mental processes" (Yoga Sutra 1.2).[12] To achieve this state of yoga, Patanjali prescribes eight components of yoga to destroy impurities and lead to "a growing light of knowledge up to Knowledge of the difference" (between Seer and seen).[13] It is therefore useful for the yoga therapist to understand the psychological and meditative nature of all eight yogic limbs: *yama* (restraints or ethics), *niyama* (observances), *asana* (postures), *pranayama* (restraint of vital currents or breath control), *pratyahara* (withdrawal of the senses or inwardness), *dharana* (concentration), *dhyana* (meditation), and *samadhi* (the state of being absorbed). (Yama and niyama, asana, and pranayama are explored in other chapters in this section.) These practices may be preparation for Vedic meditation, used as part of Vedic meditation, or stand alone as meditation for attainment of kaivalya.

The yamas and niyamas (Chapter 24) become meditation when used as cues for self-awareness, for being mindful in interactions with other people (e.g., "Is my behavior violent?") and with things (e.g., "Am I hoarding?"). The yamas and niyamas can also be used as themes in Vedic meditation.

As for asana, Patanjali treats them as a mind-body approach that enables one to overcome dualities such as profit and loss or praise and criticism: "By lessening the natural tendency (for restlessness) and meditating on the unlimited, posture becomes firm and pleasant. Seat being conquered, the dualities do not obstruct" (Yoga Sutras 2.47–48).[14]

The choice of asana or pranayama should be such that no corrections to alignment or adjustments are necessary. This approach enables clients to focus solely on changes in physical sensations and breathing, without outward concerns about the duality of success or failure in a pose. Such methods build capacity to see beyond the gross physical body to the subtler workings of the mind and to see problems more objectively.

The fourth component of yoga is pranayama, which Patanjali again relates to psychological functions: "The fourth [limb] is restraining the Prana by reflecting on external or internal object. From that, the covering to the light of the Chitta is attenuated. The mind becomes fit for Dharana" (Yoga Sutras 2.51–53).[15]

Pranayama is voluntary regulation of the autonomic nervous system and prepares practitioners for regulation of psychological functions. As Patanjali says, there is a fourth pranayama beyond inhalation, exhalation, and transition: Continuous prana reaches deep layers of consciousness, removing the covering of the light of wisdom (divine light of the Self). This means that ignorance is alleviated through pranayama practice, which is also mental preparation for more advanced meditation practices.

BOX 23.1 RESEARCH EXAMPLE

A practice combining asana and pranayama as meditation is also effective as yoga therapy. For example, professor Takakazu Oka, of the Department of Psychosomatic Medicine at the Graduate School of Medical Sciences, International University of Health and Welfare, conducted a 3-year research project in Japan. He examined how people without health complaints (n = 72), people with health issues but not seeking medical care (n = 118), and people with medical diagnoses (n = 145) perceived the benefits of yoga.[16]

The yoga intervention focused on isometric breathing exercises developed by the Japan Yoga Therapy Society. These exercises integrate asana and pranayama, combining simple movements, isometric resistance, and breathing; they are practiced as meditative exercises to enhance awareness.[17] More than 90 percent of study participants found yoga therapy helpful for promoting and maintaining health. Also in that study, approximately 88 percent of people with health concerns and diagnoses felt the yoga intervention was good for their subjective symptoms and helpful for treatment.[18]

Next is pratyahara, explained in Yoga Sutras 2.54–55: "The drawing in of the organs [of action and perception] is by their giving up their own objects and taking the form of the mind-stuff, as it were. Thence arises supreme control of the organs."[19]

Asana and pranayama are preliminary pratyahara practices, requiring restraint of the karma and jnana indriyas on a gross level. As pratyahara deepens into the subtler dimensions of human existence, attention is brought to the indriyas in the *manomaya* and *vijnanamaya koshas*.

With mastery of the senses comes dharana, which when maintained is dhyana. And samadhi is realized when the boundaries dissolve between three types of awareness—of objects, of self, and of awareness itself—and only the object shines forth.

Patanjali explains dharana, dhyana, and samadhi at the start of Chapter 3 of the *Yoga Sutras*, combining them as *samyama*. With mastery of samyama comes "the light of knowledge (*prajña*)."[20] There are meditation methods to do this, and they are used by those who wish to pursue kaivalya, which many might consider to be outside the realm of yoga therapy.

Instruction Principles and Precautions

Basic principles

Meditation addresses psychological issues, and some basic principles need to be kept in mind when using meditation in yoga therapy. (See also Chapter 13 for important considerations in the therapeutic use of yogic techniques.)

- **Individualization:** The benefit of individual meditation lies in the ability to address the cognitive errors that are unique to the individual. Group meditation settings, however, may be structured to promote accountability of the individual to the group and the formation of a *sangha* (community) whose shared values can be beneficial to behavior change.

- **Free expression:** A safe environment for free expression of feelings is necessary to uncover the cognitive errors of the buddhi (see Chapter 14).

- **Client self-determination:** Clients are the agents of change in yoga therapy. They decide how fast and far to go, and yoga therapists support the process.

- **Neutrality and equanimity:** Yoga therapists must have good self-awareness and the ability to objectively analyze their own mental functions. They should not allow their own emotions or values to interfere with the goal of supporting clients in the resolution of their own cognitive errors—one reason an ongoing personal practice is so important.

- **Acceptance:** Complete acceptance, or unconditional positive regard, of the client as a whole is required for yoga therapists to serve as a healing presence. The safe space they can then create enables clients to engage in meditation and disclose what is troubling them.
- **Confidentiality:** This is essential for the trust needed in meditative work in yoga therapy. Yoga therapists working in integrative health facilities are also subject to specific requirements around data privacy.

Preliminary steps

The following steps need to be covered before using meditation in yoga therapy.

1. **Assess the buddhi:** As part of a *panchamaya kosha* assessment, evaluation of the buddhi enables yoga therapists to determine what meditation or themes best suit clients' needs. This evaluation may include considering how the client is engaging yamas and niyamas in their daily life, as discerned through manomaya and vijnanamaya kosha; those with good discernment are presenting with a strong faculty of buddhi.

   If concentration or objectivity is a serious challenge, using asana and/or pranayama as meditation is recommended. If the buddhi is prepared to focus and analyze, then Vedic meditation can be considered.

   To analyze the buddhi's cognitive errors, it is necessary to ask about illustrative examples from the client's life. Again, open-ended questions may be useful. This line of inquiry also reveals which kleshas (ignorance, ego, attachment, aversion, the deep fear represented by instinctive self-preservation) are at work.

2. **Obtain informed consent:** Acquiring clients' consent at each step ensures that their pace and needs are respected. Yoga therapists should explain the content, purpose, expected outcome, and relevant risks when proposing next steps. It is important that clients understand that Vedic meditation examines their ways of thinking; some may be reluctant to reconsider old thought patterns, and this may suggest a need for referral. Yoga therapists need to be ready to refer to a psychotherapist rather than begin a diagnosis or treatment process beyond their scope of practice. Those working in integrative health settings will also need to adhere to institutional guidelines for consent.

Precautions

Because meditation addresses subtler human dimensions and trains the buddhi, manas, and indriyas, it is a powerful form of mind-body therapy. (See Chapter 13, Box 13.1, for red flags in mental health.)

- Yoga therapists should have solid experience as practitioners in any meditative techniques they use with clients.
- Past memories, stored in the citta in anandamaya kosha, can trigger traumatic memories or strong emotions that clients may not be prepared to handle. These situations are best addressed in conjunction with a licensed healthcare provider.
- Avoid explaining your assessment of cognitive errors, instead supporting clients to gain their own insights.
- Clients need to have the tools to handle their emotions before embarking on challenging inquiry. They should never be pressured into meditation or Vedic meditation themes.
- If a client presents with psychosis or other serious mental health concerns (severe depression or anxiety, dissociative identity disorder, schizophrenia), be ready to refer the client to a licensed healthcare provider.

Working in careful collaboration with healthcare providers may make yoga therapy possible for even those with serious mental health concerns when they are medically stabilized. The author is unaware of any conclusive literature on benefits of meditation for psychosis, but studies are beginning to indicate that mindfulness-based practices may benefit people with schizophrenia.[21]

Summary

When using meditation, yoga therapists are facilitating education of the buddhi by drawing from thousands of years of wisdom found in the Upanishads, *Bhagavad Gita*, *Yoga Sutras*, and other texts. They assess clients' mind-body conditions, then support them to see through the cognitive errors that cause distress. This helps clients approach knowledge of the difference between what is temporal and eternal, Self and non-self.

Yoga therapy could be used to simply attain a certain level of health and happiness, but if that were the goal of yoga therapy as a field, then going to see a psychologist or physical therapist might suffice. The beauty of yoga therapy is that it addresses the root cause of dis-ease. If yoga therapists themselves build their own character and continue their own study and education in yogic scriptures, they can also support clients to let the qualities of the Self shine and approach ultimate health—to attain that for which Maitreyi aimed when she asked Yajnavalkya to teach her.

Additional Resources

Following is a sample of recent meditation research and studies on adverse events and side-effects.

Cancer care

Ford, C. G., Vowles, K. E., Smith, B. W., & Kinney, A. Y. (2020). Mindfulness and meditative movement interventions for men living with cancer: A meta-analysis. *Annals of Behavioral Medicine, 54*(5), 360–373.

Nittur, A., & Raghavan, G. (2020). Pranic healing as a complimentary [sic] therapy in stage-4 metastatic cancer—A case study. *Journal of Clinical & Diagnostic Research, 14*(1), 3–4.

Cardiac care

Bokhari, S., Schneider, R. H., Salerno, J. W., Rainforth, M. V., Gaylord-King, C., & Nidich, S. I. (2019). Effects of cardiac rehabilitation with and without meditation on myocardial blood flow using quantitative positron emission tomography: A pilot study. *Journal of Nuclear Cardiology*. https://doi.org/10.1007/s12350-019-01884-9

Kretzer, K., Davis, J., Easa, D., Johnson, J., & Harrigan, R. (2007). Self identity through Ho'oponopono as adjunctive therapy for hypertension management. *Ethnicity and Disease, 17*(4), 624–628.

Packiasabapathy, S., Susheela, A. T., Mueller, A., Patxot, M., et al. (2019). Guided meditation as an adjunct to enhance postoperative recovery after cardiac surgery: Study protocol for a prospective randomized controlled feasibility trial. *Trials, 20*(1), 39.

Tarrant, J. M., Raines, N., & Blinne, W. R. (2019). The effects of meditation on twin hearts on P300 values: A repeated measures comparison of nonmeditators and the experienced. *Integrative Medicine, 18*(2), 36–41.

Viveiros, J., Chamberlain, B., O'Hare, A., & Sethares, K. A. (2019). Meditation interventions among heart failure patients: An integrative review. *European Journal of Cardiovascular Nursing, 18*(8), 720–728.

Diabetes

Xia, T., Yang, Y., Li, W., Tang, Z., et al. (2020). Meditative movements for patients with type 2 diabetes: A systematic review and meta-analysis. *Evidence-Based Complementary and Alternative Medicine, 2020*, 5745013.

Meditation precautions and concerns

Cebolla, A., Demarzo, M., Martins, P., Soler, J., & Garcia-Campayo, J. (2017). Unwanted effects: Is there a negative side of meditation? A multicentre survey. *PLoS ONE, 12*(9), e0183137.

Dyga, K., & Stupak, R. (2015). Meditation and psychosis: Trigger or cure? *Archives of Psychiatry & Psychotherapy, 17*(3), 48–58.

Kaselionyte, J., & Gumley, A. (2017). "It's like a charge—either fuses you or burns you out": An interpretative phenomenological analysis of extreme mental states in meditation context. *Mental Health, Religion & Culture, 20*(10), 986–1001.

Lindahl, J. R., & Britton, W. B. (2019). "I have this feeling of not really being here": Buddhist meditation and changes in sense of self. *Journal of Consciousness Studies, 26*(7–8), 157–183.

Lustyk, M. K. B., Chawla, N., Nolan, R. S., & Marlatt, G. A. (2009). Mindfulness meditation research: Issues of participant screening, safety procedures, and researcher training. *Advances in Mind-Body Medicine, 24*(1), 20–30.

Lutkajtis, A. (2019). "The answer to all your problems?" The overly positive presentation of meditation in the media. *Journal for the Academic Study of Religion, 32*(1), 49–71.

Schlosser, M., Sparby, T., Vörös, S., Jones, R., & Marchant, N. L. (2019). Unpleasant meditation-related experiences in regular meditators: Prevalence, predictors, and conceptual considerations. *PLoS ONE, 14*(5), e0216643.

Mental health

Frick, A., Thinnes, I., & Stangier, U. (2020). Metta-based group meditation and individual cognitive behavioral therapy (MeCBT) for chronic depression: Study protocol for a randomized controlled trial. *Trials, 21*(1), 20.

Hafenbrack, A. C., Cameron, L. D., Spreitzer, G. M., Zhang, C., Noval, L. J., & Shaffakat, S. (2020). Helping people by being in the present: Mindfulness increases prosocial behavior. *Organizational Behavior & Human Decision Processes, 159*, 21–38.

Lang, A. J., Malaktaris, A. L., Casmar, P., Baca, S. A., et al. (2019). Compassion meditation for posttraumatic stress disorder in veterans: A randomized proof of concept study. *Journal of Traumatic Stress, 32*(2), 299–309.

Shen, H., Chen, M., & Cui, D. (2020). Biological mechanism study of meditation and its application in mental disorders. *General Psychiatry, 33*(4), e100214.

Sirotina, U., & Shchebetenko, S. (2020). Loving-kindness meditation and compassion meditation: Do they affect emotions in a different way? *Mindfulness, 11*, 2519–2530.

Totzeck, C., Teismann, T., Hofmann, S. G., von Brachel, R., et al. (2020). Loving-kindness meditation promotes mental health in university students. *Mindfulness, 11*, 1623–1631.

Multiple sclerosis

Pagnini, F., Cavalera, C., Rovaris, M., Mendozzi, L., et al. (2019). Longitudinal associations between mindfulness and well-being in people with multiple sclerosis. *International Journal of Clinical and Health Psychology, 19*(1), 22–30.

Pouyanfard, S., ParviziFard, A. A., Mohammadpour, M., & Sadeghi, K. (2020). Effectiveness of mindfulness-integrated cognitive behavior therapy on anxiety, depression and hope in multiple sclerosis patients: A randomized clinical trial. *Trends in Psychiatry and Psychotherapy, 42*(1), 55–63.

Schirda, B., Duraney, E., Lee, H. K., Manglani, H. R., et al. (2020). Mindfulness training for emotion dysregulation in multiple sclerosis: A pilot randomized controlled trial. *Rehabilitation Psychology, 65*(3), 206–218.

Endnotes

1 Yoga Sutra 2.17, in Leggett, T. (2017). *Sankara on the Yoga Sutras: A full translation of the newly discovered text* (3rd ed.). Motilal Banarsidass.

2 Leggett, *Sankara* (p. 185).

3 In 2018, the World Health Organization (WHO) estimated that an annual 41 million people die of non-communicable diseases a year, making up 71 percent of all deaths globally: World Health Organization. (2018). Noncommunicable diseases. www.who.int/en/news-room/fact-sheets/detail/noncommunicable-diseases

4 Easwaran, E. (2007). *The Upanishads* (p. 81). Nilgiri Press.

5 Madhavananda, S. (1950). *The Brhadaranyaka Upanisad with the commentary of Sankaracarya* (3rd ed., p. 776). Advaita Asrama.

6 Leggett, *Sankara* (p. 52).

7 Characteristics of perfect health are given, for example, in the *Bhagavad Gita* as characteristics of divine nature (16.1–3) and in the *Caraka Saṃhitā* as the seven types of *sattvika* (*Sharira Sthana Śārīrasthnam* 4.37–49).

Japan Yoga Niketan, of which the author is the founder, holds kaivalya to be the ultimate state of health. The organization has therefore created a four-level Yoga Therapy Darshana: Level 1 is the intake interview; level 2 begins work on simple cognitive errors; level 3 addresses cognitive transformation more deeply; and level 4 is essentially Raja Yoga, introducing samyama practices for attainment of kaivalya.

8 Easwaran, E. (2007). *The Bhagavad Gita* (2nd ed., p. 96). Nilgiri Press.

9 A process like this reflects the style of yoga therapy commonly practiced by members of the Japan Yoga Therapy Society.

10 Yogeshwarananda, S. (2014). *Science of soul* (S. Jyotirmayananda, Trans.; 6th ed.). Yoga Niketan Trust.

11 Vivekananda, S. (2004). *Raja yoga, or conquering the internal nature* (p. 115). Advaita Ashrama.

12 Leggett, *Sankara* (p. 60).

13 Yoga Sutra 2.28; Leggett, *Sankara* (p. 257).

14 Vivekananda, *Raja yoga* (p. 214).

15 Vivekananda, *Raja yoga* (pp. 215–216).

16 Among the study participants' health issues and diagnoses were fatigue, backache, shoulder stiffness, hypertension, autonomic imbalance, menopause, depression, and cancer.

17 Videos of isometric breathing exercises are available on the Japan Yoga Therapy Society's YouTube channel (www.youtube.com/channel/UCHqvAjJ-4jzGdmPVy1JcBrw).

18 Oka, T. (2018, Feb. 26). *Research on the efficacy and safety of yoga therapy in integrative medicine* [in Japanese]. Report to Ministry of Health, Labour and Welfare, Japan, on 3-year grant for integrative medicine (2015–2017) from the Japan Agency for Medical Research and Development.

Note that this chapter offers meditation as presented by a highly experienced yoga therapist working primarily in one tradition (Vedic meditation) and is meant to impress upon the reader the possibilities that exist within the yoga therapy toolbox. It is useful for the beginning yoga therapist to remember that a wide variety of tools fit under the headings pratyahara, dharana, and dhyana; although they may be referred to by other names in Western research protocols, each will have relevance and use for specific conditions. As mentioned at the beginning of this chapter, contemporary research has favored forms for which a research protocol exists and for which outcomes may be more readily measurable. Creating protocols that provide the means to measure outcomes with different meditation techniques from the yogic traditions may help a broader population of healthcare providers to understand the value of these traditions.

Additionally, different clients will benefit from different meditation tools. A top-down approach may irritate one, whereas a bottom-up approach may unsettle another. Thorough intake that helps the yoga therapist to develop a keen understanding of the individual's experience with meditation as well as their needs and personality is of the utmost importance.

In some instances, meditation can prove detrimental. The articles in this chapter's Additional Resources offer more information that may be helpful for creating plans of care for diverse clients. Yoga therapists are advised to explore a variety of techniques, from loving-kindness meditations to mindfulness and mantra. Examine gentle mindful movement, precursors to meditation such as pratyahara, and dharana practices such as guided imagery and *trataka* (candle gazing) to begin to develop the skills that will support the needs of different individuals.

19 Vivekananda, *Raja yoga* (pp. 216–217).

20 Yoga Sutra 3.5; Leggett, *Sankara* (p. 284).

21 Igarashi, S., & Igarashi, M. (2014, July 4–6). Report on Instruction of Yoga Therapy for Schizophrenia [Poster presentation, in Japanese]. Annual conference of the Japan Yoga Therapy Society, Gifu, Japan.

Wang, L. Q., Chien, W. T., Yip, L. K., & Karatzias, T. (2016). A randomized controlled trial of a mindfulness-based intervention program for people with schizophrenia: 6-month follow-up. *Neuropsychiatric Disease and Treatment*, *12*, 3097–3110.

24

Yama and Niyama Therapeutic Lifestyle Practices

GINA MACAULEY AND LEIGH BLASHKI

The *yamas* and *niyamas* are the first two limbs of the eight-limbed (*ashtanga*) yoga, detailed by the sage Patanjali in the *raja* (royal) yoga treatise the *Patanjali Yoga Darshana*, more commonly known as *the Yoga Sutras of Patanjali*.[1] The *Yoga Sutras of Patanjali* were compiled in the "classical period" of yoga (100–500 CE). The text synthesizes a number of the principles of Samkhya and was influenced by ideas from Buddhism and Jainism (see Chapter 2).[2]

The placement of yama and niyama as the first two limbs indicates the importance of these foundational principles and practices that prescribe how a yoga *sadhaka* (practitioner) should behave in or relate to the world (in the case of the yamas) and relate to themselves (in the case of niyamas). The yamas and niyamas are regarded as the basis for ethical living.

The word *yama* is usually translated as "restraint." Interestingly, the word also means twin, which may point to the importance of the yamas and niyamas being practiced together. The word *niyama* is usually translated as "observance." However, the word also refers to performing set duties and restraint of the mind, the latter fitting well with the notion of twinship with the yamas.

Although each of the yamas and niyamas is described separately in the *Yoga Sutras*, in reality many arise concurrently and can therefore best be practiced as a set of principles that support one another. The yamas and niyamas form an important part of living an ethical, yogic lifestyle, but this chapter explores their use as the backbone for effective, therapeutic lifestyle interventions.

There are countless translations and interpretations of these core yogic principles. The interpretations in this chapter are informed by Frans Moors, T. K. V. Desikachar, Bernard Bouanchaud, and Deborah Adele.[3]

This chapter focuses more on the "dos" than on the "don'ts" with respect to the yamas. However, at times awareness of and attention to the practices from which one should refrain become encouraging guides. This is a form of *pratipaksha bhavanam*, or cultivation of opposite attitudes. Sutra 2.33 states that when the light of questioning is shone on attitudes, self-reflection on possible consequences of alternatives can be helpful.[4] Helping clients learn to discern when acceptance is appropriate and when they may wish to take action for change is another useful yoga therapy skill.

Yamas

Discussing the yamas provides an opportunity to engage and self-empower the client in co-development of their self-care plan. Explaining the principles and asking the client to reflect on how these are present in their life promotes self-agency in the therapeutic process.

Ahimsa—non-harm

Ahimsa translates as non-harm or non-violence. It is tempting to declare adeptness at this yama just by avoiding gross acts of violence. However, Desikachar describes ahimsa as "more than just lack of violence. It means kindness, friendliness, and thoughtful consideration of other people and things."[5] The power of ahimsa lies in actions much closer to home, starting with relationship to self. How one regards oneself and behaves toward others creates the foundation for health and well-being, as well as the foundation for all other yamas.

As a practitioner, it is important to create a safe space for both yoga therapist and client to tap into self-compassion. When starting work with a client, asking them to assess sensation and pain as a first step brings attention to the way the client relates to self. Inviting them to articulate how they feel about their situation/condition may reveal how they regard themselves in the world. In yoga therapy, practices that promote self-care and self-kindness are sound starting points. Then, from a place of authentic ahimsa follows a natural extension of kindness out into the world as the client recognizes that any harm done outside self is immediately reflected within. Nursing professor Patti Zuzelo argues that kindness can be an antidote for (among other things) fatigue and irritability in practitioners and for loneliness and disconnection in clients.[6]

Working with meditation and journaling practices can develop the self-awareness to notice the quality of self-talk and habitual thinking patterns.

This foundational awareness is a good starting place to begin a discussion about ahimsa and, if appropriate, cultivating the opposite. An example of this might be to inquire as to what the client has discovered about how they regard themselves. If the client expresses thoughts of being less than, in any way, the yoga therapist might encourage the consideration of the opposite of these statements, a practice that can be particularly helpful when the client recognizes kindness is lacking. If the initial response regarding current well-being is negative, the client can be invited to reflect on another way of looking at the situation. Perhaps they can make space for being softer or kinder, regardless of the situation. (See the practice "Having a cup of tea with yourself" in Appendix 24A.)

Satya—truthfulness

Satya, translated as speaking the truth, invites both client and yoga therapist to examine authenticity and sincerity in thought and action as well as speech. The richness of this yama goes beyond simply not telling lies. Truthfulness comes from a deeper place of honesty with oneself. Like all the yamas, satya is underpinned by ahimsa, kindly and compassionately exploring how the individual is living into their values rather than simply talking about them.

Humility is key for the yoga therapist, as the journey is the client's. The role of the yoga therapist is to create a safe container in which the client can explore wholeness and truth (see Chapter 14). Furthermore, it is important that the yoga therapist is truthful in relation to how they show up for the client. Edwards and Bess suggest that therapists need to be aware of and use their authentic self in the therapeutic relationship; the client's potential for healing is enhanced by genuine relating rather than a type of anonymous neutrality.[7] (See Chapter 13 for more on the creation of therapeutic relationship.)

Exploring a situation through the lens of satya may be painful for the client. They may not like what they discover about themselves. One role of the yoga therapist is to encourage clients to be gentle with themselves throughout the process.

A powerful way to start clients on the practice of satya is to guide them in telling the truth to something inanimate such as a tree, a deity, a symbol, or a pet. This exercise can help the client to feel safe opening up around something they have been avoiding. Journaling is another powerful practice for exploring satya. Useful questions for journaling include

- How honest are you being with yourself and your loved ones about your illness/condition?

Some clients might be acting in such a way as to avoid troubling or concerning the people around them, not asking for help when they need it. Others might not be considering the effect their illness is having on those around them.

- How honest are you with yourself in all areas of your life?
- To what extent are you living in accordance with your own values and ethics?

  Deeper inquiry can often reveal an area where the client feels uncomfortable about a situation and that they are not being true to themselves.

The practice of satya is a deeply personal exploration. The way the yoga therapist and client approach satya will point directly back to ahimsa. It is important that the client understands how to create a firm foundation in kindness and compassion before they are invited to move into the deeper work of satya.

Asteya—non-stealing

Asteya means non-stealing and refers to not taking that which is not freely given. This yama invites a balance between give and take, to not take anything without giving something in return. Often in healthcare, people expect to be given a "pill"—a quick and definitive solution to a problem—but rarely are they invited to participate in their own wellness.

As a yoga therapist, it can be very useful to ascertain how much the client is prepared to contribute to their own wellness and whether the client is more focused on what they can get or take from the yoga therapy experience. Establishing realistic short- and long-term goals will allow the client to actively participate in their wellness. They may only be able to manage 10 minutes of practice 4 days a week, in which case there is no point in asking them to do a 20-minute practice every day; likewise, incorporating yogic principles into daily life may be more realistic for some clients at some times than a stand-alone practice. Skill is involved in giving clients only practices with which they have the capacity to kindly (ahimsa) and honestly (satya) work.

Guiding the client through a meditation of gratitude can encourage acknowledgment of all the other aspects of their healthcare. Engaging the client in expressing gratitude for the assistance they have been given, including from medications, healthcare providers, and family, can create openness rather than resistance (e.g., to medication) and support healing effects from all sources.

Brahmacharya—wise use of energy

Brahmacharya is generally translated as restraint or moderation. An ability to practice moderation in all things, control of one's impulses, and discipline is conducive to spiritual development. This impulse control is often interpreted to include chastity or sexual restraint.

The interweaving of ahimsa, satya, and asteya is crucial to practicing brahmacharya. Having already established the client's relationship to their illness or circumstances through the previous three yamas, the client can now begin to effectively support their own wellness through the application of brahmacharya. How kind they are, how honest they are, and how much they give and take all affect how they use their energy toward themselves and others.

Guiding clients to recognize ways in which they may be interfering with their own wellness is fundamental to improved health and reduced over- or under-use of energy. What evidence is there of "wallowing in" unwellness? Of overplaying illness and the need for assistance? On the other hand, what evidence exists of the client being brave and soldiering on to their detriment?

For a yoga therapist, understanding the use of personal energy can have a positive or negative effect on the client's ability to participate in their wellness. Following are examples of practices to support brahmacharya:

- Invite the client to begin the morning reflecting on the things they need to do for themselves that day. Ask them to assess their energy levels and prioritize how best to utilize their energy for the day while applying the other yamas and niyamas in a way that will optimize their energy.

- *Mudra* can be an effective way to help clients work with their energy (see Chapter 21). The practice of the *prana nadi* mudra sequence of *chin*, *chinmaya*, *adi*, and *brahma* mudras (details of which can be found in Appendix 24B) may help the client sense the breath more deeply and become more attuned to their own capacity and energy for self-healing.

Aparigraha—generosity and non-possessiveness

The yama of *aparigraha*, non-possessiveness, invites generosity and non-grasping while it helps to create freedom from desire (*raga*) and greed.

When one is unwell, it can be challenging to let go of the need to grasp onto or become obsessed with that unwellness. The client may reach for more attention or become self-possessed and obsessed to the extent of hypervigilance about their illness. They may also shop around for the next thing to make them feel better.

Alternatively, they may not ask for help when it is needed, feeling weighed down by their illness as they attempt to carry it all by themselves.

Confusing their identity with the identity of the illness may hold the client back from fully embracing life. Listed below are examples of aparigraha, which can be developed through *dharana* and *dhyana*, practices of concentration and meditation, respectively, on the eightfold path (see Chapter 23):

- discerning that one is not their illness or condition
- writing a list of the things that contribute to personal wholeness
- recognizing that a present grasping can be released
- recognizing that shopping around for more and more things to fix the problem places the focus on the problem
- cultivating gratitude for what is
- committing to the practice at hand
- simply noticing the natural flow of the breath without having to hold or grasp onto it
- taking inventory of physical possessions and asking whether each item creates lightness and freedom or weight

In the words of Swami Jnaneshvara, "can you live fully in the experience of life without the burden of attachment or the need to possess?"[8]

Niyamas

The niyamas provide a useful way for clients to look at how they may be relating to their illness or condition and to themselves. Skillful use of the niyamas can empower clients to be proactive in their own care and healing.

Shaucha—purity

Shaucha means purity and cleanliness. As Desikachar explains, "Śauca has both an inner and an outer aspect. Outer cleanliness simply means keeping ourselves clean. Inner cleanliness has as much to do with the healthy, free functioning of our bodily organs as with the clarity of our mind."[9] This first niyama is an invitation to live simply—to take care of the body, mind, and environment in a way that aligns with personal truth. There are simple techniques clients can use to work with shaucha in each of these areas.

Physically, clients can use gentle *asana* and *pranayama* to help "purify" the body. Practices that gently move the spine in all directions—lateral flexion, twisting rotation, and flexion/extension—and *shatkarmas* (six purification techniques) or gentle pranayama, such as *anuloma viloma* (alternate-nostril breathing) or very gentle *kapalabhati* (skull-shining breath), are good places to start. The less complicated, the better.

Mentally, clients can begin to take the practice of watching thoughts and attitudes from the cushion to daily life by routinely checking in regarding the quality of those thoughts and attitudes. Such reflective practices may be especially useful when coupled with cultivating the opposite if there is negativity.

In terms of the client's environment, it may serve to simply open a window for fresh air or to step outside to sit in the sun or by the ocean for a few minutes. Flowers or calming music can also freshen a space.

Santosha—contentment

It may be challenging for a person suffering from an illness or injury to find *santosha*, contentment, with discomfort. However, santosha can also be regarded as being with what is, even when there exists a preference for something more comfortable.

Many clients are expressly seeking to change what is; the yoga therapist should be aware of a client's potential responses when asking them to cultivate contentment with a condition that may have prompted them to seek care in the first place. Useful practices include

- inviting the client to cultivate an appreciation for what is helpful
- acknowledging the parts of themselves that are well
- being with the part of themselves that is unwell
- simply being open to the idea of contentment with what is

A gratitude journal can be a nourishing way to explore these questions. Other techniques for working with the niyama of santosha are cultivating an inner safe haven or inner resource of ease, safety, security, and well-being (which can be a tremendous support to someone who may be undertaking intensive treatment or surgery); welcoming and accepting; and learning to listen to, embrace, and respond to the body, including while continuing to engage in supportive actions, whether that be morning tea with a friend, a walk in nature, or reading a book in a favorite chair.

Tapas—discipline

Tapas, translated as heat or discipline, encourages a disciplined effort to remove impurities in the body and mind. It is also sometimes interpreted to include asceticism.

It may seem obvious that a client needs to undertake actual yoga therapy practices to move toward greater wellness. However, not all clients have the enthusiasm or discipline to play their part in creating a positive therapeutic outcome. Although only the client can do the work, the yoga therapist can support the client in this regard in many ways.

From the outset, the yoga therapist can engage the client in the processes of *hanam* and *upayam* (priority-setting and choice of practices; see Chapter 3) to provide a sense of client ownership in developing the plan of care and commitment to the practice. Ideally, this effort would include having the client state when they are likely to do the practice and how much time they can commit to, as noted in the section on asteya.

It is helpful for clients to understand yoga therapy as a gradual process of cooking, whereby changes occur over time when the appropriate ingredients are included in the practice. Understanding this encourages clients to maintain their discipline and enthusiasm, even when changes may not be apparent day to day. Clients also need to understand that progress is not always smooth and linear. There may be times when a major change appears to be taking shape and then progress seems to plateau. These bursts of change can be uncomfortable in the short term but helpful in the longer term, just as a small, controlled burn of vegetation can prevent a devastating wildfire later.

Discipline and patience can also be supported when clients understand that their malady—or indeed any circumstance—will go through the normal five stages of birth, growth, stability, decay, and dissolution (see the section "The Five Acts or Stages of the Divine" in Chapter 5). Recognizing the stage being experienced can transform discouragement into enthusiasm.

Svadhyaya—self-study

Desikachar explains *svadhyaya* as "to get close to yourself, that is, to study yourself."[10] Any activity that encourages self-inquiry and self-reflection can be considered svadhyaya, including reflective writing and the study of foundational texts. The yoga therapist might work with this niyama as a means of dismantling *samskara* (long-held conscious or unconscious patterns), helping the client to consider unifying disparate aspects of themselves and moving toward the possibility of liberation through the experience of whole, embodied living.

The client's reaction to symptoms, as well as their beliefs about the meaning of the condition, can make any situation more worrying or upsetting in daily life. Many methods of svadhyaya can be employed to help the client better understand their true nature as something more than a collection of physical sensations and thoughts, a being that includes the mind-body but is greater than it.

One such method is cultivating witness consciousness, wherein the client can disidentify with or de-fuse from the condition and recognize the wholeness that exists behind the malady. An example of this practice can be found in Appendix 24C.

Another method is to ask the client to notice where they sense an emotion (e.g., anxiety) in the body and then to explore the nature of that sensation (texture, color, temperature, shape, etc.). The client can be asked to anthropomorphize the experience of anxiety, welcoming it in as a visitor and engaging it with questions such as "What do you need?" or "What do you want me to know?" The responses that arise can be used to better understand the genesis of, in this case, a chronic anxiety state.

Fundamental to all teachings of yoga is the importance of understanding that optimal health and well-being can only occur when a person is living in accord with their true nature and thereby fulfilling their *dharma*. No matter what malady a person is dealing with, svadhyaya, Self-reflection, can be a valuable therapeutic tool to assist a client's return to good health. Through developing an effective therapeutic relationship with clients, yoga therapists can tailor Self-reflection practices to assist the reduction of *avidya* (misperception; see Chapter 3) and encourage an intimate understanding of true Self.

Another benefit of svadhyaya as a yoga therapy tool is its ability to support and enhance all the other yamas and niyamas. Through greater Self-knowledge, clients learn how to be kind and honest with themselves and others (ahimsa and satya), how to be more discerning about energy expenditure (tapas and brahmacharya), and to know contentment (santosha). The recognition of what is sacred in life (brahmacharya) and the development of discipline (tapas) lead to appreciation of that which is greater than one's "small s" self (*ishvara pranidhana*). A suggested practice for yoga therapists can be found in Appendix 24D.

Ishvara pranidhana—attunement to the Divine

Ishvara pranidhana translates as fixing attention to and aligning with the Divine. This can be interpreted to include surrendering one's will to that of some sort of universal creative force. (These ideas could be interpreted in a multitude of ways; see Chapter 17.) Recognizing and attuning to the great mystery offers numerous benefits in therapeutic processes.

The practice of ishvara pranidhana connects closely with the yogic principle of *shraddha*, often translated as faith or trust. Faith, trust, and conviction have been shown to have a powerful positive effect on health outcomes.[11] The specific object of trust is unimportant as long as a person regards that entity as somehow higher or greater than (their perception of) themselves and imbued with some form of agency in affecting health outcomes. The practice of ishvara pranidhana is one way for clients to develop such trust.

When suffering from illness or injury, people may feel that they need to gain control over the condition and expend a lot of mental energy trying to do so. By releasing the need to control and developing trust or faith in a greater good, a person can save valuable mental energy while aligning with the greater wholeness that eventually becomes recognized as their own highest true nature as unitive consciousness.

Being an audience of the divine mystery begins to shift people out of human-constructed clock time and into divine rhythm.[12] Suggested practices for ishvara pranidhana are making a personal retreat or tuning into the rhythm of life rather than the clock and the mind's habitual expectations. Another suggested ishvara pranidhana practice can be found in Appendix 24D.

It can be tempting to regard svadhyaya and ishvara pranidhana as purely spiritual niyamas that have little to do with the therapeutic application of yoga. However, yoga regards the physical, mental, social, and spiritual as equally important aspects of well-being, all interconnected and all affecting the others; each should be considered in the application of yoga therapy. Furthermore, questions of meaning and purpose or "existential crises" often arise in the context of chronic, especially life-threatening, illness.

The application of svadhyaya and ishvara pranidhana can provide greater insight into and understanding of the nature of many physical and mental expressions of unwellness. In the *Yoga Sutras*, the *vyuha* model of healing presents four questions for the client: (1) *heyam* (What form of suffering is the client experiencing?—i.e., the presenting condition); (2) *hetu* (What is the cause of the suffering?); (3) *hanam* (What short- and long-term goals aid the client in easing or ending this suffering?); and (4) *upayam* (What are the means or tools to use?). (See Chapter 3 for more on this model.) Hetu, hanam, and upayam can all be facilitated by the careful self-reflective process of svadhyaya and aligning with a more fully conscious aspect of Self, or ishvara pranidhana.

Summary

The yamas and niyamas provide a valuable framework for yoga therapists to assess a client's ethics and lifestyle. They are the backbone for effective, therapeutic lifestyle interventions that promote self-agency in the therapeutic process.

Inviting the client to reflect on their current situation through the lens of the yamas helps them to recognize how they relate to the world around them. Reflecting on the niyamas helps clients to consider how they may be relating to themselves and their condition. Both yamas and niyamas engage clients in the co-development of their care plans.

Additional Resources

Byron, K. (2002). *Loving what is.* Harmony.

Fields, G. P. (2001). *Religious therapeutics: Body and health in yoga, ayurveda and tantra.* State University of New York Press.

Appendix 24A: Having a Cup of Tea with Yourself (Ahimsa)

This is a practice of sitting with yourself as you would sit with a dear friend over a cup of tea, listening actively and holding space for them to share with you. It is about treating yourself, sitting with yourself, in the same way, with the same love and tenderness you would offer as you sat with a friend.

- Prepare a cup of tea or favorite warm beverage. Find a comfortable seat and spend a few breaths settling into the support of the seat.
- Hold the cup at your sternum and feel its warmth seeping into your heart. Inhale the warmth. Exhale and feel the warmth radiate through your body. Take a sip and feel the physical warmth internally. Spend a few breaths experiencing the warmth.
- Allow the heart to feel warm, open, and spacious. Welcome the idea of listening to the heart with warmth, openness, and spaciousness, allowing the heart space to share what it needs to share with you today.

- Continue breathing in the warmth and sipping as you like. Feel a sense of tenderness and gentleness for yourself.
- From the warmth of your heart center, simply ask, "What do you have to tell me today?" And listen. Ask yourself, "What is my heart's purpose today?" Feel into your heart, "What gives me purpose today?" The answer may arise as a felt sense and emotion, a thought, or language.
- Sense the warmth of your own loving heart nourishing every cell. Being with whatever arises, tenderly and lovingly holding space for yourself.
- As you finish your cup of tea, let go of the idea that you need to fix or change anything. Be open to whatever insights arise.

When you feel ready, continue with your day, nourished by your own tender heart.

Appendix 24B: Prana Nadi Mudras (Brahmacharya)[13]

Prana is the energetic life force that enlivens every living thing. It is most readily available through the breath. The *nadis* are the pathway through which prana flows. This set of mudras is about directing and feeling the subtle movement of breath in each part of the torso/lungs.

The mudras can be used independently or together, although you may find the greatest benefit when using them as a set. Begin in your favorite meditation posture with the spine straight and hands resting palms down on the thighs. Beginning meditation with the palms down helps with grounding and centering before moving into the mudras. When you first begin this practice, hold each mudra for 2 minutes; over time, you can begin to extend to 5 minutes.

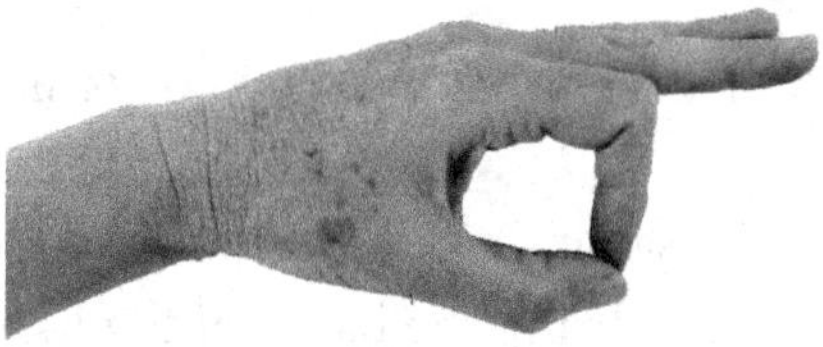

KANISHTA PRANA NADI MUDRA (OR *CHIN MUDRA*)

Bring the tips of the thumb and index fingers together, palms still facing down on the thighs. Extend the other three fingers out. Soften through the spine, arms, and shoulders as you allow your attention to be drawn to a felt sense of the breath in the lowest lobes of the lungs—front, back, and sides—maybe even down into the pelvis.

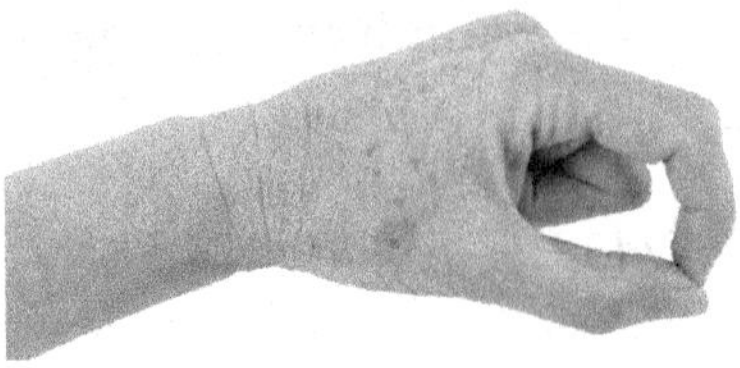

MADHYAMA PRANA NADI MUDRA (OR *CHINMAYA MUDRA*)

Keep the tips of the thumb and index fingers together as they are and the palms still facing down on the thighs. Curl the three extended fingers into the palms so that the tips of the fingers are gently pressing into the palms. Staying relaxed through the spine, arms, and shoulders, allow your attention to be drawn to a felt sense of the breath in the middle lobes of the lungs—front, back, and sides.

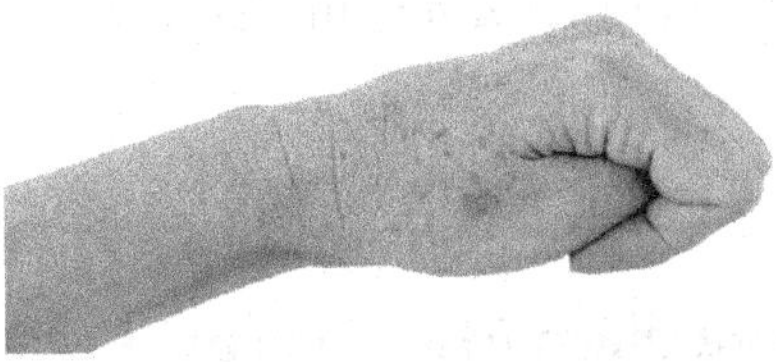

JYESTHTHA PRANA NADI MUDRA (OR *ADI MUDRA*)

Curl the thumbs into the palms and wrap the fingers around the thumbs, palms still facing down on the thighs. Staying relaxed through the spine, arms, and shoulders, allow your attention to be drawn to a felt sense of the breath in the upper lobes of the lungs, upper chest, upper back, collarbones, and shoulders.

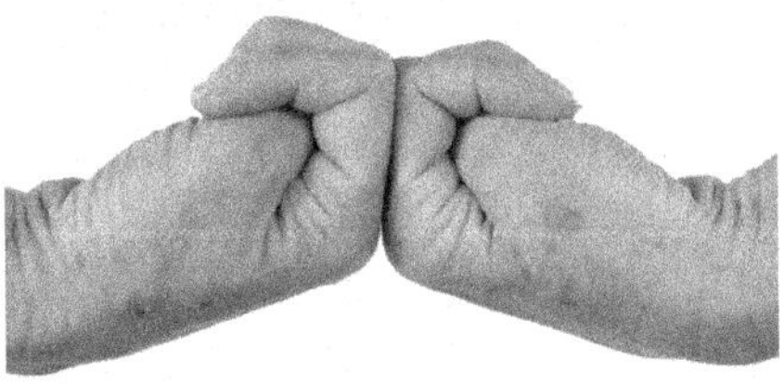

POORNA PRANA NADI MUDRA (OR *BRAHMA MUDRA*)

Keeping the hands in the same shape as *jyesththa prana nadi mudra* (fingers wrapped around the thumbs), bring the backs of the knuckles together, palms facing up now and the little fingers gently pressing into the belly below the navel. Staying relaxed through the spine, arms, and shoulders, allow your attention to be drawn to a felt sense of the breath in all lobes of the lungs—upper, middle, and lower, front and back.

Finally, release the hands back to the thighs and sit in being for as long as you like.

Appendix 24C: Witness Consciousness Self-Reflection (Svadhyaya)

Take a moment to come to total rest, putting aside all that you had been doing, and feel the presence of your physical body as it sits or lies quietly.

- Notice all the points of contact between the body and the surface on which it rests, starting from the feet and moving up.
- Now notice any leftover, unnecessary tensions or gripping and allow them to release.
- Notice the felt sense of the whole front of the body, then the felt sense of the whole back of the body.
- Now feel the whole global body as one.
- Imagine or feel that the body is out in front of you, perhaps as though it is on a stage or screen and a part of you is the audience.
- Notice how you are aware of the body, observing it as a witness.
- Then, inquire into who or what is the witness and notice that there is a deeper witnessing consciousness or awareness in which all these perceptions and sensations arise and fall away.
- If it feels okay, feel back into the felt sense of the global body and then feel back or step back as the witnessing consciousness in which everything arises and falls away.
- When ready, return to your day-to-day experience of the body and mind with the felt understanding of your Self as witnessing consciousness.

Appendix 24D: Self-Reflection on Alignment with Life Purpose (Ishvara Pranidhana)

Take a moment to come to total rest, putting aside all that you had been doing, and feel the presence of your physical body as it sits or lies quietly.

- Let yourself open to the visceral feeling of life living itself through you—the pulse, throb, or vibration of life-force (*prana*). Take your time to really feel into the sensations, perhaps in the heart center or solar plexus.

- Pose the question, "What is my deepest, heartfelt wish, desire, or mission for this life—how does life want to live itself through me?" Stay with this open question without seeking an answer in words, then pose a similar question: "What is it that would give my life purpose, meaning, and value?"
- As you sit with these questions, notice any thoughts, images, and feelings that arise and allow them to be felt in the body as sensation. Be in no hurry, as words or phrases may start to unfold, pointing toward a deep expression of your true nature and highest Self.

Let yourself feel an alignment with this highest guidance and a trust that it is an ever-present support on which you can rely and into which you can surrender.

Endnotes

1 Feuerstein, G. (1993). *Living yoga.* Tarcher Perigee.

2 Mallinson, J., & Singleton, M. (2017). *Roots of yoga.* Penguin Classics.

3 Adele, D. (2009). *The yamas & niyamas: Exploring yoga's ethical practice.* On-Word Bound Books.
Bouanchaud, B. (1997). *The essence of yoga: Reflections on the Yoga Sutras of Patanjali.* Sri Satguru Publications.
Desikachar, T. K. V. (1995). *The heart of yoga: Developing a personal practice.* Inner Traditions.
Moors, F. (2012). *Liberating isolation: The yogasutra of Patanjali.* Media Garuda.

4 Desikachar, *Heart of yoga.*

5 Desikachar, *Heart of yoga* (p. 98).

6 Zuzelo, P. R. (2016). Dosing kindness as a therapeutic intervention. *Holistic Nursing Practice, 30*(4), 241–243.

7 Edwards, J. K., & Bess, J. M. (1998). Developing effectiveness in the therapeutic use of self. *Clinical Social Work Journal, 26*, 89–105.

8 Quoted in Adele, *Yamas & niyamas* (p. 101).

9 Desikachar, *Heart of yoga* (p. 101).

10 Desikachar, *Heart of yoga* (p. 101).

11 Barefoot, J. C., Maynard, K. E., Beckham, J. C., Brummett, B. H., Hooker, K., & Siegler, I. C. (1998). Trust, health, and longevity. *Journal of Behavioral Medicine, 21*(6), 517–526.

12 Adele, *Yamas & niyamas.*

13 Shared with permission from Macauley, G. (2017). Prana nadi mudras. www.yogahara.com.au/news/2016/12/10/prana-nadi-mudras

Section IV

PROFESSIONAL PRACTICES

Beyond understanding yogic traditions to enable them to appropriately honor and contextualize the practices, and assiduously developing their clinical skills, yoga therapists will need to cultivate an ethical mindset as well as an entrepreneurial one. Together, these foundations allow for success in all dimensions of practice, including personal wellness.

In addition to offering starting points for considering one's clinical and business practices from a yogic base, this section introduces a range of health systems approaches and delivery settings to help yoga therapists to expand the reach of the profession beyond the bounds of traditional environments and to clients who may not fit culturally dominant norms of able-bodied, affluent yoga practitioners. "To put it simply," activist Jivana Heyman told us, "yoga is designed to reduce suffering through increased self-awareness. A community of people who are suffering less would be beneficial for society as a whole."

In the words of yoga therapist Tawanna Kane,

> Increasing the numbers of people who engage a pause before action can change the world. *Ahimsa* becomes the norm instead of the extraordinary. We learn to pause not only before action but before speaking as well. The cliché of kindness swells spontaneously from the heart.

Laurie Hyland Robertson and Diane Finlayson

25

Ethics in Yoga Therapy Practice

GAIL PARKER

As a healing art, yoga therapy becomes a therapeutic tool that interfaces with and becomes part of a healthcare system that is highly regulated by state and federal laws as well as professional and ethical standards of care. Although yoga therapy is a self-regulated and self-regulating profession, yoga therapists are expected to abide by standards of care and ethical guidelines that apply to yoga as therapy. The International Association of Yoga Therapists has defined a basic scope of practice and ethical guidelines that yoga therapists certified by the organization commit to following.[1] Cognitive knowledge of ethical codes, however, is not sufficient to prevent ethical missteps and can take a backseat to contextual factors and subjective interpretations of the codes and guidelines.

Subjective factors influence judgments and behaviors: Personal feelings, interpretations, and intuitions can obscure good judgment, and despite their best intentions yoga therapists can find themselves in situations where, without realizing it, they slip into ethically problematic behaviors. Examples might include failure to report a colleague one knows is sexually involved with a client, working when too distressed to be effective, working outside the scope of one's training and competence, failing to document or report when a client appears to be a threat to themselves or others, failing to adhere to strict protocols when using email or connecting with clients on social media platforms, and failing to educate clients about the privacy risks involved in communicating electronically.

In addition to presenting a code of ethics, yoga therapy education has a responsibility to help students and practitioners of yoga therapy understand the thought processes, motivations, blind spots, values, and emotions that influence their work as therapists. Ongoing self-study as part of an ethics curriculum is necessary.

What Comes First—Ethics or Practice?

Ethics are the guidelines and standards that govern conscious lives and decision-making. Ethical guidelines are important because they offer a baseline for understanding the concepts of acceptable and unacceptable behavior. Their aim is to provide a ready understanding of how to react to a certain situation long before that situation happens. One's ethics govern one's thought process so that when a problem arises or there is a need to work through a situation the solution is ethically grounded.

Many in the yoga traditions turn first to the *Yoga Sutras of Patanjali*, which outline ethical guidelines for behavior in one's relationship to others, the environment, and oneself. The sutras offer the caveat that ethical behavior is established not by memorizing guidelines but by internalizing and living them.[2]

Yoga therapists must engage in self-sustaining actions to avoid self-deception that results in acting in ethically unacceptable ways. "The whole practice of yoga is a process of examining our habitual attitudes and behaviors and their consequences."[3] It is through personal practice, then, that yoga therapists approach ethical standards—not as rules to follow, but as ways of being. Yoga and ethics are intrinsic to each other—there is no separation. It is through a consistent practice that yoga therapists become ethical, embodying the standards, not by memorizing ethical codes. It is important, however, to be familiar with the ethical standards that yoga therapists are expected to abide by.

Guidance from the *Yoga Sutras*

Chapter 24 discusses the ethical precepts of the *yamas* and *niyamas* in relation to clinical encounters. The present chapter steps back to more broadly consider this yogic guidance in terms of the countless daily thoughts and decisions yoga therapists engage in the course of business and practice. These ideas invite a return to the concepts presented in early chapters of the book for viewing through a new lens of clinical skills and therapeutic tools.

Yamas

Yamas are five attitudes that express as behavioral patterns in relationship to others and to one's surroundings:[4]

1. ***Ahimsa*** can refer to considerate behavior in relationship to others. It involves kindness, compassion, friendliness, and taking others into thoughtful consideration.

2. ***Satya*** means truthfulness, but truthfulness with discernment so as not to do harm.
3. ***Asteya*** means to take nothing that does not belong to one.
4. ***Bramacharya***, the merging of one's sensual and spiritual natures, creates balance and moderation in action.
5. ***Aparigraha*** means a willingness to let go and not cling to or take advantage of a situation for personal gain.

According to the *Yoga Sutras*, when these five behaviors become a part of one's life through a consistent and sustained comprehensive yoga practice, kindness, truthfulness, honoring of boundaries, self-regulation, and the ability to let go of what does not serve are more likely to become internalized as ways of being. At this point one's very presence can engender these qualities in others.

Niyamas

Niyama refers to one's attitudes toward oneself.[5] Yoga therapists have a responsibility to treat themselves in the way they hope clients will treat themselves; they have an ethical responsibility to model the behaviors they are teaching.

Niyamas can be considered in the context of client interactions:

1. ***Saucha*** means cleanliness, keeping one's body and surroundings clean, orderly, and esthetically pleasing.
2. ***Santosha*** means being content with who one is and what one has to offer.
3. On the physical level, ***tapas*** refers to heating the body to cleanse it to optimize health.
4. ***Svadhyaya*** means self-study and self-reflective awareness.
5. ***Ishvara pranidhana*** includes surrender to a higher power that exists beyond the limits of the thinking mind and egoic identity.

Yamas and niyamas are more than aspirational ideals or commandments to follow. To sustain living by these codes, one must embody them and commit to an understanding of oneself.

Obstacles on the Path

Behavior toward others and the environment is a subjective reflection of personality and blind spots, as well as frame of mind. Cultural conditioning—including religious beliefs; social background; racial, ethnic, and gender identity; and individual character traits, strengths, and limitations—influence yoga therapists' attitudes and the way in which they exhibit the yamas and niyamas. The subjective nature of one's personality and cultural and social conditioning, as well as state of mind, mean that attitudes and behaviors that contradict the yamas and niyamas must be examined with an intention of identifying misapprehensions that make it difficult to sustain action in accordance with these principles. When one engages in self-study and identifies the obstacles that interfere with the ability to live the yamas and niyamas, these obstacles to clear understanding dissolve and behavior toward others and the environment changes.

Yoga therapists have an ethical responsibility to engage in practices that support them in embodying these guidelines. These are not behaviors that we can expect to sustain without ongoing self-study. Self-reflective awareness through ongoing self-study helps us observe the contrary attitudes that hinder the ability to be effective in the therapeutic relationship (see Chapter 13).

Interruptions to mental clarity

According to the *Yoga Sutras*, one's state of mind is affected by obstacles that cloud judgment.[6] Clouded judgment leaves one vulnerable to ethical missteps, including mental sluggishness, persistent uncertainty, impulsiveness, excess, self-deception, lack of endurance, and backsliding. All of these interruptions become distractions that can result in choices that disregard ethical guidelines.

Other life influences shape perception as well: adverse childhood experiences (ACE) such as neglect, trauma, and abuse; childhood advantages that protect against certain difficult experiences; cultural conditioning; gender identity; racial and ethnic identity; racial, ethnic, and cultural biases; national and regional origins; and more.

Without awareness, one may assume that their perceptions of reality are factual and objective and are shared, or should be shared, by everyone. People consider their perceptions to be correct and behave accordingly, when in actuality they may be seeing through a distorted lens without realizing it and cause harm to themselves or someone else. By the same token, someone might misperceive a situation by doubting that their own perception could be accurate. In this case, they may fail to take action when action is called for.

The *Yoga Sutras* call these misapprehensions *avidya*, faulty perceptions or incorrect understanding. Avidya is best understood as the habitual ways of perceiving and behaving that one has engaged in for years. These habits, or *samskara*, are buried in the unconscious and become normalized to cloud vision. Most people do not see with clarity, as they think they do, but through a filmy layer of conditioning and past experiences. Avidya is described as superficial perception that obscures clarity of thought, but there is a deeper level of perception not obscured by avidya. The goal of yoga is to cultivate a relationship with this deep level of perception to enable clear vision and the resulting appropriate actions; this prevents ethical missteps.

Kleshas

The five main obstacles to mental clarity vary in intensity and can range from being of little or no consequence to utter blindness. The *Yoga Sutras* refer to *kleshas* as afflictions or negative mental states that cloud perception, distort reality and affect how one thinks, feels, and acts, and result in suffering (see Chapter 3).[7] Kleshas can lead to ethical missteps.

All of the kleshas are interrelated, but the first, avidya, is the source of the other four obstacles to clarity.

1. ***Avidya*** (ignorance) is the unwillingness to accept reality as it is, and instead to insist that reality is based on one's own perception of it. This false representation of reality prevents seeing beyond the obvious and exploring what one does not already know.

2. ***Asmita*** (I-am-ness or ego) is the assumption that what one thinks is a constant and unchanging source of perception that is always valid.

3. ***Raga*** (attachment), emotional bondage to any source of pleasure, is an inability to let go even when the object of attachment no longer serves or no longer exists.

4. ***Dvesha*** (aversion) is an emotional repulsion and flight from pain or difficulty that manifests as prejudice or hatred, making it impossible to learn from life's hardships or from one's own mistakes.

5. ***Abhinivesha***, often translated as fear of death, is an instinctive clinging to life that is biologically programmed but destructive when extended to the perpetuation of the ego.

The first stage of working with the kleshas is to simply acknowledge them. Self-reflective awareness supports the ability to see the kleshas and their roots as well as how they create suffering. The practice of yoga enables the recognition of avidya, and habitual patterns of perception gradually begin to change. Periods of clarity and distraction are inevitable throughout life, so vigilance is important to support increased stability in clear thinking and to avoid delusion.

The state of yoga is discovered through tapas, svadhyaya, and ishvara pranidhana. Tapas involves practicing *asana* and *pranayama*, svadhyaya involves self-refection, and ishvara pranidhana involves focusing on the quality of an action and the spirit in which an action is taken. These three ways of being—with health, self-study, and quality of action—help to reduce avidya and to prevent, avoid, and bounce back from ethical missteps.

BOX 25.1 AVOIDING ETHICAL MISSTEPS

It is not enough to know what ethical guidelines are intellectually. Despite our best intentions we may find ourselves in situations where we unwittingly slip into ethically problematic behaviors that could have been prevented. As part of your preparation for avoiding ethical missteps and moving toward ethical excellence, answer the following questions:

1. Why have you chosen to be a yoga therapist?
2. How can serving as a yoga therapist foster positive change in the clients you see?
3. How can you as a yoga therapist have a positive impact on the perceptions of yoga as a healing modality?
4. What are four core professional values that you rely on to guide your behavior and decision-making process as a yoga therapist?
5. What are your emotional strengths?
6. What are your emotional weaknesses?
7. What are your abilities as a yoga therapist?
8. What are your limitations?
9. What are your self-care practices?

Additional Resources

Edge, R. S., & Groves, J. R. (2017). *Ethics of health care: A guide for clinical practice* (4th ed.). Cengage Learning.

Sohnen-Moe, C. M., & Benjamin, B. E. (2013). *The ethics of touch: The hands-on practitioner's guide to creating a professional, safe and enduring practice* (2nd ed.). Sohnen-Moe Associates.

Sullivan, M., & Robertson, L. C. H. (2020). Dharma, ethics and right action. In *Understanding yoga therapy: Applied philosophy and science for health and well-being* (pp. 30–48). Routledge.

Endnotes

1 International Association of Yoga Therapists. (2020). IAYT code of ethics and professional responsibilities. https://cdn.ymaws.com/www.iayt.org/resource/resmgr/docs_certification_all/2020_updates_scope_ethics/2020-09_code_of_ethics_v2.pdf

2 Desikachar, T. K. V. (1995). *The heart of yoga: Developing a personal practice*. Inner Traditions.

3 Desikachar, *Heart of yoga* (p. 97).

4 Yoga Sutra 2.30, in Desikachar, *Heart of yoga* (p. 175).

5 Yoga Sutra 2.31, in Desikachar, *Heart of yoga* (pp. 175–176).

6 Yoga Sutra 1.30, in Desikachar, *Heart of yoga* (p. 158).

7 Yoga Sutra 2.3–9, in Desikachar, *Heart of yoga* (pp. 166–167).

26

The Business of Yoga Therapy

MARSHA D. BANKS-HAROLD, THERESA CONROY, MOLLY MCMANUS, MELINDA ATKINS, AND LAURIE HYLAND ROBERTSON

It is not only appropriate to run a yoga therapy practice like the business it is, but also a sustainable way forward for the profession. Upholding yogic principles while providing transformational potential for clients and a decent living for yoga therapists themselves is possible given a well-considered foundation that builds on the discipline of *tapas* and the unflinching self-study of *svadhyaya*.

Additional essential foundations of successful yoga therapy practice include scrupulous adherence to scope of practice and avoiding direct competition with pathogenesis-oriented providers. Yoga therapists instead provide support that helps people to increase their self-agency and be their best selves, regardless of their clinical conditions; they do not treat pathology or address symptoms. They need to learn the appropriate specific language to work alongside particular types of medical providers so they can complement a disease-driven model with one that supports well-being. Yoga therapists' ability to care for the psychosocial and spiritual elements of health distinguishes the practice from other modalities.

This chapter offers a strategic framework for cultivating an entrepreneurial mindset in yoga therapy practice, which applies regardless of the business model chosen and whether the entity is for-profit or non-profit. More specific, detailed resources and planning instruments abound. Additional Resources at the end of this chapter lists some of these tools.

An Entrepreneurial Mindset

Entrepreneurs in any field must cultivate skills for selling their ideas, services, and products, networking, and competing or collaborating with other businesses. Most entrepreneurs, with the goal of success driving their decisions, create business plans based on specific financial and market-driven data.

Yoga therapy entrepreneurs are additionally tasked with the overarching goal of supporting people to progress toward improved health and well-being. Helping others to improve their self-agency, a heart-driven and service-oriented goal, differentiates yoga therapists from most other entrepreneurs. Accepting the calling to serve is rooted in *sankalpa*, a Tantric concept that encompasses a singular intention or resolve that can help to guide action.

Yoga therapy entrepreneurs, focused on the goal of serving others, may struggle with the business of being a yoga therapist. Some yoga therapy entrepreneurs even contemplate whether yoga professionals should be financially compensated at all. Consciously allowing the attitudes of the *bhavas* to guide one's state of mind can help to sort through such complex questions. For example, contemplating the bhava of non-attachment (*vairagya*) as "a state of being in the world but not of the world" may be useful; "[n]on-attachment involves humility, objectivity, faith, ego reduction, acceptance, and surrender to a larger reality."[1]

Being in the world requires all entrepreneurs, including yoga therapists, to prioritize their own well-being and that of those they serve. Underpinned by *dharma*—"action that supports individual spiritual development and the well-being of the larger community"[2]—this idea points toward health in all aspects of life, physically, intellectually, emotionally, and spiritually. Without prioritizing their own well-being, yoga therapists may succumb to the pressures of the many responsibilities of being an entrepreneur and experience anxiety, depression, and low self-esteem. Such impediments may negatively impact the ability to successfully oversee the stability and growth of a business.

Competing priorities

Handling the numerous responsibilities associated with being an entrepreneur while maintaining a positive presence for those served may generate internal conflict. Many entrepreneurs radiate positivity publicly when the business thrives and struggle to mirror this mood privately, or they suffer quietly as they attempt to hold space for themselves and others during less successful times. Remaining aware that the journey of entrepreneurship can encompass despair and positivity sets a realistic stage for sustainability.

Change is inevitable when managing a yoga therapy business. The practical requirements, if not addressed, will prohibit yoga therapists from staying present and focused amid necessary transitions and carrying out their dharma:

> Dharma is the foundation of this world; and there is nothing of greater value than dharma. But undoubtedly dharma requires money. Always, dharma is a factor in wealth; but wealth is to be grasped for securing the ends of dharma... And money cannot be had by begging, or by cowardice, much less by concentrating on dharma alone.[3]

Personally taking advantage of the tools and practices that also empower clients and committing to consistently connecting with an uplifting community facilitate perseverance through both thriving and trying times. The well-being of the yoga therapist and those they serve requires the development of "the consciousness and skills to attract whatever is needed to fulfill our dharma or higher purpose."[4]

Fortunately, yoga therapists can tap into the foundational practices of contentment, surrender, and self-study to enable them to serve from a place of abundance and prosperity. Note that "Prosperity is more than financial success and material comfort... True prosperity is experienced in a spiritual context."[5] Like *prana*, money represents the flow of energy through systems and is not an inherently evil—or good—concept.

When the yoga therapy entrepreneur accepts (1) the calling to serve and (2) the responsibility of managing a business, the resulting prosperity is the blessing needed to ensure the financial resources to carry out one's dharma. *Artha*, the pursuit of sufficient material comfort to support the dharmic path, is a basic goal of human life: "The aim of artha is to prosper in every way."[6]

BOX 26.1 ALIGNING PERSONAL STRENGTHS AND MARKET NEEDS

MARSHA D. BANKS-HAROLD

Meeting market needs usually involves the identification of unaddressed areas and the creation of a service or product that fills those gaps. This strategy falls short for yoga therapists who see their personal strengths and skills in opposition to market needs. They may feel they have to choose between aligning with their personal strengths and meeting those demands.

Consciously bridging personal strengths and market needs, on the other hand, can be effective and rewarding. My lived experiences as a Black woman engineer and as a yoga studio owner and trainer of yoga teachers and yoga therapists, combined with self-study, manifested the platform for me to showcase resilience, encourage self-empowerment, and build community. I established PIES Fitness Yoga Studio—PIES stands for physical, intellectual, emotional, and spiritual peace—as an inclusive, safe, and diverse community. Knowing personally the impact of *not* feeling included, I responded to the market's need for a community where socioeconomic status, race, ethnicity, gender, sex, sexual orientation, age, physical ability, and religion did not prevent access to the healing benefits of yoga and yoga therapy. Self-study promotes increased awareness of the thoughts and beliefs that drive actions. Ultimately, yoga therapists who assess who they are at the core will be able to use this knowledge to identify the clients they most authentically feel comfortable serving.

The strategy of self-study is an essential preparation for attracting the clients who will resonate with each yoga therapist. My own introduction to yoga was life-transforming but extremely uncomfortable because I had no idea what to expect; based on early experiences as a student, teacher, and yoga therapist, I recognized that I was not alone. Self-study prepared me to hold space for those who were new to yoga, felt intimidated, or thought that they were not flexible enough to benefit from the practices: I created "My Body Don't Bend that Way," a class designed for every being, but especially for those who believe themselves to be too inflexible for yoga and those seeking a fun, unassuming class where questions are always welcome and judgment is not.

Given the necessary groundwork to stand confidently in who they are and who they are called to serve, market needs will tend to align with the yoga therapist's strengths—or viable opportunities will tend to become easier to identify. Assuming the ongoing development of appropriate clinical skills, the yoga therapist will be more than prepared to serve the clients who appear based on the work they have done to connect with their authentic self. These clients will be the ones seeking exactly what the yoga therapist's journey has revealed to them.

Self-study must include articulation of one's "ideal client" and inquiry into their needs and characteristics. Such inquiry may involve both formal and informal research at the level of individual clients and groups of clients alongside research into the conditions of local markets (and, depending on the business model, perhaps regional, national, or international markets). The resulting insights will enable the yoga therapist to thrive, with an integrated perspective of authentic alignment between personal strengths and skills and the needs of the market—that is, what would benefit the health and well-being of their ideal client(s). From this space the yoga therapist will more reliably be able to honor the broader goal of guiding people toward self-engendered health.

BOX 26.2 MARKET YOURSELF WITH EFFECTIVE, AUTHENTIC POSITIONING

THERESA CONROY

Self-definition

As writer Anne Lamott said, "Lighthouses don't go running all over an island looking for boats to save; they just stand there shining."[7]

Be the lighthouse. Find a comfortable cove within the profession—one that makes room for your personality, passions, and vision for your dream career—then guide your ideal clients to your shore.

Being specific about your skills and interests will help you reach and engage your target audience much more effectively than trying to be everything for everyone. According to yoga therapist and business coach Laura Kupperman, when asked to define their offerings too many yoga therapists offer a statement like "I give people customized tools for increasing well-being."[8]

Potential clients, however, do not "wake up and say, 'I need customized tools,'" then search online for that term. Instead, people say, "'My back hurts,' or, 'I need someone to help me work through this grief.' They don't search for a specialist in 'living radiantly.'"[9]

Creating a yoga therapy niche not only establishes your expertise, interests, and talents, but also focuses your marketing and enables clients to find you more easily. People are willing to pay for help with an area causing them discomfort, such as insomnia or anxiety. Although yoga therapists work in a holistic way, clients typically seek a solution to an issue, searching for their particular problem online or consulting first with more traditional healthcare practitioners.[10]

Settling on a niche requires self-study to honestly design boundaries around your skills and passions while editing out the elements that do not align. Similar to *neti neti* meditation of identifying with "not this, not that," the process of introspection can help to elucidate exactly who you are as a yoga therapist by revealing who you are not.

Remember that it is not necessary to do every job yourself, follow every social media trend or marketing recommendation, or take on every client who presents to your practice. Similar to referring to a colleague those clients who are not a good fit for your practice, hiring out tasks for which you lack expertise or interest (e.g., website design, IT services) supports the community as a whole and frees the yoga therapist to focus on their dharma.

One of the most enlightening and stabilizing ways of defining yourself is to write a business plan, as discussed further below. Begin the business plan with a mission statement—a sankalpa not only for your business, but for your personal path. Answer these questions:

- Who do I want to serve?
- What problems can I help solve?
- How do I want to offer those solutions?

As with any workable intention, the mission statement should be constructed in the present tense, as if it were already true. My own mission statement is "I work individually and in small groups helping clients with neurological disorders improve their daily lives." I often use variations on this easy-to-understand statement to tell friends, colleagues, and family members—in person and on social media—what I do and how I can help them or their friends.

I found this niche thanks to my first client with Parkinson's disease (PD). That client told his neurologist about me. That neurologist was impressed with our results and began using his prescription pad to "prescribe" my practice to patients. Those clients began to tell their other practitioners about me, and soon I was receiving referrals from physical, occupational, and speech therapists. I now train other yoga teachers and yoga therapists to work with this population.

Although my niche was not what I had expected it to be, I opened easily to it as I felt the momentum build. My client base in that specialty expanded as my reputation among healthcare professionals grew. The more people I met with these conditions, the more personally invested I became in my niche. I also work with anxiety and chronic pain—also symptoms of some neurological disorders—but I became known and built the foundation of my practice by clinging to that little cove next to my lighthouse.

Referral success

The most powerful step I took to market my yoga therapy practice was networking with healthcare professionals who work with my target audience. I found those contacts through local support groups, social media pages, doctors' offices, physical and occupational therapy practices, psychologists, chiropractors, acupuncturists, and other yoga teachers.

The key to establishing a relationship with another practitioner is to make it mutually beneficial. Loren Fishman, yoga therapist and medical director of Manhattan Physical Medicine and Rehabilitation, said that an effective way to obtain referrals is to refer out yourself. "Then, when you get a referral back, do your best to help."[11]

That one neurologist from my first PD client is largely responsible for helping to build my entire practice and reputation in the field. I now even receive referrals from health professionals I have never met but who heard about my work through a chain that can be traced back to that physician.

After referring clients back to a local physical therapist, my group Yoga for Parkinson's class began to fill up with the patients she sent back to me. Even some of the practitioners I see for my own health have referred clients to me after casual discussions about my work.

Dozens of referral sources are not necessary—a few quality professional relationships can fill your work days with interesting, engaged clients. Making those business connections beneficial requires planning, professionalism, and a willingness to gently educate others about the burgeoning field of yoga therapy.

Positioning yoga therapy as something that complements another professional's work can be helpful. Yoga therapists are not replacements for physical therapists or talk therapists, but instead often serve as adjuncts and enhancements to necessary medication or medical treatment. The yoga therapy approach offers the benefit of seeing the whole person and working with each *kosha*—a practice not usually present in the Western medical model.

Making clear to health professionals exactly what yoga therapy is—and is not—accomplishes a few important goals: Such an approach establishes the professionalism and competence of the field, creates an atmosphere of collaboration instead of competition, and clearly defines the yoga therapist's scope of practice.

Success here, however, requires action as well. Ask clients to update their healthcare workers on their success and satisfaction with your work. With the clients' permission, share copies of your care plans with their physical therapists. Invite the practitioner for a free private session. And, as Fishman recommended, always refer clients back to them.

Once the connection is made, continue to nurture those relationships as you would a friendship. Keep in touch. Send holiday gifts and cards. Keep them informed about patients' progress (again with express written permission). Consider these providers mentors, teachers, and bridges to others.

When meeting with someone friendly and willing to help, Kupperman recommends asking whether there is someone else you should talk to, and whether you may use their name when you do so: "Just that simple act has filled my practice."[12]

Business Planning

Regardless of the shape one's dharma takes, the business of yoga therapy can require complex planning. A diversified revenue strategy may entail a variety of offerings, including hosting local classes and workshops, private and small-group sessions, and education for other professionals and the public.

Although business planning in this context may not be easy, as noted above, this work also offers an opportunity for self-study. Developing the mission and vision of a yoga therapy business must begin with identification of one's professional dharma—what is uniquely yours to do in this lifetime as an organization. From such a place of clarity, it is easier to articulate one's values and to develop a strategy to accomplish it—from the yogic perspective, laying out the path for artha, the means by which that dharma will be accomplished.

Non-profit business entities may be perceived as more accustomed to deliberately understanding themselves as an organization and being able to clearly articulate values, mission, and vision. Still, when approached consciously, such dharmic work will help non-profits to identify compatible funding options and better tailor grant writing. For-profits can use these same skills to clarify their organizational structures, qualify their lines of business, and do the work they are meant to do rather than getting swept up in trends or impulsive changes.[13]

Values

Identifying an organization's passion and its niche[14] can help in the expression of the dharma that arises from being clear and current, from understanding the "why" of the business. Once the organization's values are clearly identified, they can be used to tell the story of an organizational identity. They can also be used to measure success and even consulted to aid in decisions such as the hiring, promoting, or releasing of employees.

Succinct values statements allow organizational members to create sutra-like declarations that easily convey their dharma. This clarity is important for mission-based providers whether they have for-profit or non-profit structures because many similar services will likely be available to potential clients. Clearly stating the "why" of an organization and articulating what these values enable it to do aids in creating relationships with other providers, clients, potential employers, and collaborators.

Vision

Specific benchmarks with time-staggered goals characterize a strong vision. At the end of the day, many look back on their to-do lists and the course of their hours and see that their various choices have sent them in many—perhaps less than functional—directions. They may have mistaken individual tactics, which are part of any strategy, for the strategy itself, which is always guided by a sound plan.

Many thriving organizations develop a simple 10-year target statement that helps them identify a big-picture vision and the steps needed over those years to reach that point.[15] This target might take the form of a financial goal or number of clients served; the only real requirement is that the target be measurable. The organization then moves toward its big-picture goal by identifying and completing smaller, incremental plans. Those plans, too, are completed incrementally by committing to completing specific short-term (e.g., 90-day) tasks. These accomplishments provide day-to-day momentum to reach 1-, 3-, and ultimately 10-year targets.

Mission

A robust business plan should be as simple and straightforward as possible. When informed by such a plan, decisions and daily actions become natural outcomes of a mission-based mindset rather than resulting from indiscriminate attempts to just get things done. Perhaps counterintuitively, having a plan also allows for flexibility, particularly to quickly adjust to inevitable unexpected events. A plan that supports movement while creating a clear flow of action enables yoga therapists to accommodate both adversity and opportunity as they arise.

BOX 26.3 TANGIBLE BENEFITS OF CLEARLY ARTICULATED VALUES: TWO EXAMPLES

MOLLY MCMANUS

Yoga North International Soma Yoga Institute

The business I co-own had long wanted to establish a non-profit division to reach people who would not otherwise have access to yoga. We have done this on our own with scholarships, community outreach, donating services, hiring professionals to help with grant writing, and even getting a fiscal agent to allow us to take on funding. Each attempt met with little success and created minimal impact in our community while taxing our limited personal and professional resources.

Change came when a local organization whose main work is to bring integrative healthcare services to unserved communities in our city learned of our values and mission. A member of the organization approached us for partnership, and we were able to quickly create synergy to bring the visions of both organizations to fruition by combining our efforts.

A volunteer committee

During my tenure on the Accreditation Committee for the International Association of Yoga Therapists (IAYT), we also used simple planning tools[16] to help to unify and organize a group of diverse individuals from around the world, all volunteers for a time- and labor-intensive mission. We were responsible for ensuring that the professional standards established around yoga therapy were being followed and taught in yoga therapy certification programs worldwide.

Identifying and adhering to a structure allowed us to make cohesive decisions based on the values of the overarching mission of IAYT and on the true heart of each professional woman who had given of her time to support the development of the profession. Some of the best results from our work using this planning process were the core values the group articulated for guiding accreditation decisions:

- Committing to **trust** in the programs applying for accreditation and remembering an **environment of positive intent** helped us to stay connected to the fact that each program was presenting its best work with a commitment to the field of yoga therapy.
- **Respect and inclusivity** toward each member of the committee as well as each program director were important when decisions became difficult.
- We called on the **courage to lead and learn** often as we faced areas of our service as a committee that required change as a result of simple mistakes, progression of the field, or process overhauls for efficiency and effectiveness.

Our work with the values developed under this simple plan helped us to move step by step toward what is now a more robust and efficient team.

Business Strategy

As noted above, attending to daily business demands can result in frenetic activity with limited substantial progress. The guidance of a sound, values-based plan can help yoga therapists to wisely target their efforts for new projects.

When considering strategies for bridging personal strengths/skills and market needs to engender success in projects and partnerships, analysis models are helpful. Two instruments are often used: the SOAR model, which identifies strengths, opportunities, aspirations, and results; and SWOT analysis, which focuses on strengths, weaknesses, opportunities, and threats.

For yoga therapists, the SOAR analysis strategic planning tool can help to establish a particularly enlightening path to prosperity. With its proactive focus, SOAR analysis is useful for identifying and focusing on current strengths while visualizing longer-term strategic goals. The more restrictive SWOT analysis dwells on weaknesses that can sometimes be outside one's control; protecting against threats cannot change their presence, and expending vitality to address them can inhibit strengths and skills from growing and flowing energetically.

To understand the application of SOAR analysis, it is important to delve into the nuances of each part of the acronym (see Box 26.4):

- **strengths:** taking into account an individual's or organization's resources, their potential, and their considerable achievements, including what they easily do successfully
- **opportunities:** independent or organizational prospects that could develop into resources to meet client needs (i.e., reframing and shifting risks and vulnerability into potentiality)
- **aspirations:** what the individual or organization is capable of and what they strive to be acknowledged for
- **results:** measurable, tangible results that demonstrate the accomplishment of intentions and objectives

When partnering with other organizations, a professional approach that shows you are conversant not only with the culture of the organization but also with basic financial terminology and metrics inspires confidence. As discussed in Box 26.2, both individual clients and potential partner groups are likely to respond more positively when yoga therapists identify pain points and succinctly communicate how those problems will be addressed than when they simply present their qualifications.

BOX 26.4 KRAMA CONSIDERATIONS OF SOAR ANALYSIS FOR INDIVIDUAL/ORGANIZATIONAL PROJECTS: LEARNINGS FROM THE NON-PROFIT WORLD

MELINDA ATKINS

Building on the SOAR analysis, individuals or organizations can apply ten *kramas*, or steps, for maximum success. When contemplating a yoga therapy business idea or undertaking a project, completing each krama in turn allows for identification and bridging of personal strengths and market needs. Although the below discussion focuses on examples from the non-profit setting of my business AUM hOMe Shala, this framework can also be used by individual yoga therapists and for-profit entities; the carefully mapped principles described apply to sound decision-making in a range of situations.[17] As in any business venture, cultivating an understanding of the organizational and professional culture (e.g., a hospital's reporting structure, the language used by rehab facilities) is key to a successful outcome.

Krama one: Determine the cooperating partners of the project, who could be individuals, organizations, or both. If your partners are organizations, determine which team members from each organization will be responsible for making decisions and carrying out the terms of the partnership.

For instance, imagine a scenario in which a yoga therapy non-profit wants to launch a project to benefit those with neuromotor degenerative disorders in a predominantly Latinx Hispanic community whose members face healthcare barriers due to an inability to understand English. The yoga therapy non-profit can establish a partnership with a national organization, such as The Y or Easterseals, that has well-equipped facilities and high marketing visibility in a high-density Spanish-speaking area of the county. The yoga therapy non-profit can offer free or low-cost Spanish-language group classes for community members with neurodegenerative disorders, and, in return, the larger non-profit can allow the yoga therapy organization to use its facilities free of charge.

Facility directors tend to make good partners, as they are willing (and often enthusiastic) to work with other organizations that fit their mission without taxing their financial resources. To financially support the class series, the yoga therapy non-profit can identify and apply for grants, including in each application a letter from the non-profit facility host acknowledging the partnership. Grant committees have an affinity for non-profit partnerships, especially those between small and national organizational non-profits, which may increase the odds of successful grant funding.

This krama methodology is equally applicable for individuals. For instance, a yoga therapist wanting to bridge their personal strengths with needs they have identified in their community might identify a non-profit to work with and then apply for a grant as cooperating partners.

Krama two: Determine the format and regularity of partner meetings. You could choose to hold a single extensive meeting, like a workshop; a series of briefer, more specific meetings; a virtual meeting; or any combination of the above. Regardless of their format and schedule, meetings should incorporate all levels of the organization at the appropriate stages and representatives from all practical operations.

When coordinating among various levels of partners, it is helpful to lay out how and when each meeting will occur. For instance, the yoga therapy non-profit would ideally want to plan an initial face-to-face meeting with the facility director to pitch the idea for the partnership. This introductory meeting would enlist members from various levels of the facility's organization, resulting in innovation, inclusion, and the development of an effective plan. Such sessions help everyone involved to become vested in the intentions they will be holding in their work, from the early stages of the partnership to the end results.

Krama three: Establish survey questions or other instruments for collecting data about key partners' strengths, missions, and ambitions. Data is a tool to reveal whether a decision was beneficial, whether your goals were attained, and what adjustments are needed for progress. Partners can take that data into account to adapt strategic planning, meet individual needs, and support program growth.

In particular, improvement-based analyses allow for specific feedback from a large number of individuals. For instance, our yoga therapy non-profit was awarded funding to work with 8th-grade students in a Title 1 school to help improve study and focus skills prior to state-mandated testing. (Title 1 schools serve a high proportion of economically disadvantaged students.) As part of our data collection, students completed a lengthy survey about their study habits, work environment, test anxiety, and other topics pertinent to classroom success. Analyzing the responses enabled us to focus on specific areas of improvement that were relevant to the majority of the class. By taking the time to thoroughly evaluate the knowledge collected, we were able to implement the fundamental kramas to determine issues and identify and apply solutions.

Data-collection methods should be accessible to all partners. In the case of the 8th-graders, 92 percent were Hispanic, with English as their second language. Many struggled with speaking, reading, and writing in English, leading to anxiety and lower test scores. The survey was therefore presented in both English and Spanish to ensure that a language barrier would not impede successful data collection.

Krama four: Enlist partners' input and feedback to explore what worked. Partners could include teachers, trainers, staff, clients, case-study participants, colleagues, administrators, and staff from other organizations. Exploring what tactics and strategies generated the most success enables a focus on identifying strengths to build on rather than becoming bogged down by what went wrong. This approach also engages partners, builds team spirit, and gives everyone helpful encouragement.

A three-step postassessment process is often most beneficial when it asks partners, as a first step, something as simple as "What did you appreciate most about the protocol/class series/project/grant execution?" For example, in the case of a group protocol delivery, the facilitator asks the lead teacher what they appreciated most about delivering the protocol. The facilitator next listens without responding, then asks each participant what they most appreciated about the protocol; responses focus on appreciation and strengths rather than advice and recommendations. The final step involves the facilitator closing the process by sharing what *they* appreciated most about the delivery.

A yoga therapy testimonial instrument is another useful tool for identifying strengths. A one-page, five-question form with items on a five-point scale and a blank space for comments is quick and easy to complete. Student "partners" are encouraged to share a few sincere words at the end about what aspect of the class was most helpful for them. In the case of a grant-based series, these comments are passed on to the grantor by means of mid- and post-grant reports. The comments are also shared with the team of teachers and assistants, as well as the venue administrator and staff, who in turn pass the feedback on to their national organization if one is involved. Finally, testimonial comments can be shared on a program's website and through social media, as long as those completing the form provide permission for their words and initials to be shared online.

Krama five: Outline the individual's or organization's specific foundational mission, resources, strengths, and potential. Compose a list of unique qualifications, including an inventory of resources and strengths. Guided by the individual's or organization's overarching values, this practice stimulates the potential for future success and creates an opportunity to assimilate ideas and knowledge.

Krama six: Determine objectives and goals that build a vision of the future and influence the status quo. Identifying where one has excelled in the past helps when envisioning potential. By building on the foundation of past success, the entity can reach new levels and growth.

For instance, several years ago, I identified an organization that was offering several grants that I felt might be a good fit for our organization. I soon realized that time only allowed for us to focus on one of the grant options rather than spread ourselves thin by applying for all of them. Even if the applications had all been successful, our organization did not yet have the experience and resources to handle more than one grant at a time. With an eye to the future, however, we learned to manage one grant effectively. Two years later, another multi-grant opportunity arose, and we were able to draw on our past grant success to apply for and manage the new awards with confidence.

Krama seven: Concentrate on what is desired as opposed to what is undesired. Vulnerabilities or complications need not be seen as intimidating blockages, but rather opportunities for transformation. Furthermore, looking to other organizations' models and accomplishments can be both overwhelming and discouraging. Reform habits of comparison by shifting the focus to the similarities of strengths between entities rather than what might be missing or inadequate in yourself. Honest assessment is important, but bringing positive aspects to the forefront aids growth; what initially may have been missing or considered a weakness will be transformed through the collective energy of the relevant strengths.

Krama eight: Identify intentions and discover paths to get there. Building on the results from the previous krama, compose descriptive intentions for each potential growth area, then evaluate which path(s) will best support the organization's sustainability.

During this process, write several descriptive outcomes of what the manifested intention will look like in practice, and explore various pathways to achievement. For example, our organization created a grant-funded group class targeting increased neuroplasticity for seniors. In past years, we had offered grant-funded community classes for those with Alzheimer's disease, and we were interested in working with seniors who had not been diagnosed with Alzheimer's or dementia but who wanted to proactively increase neuroplasticity to stave off these conditions. The class series became popular, and a waitlist for the next series—for which we did not yet have funding—quickly formed via word of mouth.

Using a SOAR analysis, we identified a list of potential non-profit partners—ultimately settling on the Coral Gables Adult Center—and generated descriptive intentions to help us determine the best path toward expansion and sustainability. Additionally, we partnered with the Department of Communication Sciences & Disorders at Louisiana State University to create a study of the effectiveness of our class series. To secure additional funding after initial funding ran out, we considered capitalizing on our success by applying for an additional Alzheimer's grant to expand the model. This approach would enable marketing of the class as preventive for dementia and cognitive decline while leveraging Alzheimer's funding resources, allowing us to extend the class to those not affected by the disease.

Krama nine: Identify the target market and use the SOAR analysis model as a tool for success. By determining what events and practices hold the greatest potential for success, an individual or organization can effectively direct energy. Writing goal statements for each of these potentially successful aspects of a project and identifying strengths that will help measure the organization's results are especially beneficial practices.

For instance, our non-profit applied for a highly competitive Parkinson's Foundation grant in 2018. Until that point, we had conducted all of our classes for those with Parkinson's disease (PD) from a small yoga school situated on the perimeter of a walking community, where parking was sparse and expensive. PD clients would often have to park a block away and walk to the school or have caregivers drop them off. Rainy days presented particular problems. In the process of examining our list of goals for program expansion, we recognized that we needed to improve parking. In addition, although the space was adequate for the current clientele, a larger venue was needed to accommodate growth.

With these considerations in mind, we decided to partner with another non-profit community organization in our county with a brick-and-mortar facility that could serve as a sustainable venue for our projected growth. In researching which non-profit would meet the needs of our demographic, data analyses of county-wide statistics revealed where neurologists' offices that specialized in PD were clustered, as well as hospital and university facilities that cared for and studied neuromotor degenerative disorders, specifically PD. We also looked at demographic data, targeting the largest segment of an underserved PD population—primarily Miami-Dade County's 69.1 percent Hispanic/Latinx community. Drawing on these data, we identified areas of the county that would be best served by our PD program.

We next determined which local non-profit organizations had missions that aligned with our own. We also looked at their facilities: location; accessible parking; amenities such as gyms, pools, class space, and classrooms for lectures; and types and frequency of classes already offered. Ultimately, we identified the South Dade YMCA Family Center for its state-of-the-art facility and mission—"to provide programs that build healthy spirit, mind and body for all"—which deeply resonated with our own. Furthermore, the South Dade YMCA is located in a densely Hispanic/Latinx neighborhood a couple of miles from Miami-Dade County's largest hospital, with many neurologists' offices close by.

Using the SOAR analysis model, we felt confident that the YMCA would make an excellent partner in our goal of program expansion. After we reached out with the opportunity, the YMCA not only offered us free space for our classes, but also promoted the classes in their newsletter and monthly calendar and waived membership fees for PD clients and their caregivers. In return, we provided a quality program and promoted it by creating bridges with area neurologists and hospital support groups, as well as through the Parkinson's Foundation (another partner in this project). Some of the PD patients we reached through these channels had never visited the South Dade YMCA. Impressed with the facility and range of classes, many joined the YMCA, increasing the partnership's sustainability.

Krama ten: Formulate a plan of action for each intention. Once a target market has been identified and descriptive intentions for key contingencies established, it is time to put forth a realistic plan of action. To meet economic needs and ensure that a project is sustainable, adaptability is essential. A framework constructed on the stability of existing accomplishments yields better outcomes than concentrating efforts on trying to right shortcomings.

Following the easy-to-apply ten kramas of the SOAR analysis has enabled our small non-profit to create an inclusive team atmosphere and expand our reach through partnerships with like-minded, mission-driven non-profits. Employing SOAR analysis—with its focus on strengths, opportunities, aspirations, and results—can help organizations of all specialties and sizes build sustainability and discover the power of effective collaborations.

Summary

At this stage in the evolution of the field, yoga therapists—even those who are fully employed by other organizations—must adopt an entrepreneurial mindset. As it would an entrepreneur in any other setting, becoming accustomed to adaptation will serve the yoga therapist well. The structure of a plan, regardless of the exact form it takes or the tools used, supports flexibility and sustainability.

For example, many yoga therapists never considered offering their services remotely until the spring of 2020 when the COVID-19 pandemic began. Those with an existing values-based strategy were able to call on their previously defined strengths and interests to continue to connect with clients virtually, sustaining themselves even amid rapidly shifting external circumstances. Flexibility need not impede progress toward significant or long-range goals.

Similarly, the professionalism inherent in a successful entrepreneurial mindset will serve yoga therapists as they navigate inevitable unexpected events. To continue the pandemic example, those who were able to identify and connect with legitimate information sources (e.g., the US Centers for Disease Control and Prevention, local health departments) likely found a smoother path forward when faced with questions about cleaning protocols and reopening guidelines than those who relied on word of mouth or secondary sources.

Yoga therapy is an extraordinary calling, but it is not exempt from the regulatory and market forces that shape other professions. Authentic reflection on dharma and values is a useful way of determining one's ideal client(s). Identifying and leveraging strengths and unique gifts, deliberate planning and strategizing, assiduously following through, and regularly assessing outcomes will set yoga therapy businesses apart.

Additional Resources

Betenson, T. (n.d.). The key elements of the financial plan. http://articles.bplans.com/the-key-elements-of-the-financial-plan

Godin, S. (2018). *This is marketing: You can't be seen until you learn to see*. Portfolio.

Johnson, M. C. (n.d.). Put your yoga in action to create a just world: A training on equity and justice in the yoga studio and beyond. https://yogainternational.com/ecourse/put-your-yoga-in-action-to-create-a-just-world

Kissiah, G. (2013). *Light on law for yoga studios: A guide to legal wellness* (2nd ed.). Independently published.

Kupperman, L. (2017). What we talk about when we talk about money. *Yoga Therapy Today*, Summer, 36–37, 56.

Kupperman, L. (2018). Key distinctions to help you grow your business. *Yoga Therapy Today*, Spring, 22–23.

Rockport Institute. (n.d.). How to write a masterpiece of a resume. https://rockportinstitute.com/resources/how-to-write-a-masterpiece-of-a-resume

Stavros, J., & Cole, M. L. (2013). SOARing towards positive transformation and change. *Development Policy Review, 1*, 10–34.

Stavros, J., & Hinrichs, G. (2009). *Thin book of SOAR: Building strengths-based strategy* (2nd ed.). Thin Book Publishing Co.

Taylor, M., & Oppenheim, J. (2020). *Sales as serving others: Ethical sales skills for the yoga professional.* Blurb Books.

US Small Business Administration. (n.d.). 10 steps to start your business. Available at www.sba.gov/content/follow-these-steps-starting-business

Wickman, G. (2012). *Traction: Get a grip on your business.* BenBella Books.

Endnotes

1 Butera, R. (2010). *The pure heart of yoga: Ten essential steps for personal transformation* (p. 40). Llwellyn.

2 O'Brian, E. G. (2018). *The jewel of abundance: Finding prosperity through the ancient wisdom of yoga* (p. xiv). New World Library.

3 *The Mahabharata*, quoted in O'Brian, *Jewel of abundance* (p. 11).

4 O'Brian, *Jewel of abundance* (p. 3).

5 O'Brian, *Jewel of abundance* (p. 3).

6 O'Brian, *Jewel of abundance* (p. 3).

7 Lamott, A. (1995). *Bird by bird: Some instructions on writing and life* (p. 218). Anchor.

8 Kupperman, L. Personal communication, March 17, 2020.

9 Kupperman, L. Personal communication, March 17, 2020.

10 Kupperman, L. Personal communication, March 17, 2020.

11 Fishman, L. Personal communication, Feb. 4, 2020.

12 Kupperman, L. Personal communication, March 17, 2020.

13 When making decisions about business structure, consulting with a tax and/or legal professional is recommended. The most common entities in the United States are sole proprietorships, partnerships, limited liability companies, and corporations. For basic distinctions among these business types, see US Internal Revenue Service. (2020, July 31). Business structures. www.irs.gov/businesses/small-businesses-self-employed/business-structures. For basic information on non-profit and traditional business structures, see Heaslip, E. (2020, March 30). Non-profit vs. not-for-profit vs. for-profit: What's the difference? CO (US Chamber of Commerce). www.uschamber.com/co/start/strategy/non-profit-vs-not-for-profit-vs-for-profit

14 Wickman, G. (2012). *Traction: Get a grip on your business.* BenBella Books.

15 Wickman, *Traction.*

16 Wickman, *Traction.*

17 When applying the ten kramas to for-profit businesses, a partnership between a for-profit and a non-profit (e.g., a community foundation) would typically be involved; the for-profit would write the grant under the non-profit's umbrella. Although not all grant opportunities require applicants to be non-profit entities, teaming with non-profits seeking to expand their course offerings can provide rewarding partnerships for for-profit partners. For transparency, it is advisable to determine the logistics and responsibilities of grant reporting prior to applying for the grant. In addition, the non-profit will receive the funding for a successful grant and will be responsible for directing resources to the proposed project, so it is important for the for-profit to clearly understand how funds will be disbursed.

Throughout the SOAR analysis, it is key for the for-profit to prioritize promoting and uplifting the mission of the non-profit. A successful grant written through a for-profit/non-profit partnership is less about the benefit to the for-profit and more about the realization of the non-profit's mission—a goal for which the for-profit serves as a vehicle.

27

Systems Health: Yoga Therapy Beyond the Studio

In a world more connected than ever yet paradoxically isolating, yoga therapists are increasingly setting out to broaden the scope of the transformations made possible through their practices. Many have found ways to begin to address social justice concerns, including iniquities rooted in superficial differences—societal *samskara* that oppress some groups while elevating others.

As a public health intervention, yoga has tools to address these forms of suffering; yoga therapy has the potential to effect not only individual transformation but also large-scale population-based healing. However, the liberation, *moksha*, promised by yoga requires change. Systems that remain rooted in old patterns of relating to the world make transformation impossible.

This chapter explores how visionary yoga therapists are reaching diverse populations to reimagine flawed systems. Both personal and practical lessons they have learned in the course of their work are shared here.

A Salutogenic Approach to Chronic Illness and Dis-Ease

In the United States, six in ten adults now have a chronic illness; four in ten have two or more such conditions, including cancer, heart disease, stroke, chronic lung disease, diabetes, and chronic kidney disease.

Conventional Western medical approaches use the paradigm of health versus disease: When a system breaks down (disease), it must be fixed to return to its original state (health). This pathogenic approach is highly effective for treating acute conditions, but less so for those living with chronic disease. The salutogenic paradigm of yoga therapy seeks to ease suffering and create possibilities that allow people to uncover their inherent wellness and to navigate their embodied experience with equanimity regardless of health condition.

Lifestyle choices that exacerbate chronic conditions include tobacco use, poor nutrition, and excessive alcohol or drug use. With the exception of poor nutrition, which could be socioeconomically driven, the remaining factors are forms of self-medication that alter the individual's state and provide a means of relieving stress. Even a carbohydrate-rich meal can achieve this goal temporarily.

This raises the question of what causes these levels of stress: primarily *avidya*, separation of self from source. When a society becomes stratified, the "haves" possess thousands of times more than the "have-nots" and few or no social supports exist for the bulk of the population. Distress is followed by disease (and dis-ease) and the sort of public health crises the global population is experiencing today.

People separated from source feel that they must be the hero of their drama (*asmita*) and begin to set up parameters for what is desirable and undesirable (*raga/dvesha*). This misperception leads to glorification of the body (physical *asana* classes included), as one discards the belief that anything beyond the body is real (*abhinivesha*). At its best, yoga therapy offers individuals whole-person interventions that allow each to return to their optimum, connected state and to advocate for themselves in a world that often lacks interest in diverse voices.

As yoga therapy students find their way into practice, these stories can guide them to consider ways in which implicit bias may influence their work and provide a means for self-reflection and course correction. This may include consideration of new populations and work venues.

Disaster Recovery and PTSD in the Field

Keishin Kimura • Japan Yoga Therapy Society
(translated by Madoka Chase Onizuka)

Because of yoga's ability to help people cultivate self-regulation and resilience, therapeutic asana and pranayama are effective ways to support disaster victims and those dealing with addictions, trauma, or posttraumatic stress disorder (PTSD). At the Japan Yoga Therapy Society (JYTS), we have successfully offered yoga therapy to survivors of child abuse, natural disasters such as earthquakes and tsunami, and nuclear accidents.

Many people suffering from addictions have trauma from childhood abuse. In Japan, people with drug or alcohol addictions sometimes enter private medical facilities or support groups after serving prison sentences. JYTS negotiates with these facilities, explaining the effectiveness of yoga therapy, and then arranges yoga therapy instruction there. Medical facilities provide remuneration for instructors, but those in private support groups are volunteers. In cases where instructors are not paid by the support group, JYTS covers their transportation from home and provides an allowance for post-practice snacks, an activity we've found effective for relationship building.

Our yoga therapists have also gone into areas where there have been earthquakes, tsunami, floods, and landslides—a need that will increase as a result of climate change. With the permission of the local authorities managing evacuation centers, we have provided yoga therapy to victims still living there. Even in the immediate aftermath of emergency, we've seen anxiety and the resulting increases in blood pressure alleviated.

When considering offering instruction at an evacuation center, a representative JYTS member first evaluates the site. Yoga therapists who live close to the affected areas also contact each other to coordinate work at the centers. Yoga therapists familiar with the conditions in the disaster-affected areas—some survivors themselves—create an environment conducive to yoga therapy, arranging venue and times, notifying potential participants, and so on, and making sure that yoga therapy instruction can begin as soon as others arrive on site.

Symptoms of trauma may arise from the psychological shock of large-scale disasters, so we prioritize bringing attention to the shifts between tension and relaxation in the physical body, enabling people to reconnect with themselves. Sometimes disaster victims become afraid of moving or feel helpless and just sit in evacuation centers. If the sedentary behavior continues, deep vein thrombosis and consequent pulmonary embolism are a danger, so the work sometimes includes large, whole-body movements. When things have settled down, generally after a few months, JYTS yoga therapists conduct "yoga therapy darshana"—non-directive psychological counseling that employs yogic psychology, primarily from the Upanishads, *Yoga Sutras*, and *Bhagavad Gita*. This ultimately enables victims to recount their experiences with a new, healthy interpretation and thus facilitates posttraumatic growth. We have also found consistent yoga therapy of this type to be effective for processing PTSD. In some cases, people have continued monthly yoga therapy for 10 years.

If yoga therapists working in disaster areas have not processed their own various types of grief, they might find themselves caught up in their own past traumatic experiences. We ensure that the leaders of the regional associations that support JYTS carefully select the yoga therapists to provide support in disaster-affected areas.

In Japan, we experienced wanton destruction and exposure to radiation after the World War II Hiroshima and Nagasaki bombings, so it was not difficult for us to understand the mental and emotional conditions of victims of the 1986 Chernobyl nuclear disaster. I met a doctor from nearby Kiev during his visit to Japan in 2008, and with his introduction visited an organization supporting Chernobyl victims. JYTS began providing yoga therapy in Kiev in 2009.

As in Hiroshima and Nagasaki, researchers in Kiev were only collecting basic data on the amount of radiation exposure, cancer rates, and other health problems. No one was investigating ways to restore the health of those exposed to radiation, so I was not surprised when the welcome on our first visit to Kiev was not very warm. We began by teaching simple yoga therapy exercises the Chernobyl victims could do at home. Those who continued the practices saw their health improve. In particular, cardiovascular patients noticed a dramatic reduction in the number of times they had to call an ambulance at night and a decrease in the amount of medication they needed for high blood pressure.

Each year, we taught yoga therapy for a week in Kiev, and the attitude of our host organization's leader softened every time. The third year, having established more trust, two Japanese doctors who accompanied us compiled data over two visits with yoga therapy participants. The data showed physiological changes, including a decline in levels of reactive oxygen species, over the 6 months between visits. These positive outcomes further softened the attitude of the organization head.

Beginning in about 2015, we began training victims and their supporters to offer basic yoga therapy instruction themselves. The course fees paid by Ukrainian participants go to the Chernobyl victim support group in Kiev, where graduates can teach therapeutic yoga. In 2019, JYTS also began budgeting around US$10,000 (1 million yen) annually to support local therapeutic yoga teachers educated directly by us: When they teach at various facilities, JYTS pays them $5 per lesson. The yoga teachers might instruct 10 to 20 classes a month, and we hope that in the Ukraine, where wages are low, our assistance can help their livelihood while promoting more awareness of the benefits of yoga therapy. We also hope that Ukrainian yoga teachers will participate in our longer training courses and continue to learn more about the theory and practice of yoga therapy.

It is possible to contribute to society with yoga therapy in many other areas, such as prisons, juvenile correctional facilities, and domestic violence shelters. Our experiences in these settings indicate that continued yoga therapy practice can help victims of both personal and societal disasters evolve into posttraumatic growth.

Underserved Senior Populations

Jana Long, C-IAYT, E-RYT 500 • Private practice

I work primarily with adults 60 years and older, offering practices in the therapeutic application of yoga for acute and chronic disease management. I also create and facilitate trainings in contemplative and restorative yoga practices for individuals living in dysfunctional environments caused by myriad forms of violence and historical and/or complex trauma.

The primary yogic tools I use are rooted in five of Patanjali's eight-limbed system: niyama, asana, pranayama, pratyahara, and dharana. I deliver these in group lectures, experiential workshops, sharing circles, and through a variety of therapeutic and restorative Hatha Yoga practices in community and private settings.

As with many populations, I've found that the key barriers preventing these seniors from accessing yoga are location, cost, and fear, or lack of knowledge about the practice. To overcome these barriers, we must first clearly define the yogic practices. How narrowly or expansively is yoga defined? Next, to effectively engage individuals with the practices, we need to know whether *they* desire them so as not to impose, or assume that everyone wants yoga. This population-wide promise creates an opportunity to forge energetic connections around a common activity from which people can build—or rebuild—and strengthen a sense of both self and union within community.

The value or gain from this work is first for the individual, and to the extent that individuals create the experience of society, I cannot yet foresee what society as a whole will gain. Although I don't expect yoga to change the world, more people than ever are now practicing yoga and our society is undergoing an awakening; what we create from this awakening remains to be seen.

My own efforts are threefold: (1) educating older adults about yoga, ayurveda, and gardening as part of their managed self-care; (2) providing yoga teacher training for more older adults who can in turn offer yoga to their peers; and (3) supporting the educational and professional development of Black yoga teachers taking yoga into communities where yoga has previously been inaccessible. Capacity building requires the development of alliances and partnerships with individuals and organizations whose missions align with my work. Scaling up this work also means raising funds for educational scholarships, program development and implementation, event coordination, and administrative support.

Incorporating Yoga into Healthcare Provider Education

Laura Schmalzl, PhD, RYT-500* • *Formerly co-editor-in-chief,* International Journal of Yoga Therapy; *research scientist, University of California Santa Diego; associate professor, Southern California University of Health Sciences

As an associate professor at Southern California University of Health Sciences (SCUHS), I had the opportunity to implement yoga as an educational tool in the core curricula of graduate programs of chiropractors, acupuncturists, and physician assistants. One of the core principles of SCUHS is interprofessional education: Students of all programs take foundational science and clinical reasoning classes together, which allows them to learn directly about other disciplines. This kind of education also fosters openness to the integration of complementary modalities into healthcare.

I chose to make yoga a primary component of my weekly 2-hour neuroscience lab. Every week, the first hour consisted of a yoga class that included posture sequences, breath regulation, and cultivation of focus. During the second hour, we delved into the neurophysiological mechanisms underlying the movement, respiration, and attention they'd experienced, as well as the self-regulatory potential of yoga practice as a whole. In the process of giving the students a platform for experiential learning, I was able to enhance their own wellness and stress resilience while expanding the complementary therapeutic approaches they would have available for their future patients.

Assuming that school administrators understand the value of mind-body tools, the main barriers to accessing yoga outside the academic schedule are time and finances. Integrating classes into the core curriculum without adding time or cost—for students or universities—is key.

Western medical education approaches often heavily focus on factual knowledge about disease and treatment while overlooking training in the self-regulatory skills necessary for providers themselves to maintain health and well-being while working in complex, taxing environments. Implementing educational programs that address clinician burnout, foster professional resilience and well-being, and assist in individual flourishing benefit not only students but also, most importantly, their future patients. If more institutions take steps toward these goals, there is a potential for large-scale improvement of our healthcare systems.

Implementing a program such as this requires few material resources aside from qualified instructors—literally just a classroom with movable tables and yoga mats. I believe that what made the SCUHS program work especially well is that it was taught by a core faculty member, not an instructor brought on solely for the purpose of adding yoga or meditation to the schedule. This setup facilitated the experience of yoga practice as an integrated part of the curriculum and student life rather than an add-on. The same kind of program could be implemented in the context of other classes, such as anatomy or psychology. Offering yoga and meditation training programs to educators, so that they can in turn implement these practices in their teaching, would be a great investment in societal health and well-being.

Serving Incarcerated Individuals

Reverend Lakshmi Barsel, PhD • Satchidananda Prison Project

The Satchidananda Prison Project serves incarcerated individuals throughout the United States by supporting their religious and spiritual needs. Most of the people who contact us have written us directly and are sincerely seeking to change their lives. Usually, they are interested in yoga and Eastern religions. A few who are already familiar with yoga are looking to improve their health and reduce the anxiety and stress they experience living in a prison atmosphere.

Since 2007, our primary service has been answering these letters by addressing their spiritual questions and sending books and other printed information on yoga, Eastern religions, and meditation. Over the years, we have developed two free correspondence courses, one on the *Yoga Sutras of Patanjali* and the other on the *Bhagavad Gita*. We also offer free malas (Eastern prayer beads) to individuals and groups and have been able to provide reading and audiovisual materials and yoga mats to Eastern religion, yoga, and meditation groups.

In sending out these materials, and also in setting up classes in prison, our biggest challenge is understanding the rules and regulations of each prison and how to work with the different departments and personalities within the state and federal systems.

Probably the single greatest benefit that those who write us receive is the kindness of having someone respond to their letters and offer them some assistance. They also receive the universal teachings of yoga philosophy, which give them hope along with simple and profound guidance on how to live an easeful, peaceful, and useful life; rise above fear, anger, and depression; and live harmoniously with others. If they practice the yoga asana, they almost always experience a reduction in stress, balancing of the emotions, opening of the heart, and improvement in overall health. We have also found Hatha Yoga, pranayama, and meditation to be instrumental in overcoming the addictions that afflict so many in prison settings.

In our experience, those who practice yoga while incarcerated are known for becoming model prisoners. All of the yogic tools create happier, healthier, and more integrated individuals who, when released, are in a much better position to succeed out in the world and serve the communities to which they return.

Urban Adolescents

Tawanna J. A. Kane, RYT-500 • Inner Resources Project

I am committed to working with underserved populations, to expose them to yoga and mindfulness and offer tools that might assist in living with greater ease. More than 60 percent of my work is with urban adolescent populations.

From my own cultivation of presence and commitment to practice, I am able to be with them authentically. My primary goal is to "see" these students—and to let them know that someone truly hears them. Even when I train other teachers to share these tools, we spend more time with embodiment than anything else.

I am also willing to express my own vulnerability by appropriately sharing why I am committed to this path. Once we build trust through connection, I offer students yogic tools in a way that is culturally relevant and directly applicable. I bring in scenarios with which they are familiar, and I reference famous people they respect who also use these practices. I draw in music, poetry, storytelling, and mindfulness activities to demonstrate how they can practice in their everyday lives.

The barriers to urban youth accessing yoga are both self-imposed and societal. Yoga classes or retreats are cost-prohibitive to many. Even when they do gain access, the spaces are often not diverse; it is difficult to feel at home in even the most welcoming community when you don't see yourself reflected there.

Many still negatively associate yoga with religion. Recently, when I tried to recruit a group of West African immigrant women for a mindfulness study, more than half refused to participate in the meditations, believing that an idle mind makes space for the devil. Instead of trying to eradicate this belief, I worked with it. We talked about how the mind is actually not idle in meditation or yoga, that we're acutely focusing attention on our breath, our bodies, or our responses to the practices. Offering this framework helps to slowly invite exploration. The practices then usually speak for themselves.

I believe that yoga and meditation allow young people to connect with their own humanity and awaken consciousness to the human condition. This increased awareness stands to decrease the potential harm they might do to themselves and others. Furthermore, the class sangha is often these students' first taste of intimacy within a community; they begin to see themselves in one another.

I have been part of more than a dozen randomized controlled trials demonstrating the efficacy of mindfulness with underserved adolescent populations, from those who are HIV-infected to those with severe depression or living in declining neighborhoods. Every study has found meaningful shifts over 12 weeks. However, when the intervention ends, the students are left with a lack of resources. Funding to continue long-term exposure to the practices would benefit not only the adolescents but also their communities.

Researching Yoga

Crystal L. Park, PhD • Professor, Department of Psychological Sciences, University of Connecticut

As a researcher, I study many aspects of yoga, including yoga interventions—primarily pranayama and asana for back pain patients and college students with alcohol problems—in small-group settings.

In research settings, we often don't face the barriers to accessing yoga seen in the real world—expense, inconvenient class times, transportation, and so on. Clinical trials come with their own obstacles, though, such as obtaining funding for studies (even the smallest randomized controlled trial can cost hundreds of thousands of dollars to implement), recruiting sufficient numbers of study participants, maintaining consistency in how the practices are instructed, keeping participants in the study, and many more.

If we can continue to build the evidence base for yoga, individuals stand to experience pain relief, and then, ideally, emotional regulation, well-being, and some spiritual peace. Society as a whole stands to benefit from more productive citizens, decreased opioid use, and, again, more peace.

In the United States, a major funder of non-pharmaceutical research is the National Institutes of Health (NIH). Although the National Center for Complementary and Integrative Health is the NIH center charged specifically with supporting investigation of mind-body practices, therapeutic yoga is also relevant to the missions of other agencies such as the National Cancer Institute and the National Institute of Mental Health.

My own work involves conducting trials but also survey research and other types of studies. Much of this work requires external funding support, which means writing grant applications that are as strong as we can make them. Funding is very competitive, and often our proposals fail to get support. This means we either drop that particular line of work or revise the funding proposal and try again. In implementing the research, I supervise a team. Together, we carry out all the steps in research, from conceptualizing the study and refining the ideas to collecting and analyzing the data and writing manuscripts for publication.

To me, the big question is who will fund yoga classes in the community to make the practices accessible while still paying a living wage for therapeutic yoga teachers. My hope is that eventually the scientific base of evidence will be strong enough that insurance companies, healthcare agencies, and the government will be willing to pay for yoga as therapy.

Wide Reach Through a Non-Profit

Jivana Heyman, C-IAYT, E-RYT 500 • Accessible Yoga

My work with Accessible Yoga, the non-profit organization I founded and now direct, is about reaching a broad population—basically anyone who thinks yoga isn't for them. Yoga studios tend to be exclusive environments that aren't welcoming to people who have disabilities, larger bodies, older people, or people who are not physically active. I'm interested in making the practices and teachings of yoga work for those who aren't comfortable going to a studio or attending a regular class.

My work focuses on education, advocacy, and community building. In terms of education, I'm interested in supporting yoga teachers and yoga therapists in expanding their skills and understanding of how to make yoga applicable and accessible to a wider audience. I lead trainings, speak, and write about the myriad creative ways yoga practices can be adapted and shared.

The primary goal of yoga educators is to keep students safe and to offer them effective practices, so we have to begin by examining the content we're sharing as well as the structure we're using to do so. This means reflecting on how we are teaching as well as what we teach.

Asana is by nature practical and accessible, but we've created a false hierarchy of "advanced" poses within asana practice. This misrepresents yoga's underlying philosophy of cultivating peace of mind.

Another obstacle to wide adoption of yogic practice is the power dynamic within yoga communities. If we examine the teacher/student relationship, for example, we find a dangerous opportunity for disempowerment and even abuse. The ultimate goal of the teacher or therapist should be to lift up the student and even have them surpass the teacher.

If the larger population could be exposed to the truth of yoga—rather than a watered-down, appropriated version—the societal impact would be tremendously beneficial. I believe improved training for yoga teachers and therapists in areas that have previously been ignored—among them accessibility, cultural appropriation, racism, and consent—would be the best way to appropriately serve a larger audience.

Addressing the issues that either keep people away from yoga or cause injury within yoga spaces would help us to scale up this work. Further dialog within the yoga community is essential to create a shared understanding of the importance of these topics and how they affect our work. These are difficult conversations to have, and it will take effective leadership to move us forward. In the end, each of us needs to examine our own prejudices and our own privilege to understand how we can best serve in the world.

Yoga in National Health Systems

Göran Boll • Swedish healthcare

I work as a yoga therapist with all categories of patients within the Swedish healthcare system—in primary care, cardiac health, pain management, psychiatry, rehabilitation, oncology, palliative care, and so on.

Since 1998, three Swedish researchers have received their PhDs testing my yoga programs in more than a dozen studies at some of Sweden's most prestigious research institutions. For example, I helped the Karolinska Institute (KI) conduct the first study on yoga in Sweden, on unspecified spine problems.[1]

Through the MediYoga Institute, the organization I founded, my strategy since 2006 has been to attract medical personnel with experience of doing yoga, educating them to become yoga instructors and therapists. These people are already trained health professionals, already "inside" the health system with access to patients. In combination with my available research and a lot of positive public media coverage—TV, radio, newspapers, magazines, and social media—this approach created a synergistic effect that broke down barriers. Just 3 years after the first instructor training, Danderyd Hospital in Stockholm started using my programs as a regular rehab method for heart-attack patients.

If programs like this are broadly adopted, people stand to gain easily accessible tools that promote self-efficacy and self-healing. Patients with atrial fibrillation have told me they can stop the symptoms themselves through pranayama, avoiding the need to visit the hospital. In one of its studies, KI said that it would be very cost-efficient for society as a whole if more spine patients could be taught to use yoga for pain management.

I have managed to scale up my programs with limited resources by taking advantage of a wonderful snowball effect, so I feel that this approach is possible in many other settings around the world. I started training trainers in 2008; they in turn led trainings all over the country, and the first group of six students in 2007 has now grown to some 3,000 certified instructors and therapists in Sweden. In 2010, one unit in the healthcare system was "yogic"; 6 years later we had 150 yoga-integrated units, and by the end of 2020 the figure was nearly 300, representing approximately 20 percent of all of the Swedish health service's medical units.

Survivors of Severe Abuse

Erin Byron, MA, RP, C-IAYT, E-RYT 500 • Private practice in mental health

In its quest for the true Self, yoga philosophy provides the key foundation for my therapeutic work. The *Yoga Sutras* clearly define yoga as a union with the ultimate truth of a person. Conversely, trauma isolates us from a sense of self and hinders our ability to connect with others. Helping clients to develop curiosity around questions of "who am I really?" therefore directs the actionable course of our work together. Session by session, week by week, people take steps to reclaim a connection to Self and to build a life of authenticity, peace, and even joy.

Breathing and somatic practices such as asana and relaxation are key in reprogramming the chronically aroused autonomic nervous system and promoting the neuroplastic changes required to alleviate (post)traumatic symptoms. Concentration practices that promote uplifted, equanimous thinking help mitigate the negativity that alters mood and belief in those who have lived through trauma.

Understandably, people who have been traumatized may have a difficult time trusting others. There may be resistance to trying new techniques, especially because practices that ultimately support trauma recovery are triggering at first. For example, grounding exercises eventually cultivate a sense of presence and safety. Initially, however, becoming present to our thoughts, feelings, and physical self connects us to the reality of current emotional and physical discomfort due to trauma. Furthermore, the anxiety associated with posttraumatic stress can make reaching out for help or leaving the house to attend sessions and classes very frightening.

Yogic practices and philosophy have been shown to reduce and even end PTSD symptomatology. The practices also have ripple effects: The less we are dealing with active trauma, the less likely we are to wound or traumatize others. Transcending the experience of trauma also leaves us with greater capacity for compassion and tolerance, which in turn affects the way we treat others on a day-to-day basis. As we become less reactive and better able to recognize our own agency, we are driven to take action to shift society in the direction of equality and true justice.

More highly targeted inpatient and outpatient programs would systematize the delivery of these effective trauma-recovery methods. Ensuring specialized training for yoga therapists, counselors, psychiatrists, and general practitioners would limit misdiagnoses and ineffective or counterproductive treatment while enabling providers to offer useful fundamental tools of trauma recovery, such as conscious breathing and mindful attention. It is also important for yoga therapists to find effective ways of sharing the benefits of practices with survivors and providers, and methods of recruiting participants in a context of hope and safety.

Yoga Therapy in Australia

Leigh Blashki, C-IAYT • Australian Institute of Yoga Therapy

Although it is difficult to determine when yoga therapy was first formally offered in Australia, it is fair to say that it took root following the founding of the Australian Institute of Yoga Therapy in 1991. By 2006, when the Australasian Association of Yoga Therapists was formed, along with the first set of competency standards for yoga therapists anywhere in the world, the profession was well-established. These standards became the point of reference for the development of IAYT's Educational Standards.

The profession of yoga therapy in Australia has retained its close links to the profession of yoga teaching, generally resisting the pull to become more closely allied to the mainstream healthcare system as has occurred in other parts of the world.

To inform this report, I informally surveyed 100 Australian yoga therapists in 2019. The practice of yoga therapy typically accounts for approximately 40 percent of their working hours; 65 percent practice from their home, 52 percent from their or another person's yoga studio, 10 percent in the client's home, and 9 percent in a healthcare setting. Twenty-four percent reported having a qualification in another well-being or health modality, most commonly massage.

In our country, the majority of yoga therapy is provided one-to-one; group yoga therapy sessions are uncommon. The most common presentations yoga therapists work with include chronic pain, back care, sleep disturbances, fatigue and fibromyalgia, anxiety and depression, cancer of various types and stages, and hypertension.

Despite the small percentage of yoga therapy delivery in clinic settings, licensed healthcare providers do regularly recommend yoga as a therapy to their patients. Furthermore, as integrative health finds its way into more hospitals, yoga therapy is being included in the programs on offer. Two examples are the Olivia Newton-

John Cancer Wellness & Research Centre at Austin Hospital in Melbourne and Sydney Children's Hospital, Randwick.

In recent years, there has also been growing interest in yoga and yoga therapy for mental health. A number of short courses are now available to train yoga therapists to better understand mental health. Some of these courses include a broad perspective on mental health generally, whereas others focus on depression and anxiety.

Yoga therapists are well-supported by two associations in Australia. Yoga Australia, an umbrella organization for all yoga professionals, provides an internationally respected registration, online visibility, and regular professional development and community networking opportunities. The Australasian Association of Yoga Therapists is smaller and dedicated entirely to yoga therapy and supporting practitioners. Both organizations continue to work toward educating the public about yoga therapy, in particular developing targeted education and promotion of yoga therapy for the healthcare sector.

Chronic Fatigue Syndrome and Fibromyalgia

Takakazu Oka, MD, PhD • Outpatient and hospital settings

I am a specialist in psychosomatic medicine, exclusively seeing patients with stress-related diseases. My practice includes many people with myalgic encephalomyelitis/chronic fatigue syndrome (ME/CFS) and fibromyalgia (FM) because, in some patients, stress exacerbates their symptoms and appropriate coping strategies improve outcomes.

To treat these diseases, comprehensive and integrative interventions are necessary. One such option is yoga. In collaboration with the Japan Yoga Therapy Society, I developed isometric yoga programs for patients with ME/CFS and FM, taking into consideration the pathophysiological characteristics of these diseases and patients' limitations, which can be severe.

In my outpatient clinic, patients receive instruction on self-help strategies, pharmacotherapy, and psychotherapy, if necessary. In cases where sufficient improvement is not achieved, we introduce yoga if the patient's illness and motivation make it an appropriate choice. When they visit the hospital (usually once per month), patients practice isometric yoga (for 20–30 minutes) with a yoga therapist one-to-one. They also practice at home with the guidance of booklets and online videos (e.g., www.youtube.com/watch?v=tuQngCHfrvk&t=945s). The program instructor is an experienced yoga therapist who has knowledge of their conditions.

Several barriers may prevent these patients from accessing yoga. First, most doctors do not fully understand what yoga is and how therapeutic yoga works for patients with ME/CFS or FM. Second, the number of yoga instructors with knowledge of these specific diseases and sufficient patient experience is quite limited. Third, in Japan, as elsewhere, yoga therapy is not a licensed profession and yoga is not covered by health insurance. These factors also hinder the establishment of critically important therapeutic relationships among doctors, patients, and yoga therapists. If these difficulties can be overcome, yoga may become more widely accepted as an efficient self-help tool for coping with ME/CFS or FM.

At many Japanese hospitals, yoga therapists teach yoga as volunteers; in my case, a research grant provides funding. When teaching in hospitals, yoga therapists must have disease-specific knowledge to prevent adverse events. I have conducted workshops to help provide this education, but more workshops, held more regularly, are necessary to enable the efficient and safe provision of what we refer to as "remedial yoga." Additional well-designed clinical trials and basic research are also needed. To conduct these studies, support from research grants or other means will be crucial.

Women's Well-Being

Uma Dinsmore-Tuli, PhD, C-IAYT • Total Yoga Nidra and Santosa Living Yoga and Bhakti Camp

Since 1998, I have been supporting women's well-being through individual and group yoga therapy in women's circles and other venues. My practice is rooted in respect for Shakti manifesting in cyclical rhythms and integrates menstruality consciousness with yoga therapy in seasonal and social contexts. This nurturing approach to yoga therapy uses intuitive methods of inquiry to empower women's health throughout their lives.

The efficacy of yoga nidra as yoga therapy for women's health issues primarily resides in its capacity to empower women to welcome all that arises, to dignify the integrity of these experiences as powerful siddhis signaling the potential for spiritual initiations into power, and to regulate their nervous systems, thereby opening space to rest in every bodily system and dimension of being. I can testify personally to this practice as an effective means to manage the pain of uterine contractions during three vaginal homebirths, two miscarriages, and 20 years of monthly menstruations.

I am determined to share yoga nidra's benefits as widely as possible, beyond the confines possible in my own teaching and private practice. One of the venues where I offer the postlineage style of Total Yoga Nidra is the Santosa Camp I have run at least annually in the British countryside since 2005. Begun as a peaceful, supportive place for yogis of all ages to practice all kinds of yoga, the gathering offers yoga nidra sessions several times each day, alongside Acro Yoga, Kundalini Yoga, Yin Yoga, and many others. Another way I expand the reach of the practices is by sharing, through the Total Yoga Nidra Network, free recordings in a variety of languages from teachers who have studied with us.

During the first 2 months of the COVID-19 pandemic in spring 2020, each day I shared 30 minutes of co-creative Total Yoga Nidra live online. (I also continued to practice twice daily myself.) The overwhelmingly grateful response from the thousands of people who listened in to practice together in our virtual circles of belonging was deeply moving, confirming for me that yoga nidra is a potent mode of healing. The practices we co-created during that time offered opportunities to pause, rest, and integrate the unimaginable truth of all that was happening and to welcome feelings of grief, anger, frustration, fear, and, for many, deep relief that the relentless busyness of their lives had been stopped overnight.

Terminal Illness

Lucia Plata, C-IAYT • Private practice in palliative care

Many years ago, I decided to help and accompany clients with terminal diseases such as cancer and amyotrophic lateral sclerosis. Yoga therapy gives me the chance to offer these clients self-agency from the moment of diagnosis on, alleviating symptoms of both the disease and treatments.

Although this meaningful work is of great help, I had the feeling that something was missing. Hospitals frequently send these patients home when no further clinical procedure is available, telling them "nothing else can be done" and discouraging both family members and patients.

I decided to seek training in palliative care, which, together with my yoga therapy training, allows me to provide comfort by saying honestly, "There is still a lot to be done." Restorative poses, gentle stretches, and breathing exercises can help to bring relief from a place of patience and loving kindness. I ask clients to use their bodies as a laboratory of experimentation to find the most comfortable posture, being kind and loving with themselves. My presence is an opportunity to heal without trying to fix anything.

We know we are all subject to suffering, getting sick, getting old, and dying. To facilitate doing it all well, with mindfulness of ethics and human rights, it has been helpful for me as a therapist and for clients at the end of life to embrace the yamas and niyamas; these precepts drive us all safely to "suffer less."

I do my best to recognize my physical, mental, and emotional limits in each moment. Disciplined meditation is the source from which I obtain peace, strength, and an ability to let go so as to get on with each day. I sometimes do not have the opportunity to see a client more than once, and the non-grasping of *aparigraha* reminds me that every moment is precious. The opportunity is always in the now; one interview can change it all.

The principle of non-harming (*ahimsa*) guides me to deep respect and protection of clients when their decision-making capacity is limited. Even when clients are unable to express their wishes in the moment, good communication with close relatives and physicians helps me to respect their agency at all times.

Satya reminds me that clients always have the right to know the truth about their health, treatment, and prognosis. This gives them the chance to work with their reality more efficiently and helps them to feel supported and less alone.

I take care, through neat presentation (*shaucha*) and colorful dress, to show clients that in each moment we are celebrating life.

I teach clients about the importance of breath and how each respiration can contact their nervous systems to cultivate peace and regulate emotions. I illustrate gentle movements to relieve pain and tension in bed or a chair. I let those who cannot move know about mudras. Meditation becomes a beautiful tool to pacify our minds and souls. We cultivate tapas, practicing at every opportunity. At clients' homes I promote establishing discipline without sacrifice, setting a time for daily meditation, balanced healthy eating, waking and sleeping, and mild asana to move each personal rhythm toward balance during difficult times.

At the end, we surrender ourselves to the wisdom of uncertainty, to the unknown, because all that we know corresponds to the past; through *ishvara pranidhana* we let it go into a present that transforms and heals.

Endnote

1 Aboagye E., Karlsson, M. L., Hagberg, J., & Jensen, I. (2015). Cost-effectiveness of early interventions for non-specific low back pain: A randomized controlled study investigating medical yoga, exercise therapy and self-care advice. *Journal of Rehabilitation Medicine*, 47, 167–173.

28

Career Development: Yoga Therapy Delivery Settings

Yoga therapy has been historically considered an entrepreneurial field. As recently as the mid-2010s, the only professional avenue for graduates of yoga therapy training programs was solo private practice.

Yoga therapy is shifting from a developing to an emerging role in integrative health. Licensed healthcare professionals have begun to recognize the value of yoga in the lives of their patients and clients and have become more willing to recommend yoga—and perhaps to directly offer yoga-based methods themselves. A steady stream of research and education on the value of yoga has resulted in institutions as diverse as the Veterans Administration and Simon Cancer Center being willing to hire yoga therapists as either employees or contractors. Still, yoga professionals delivering care to diverse populations must remain open to educating the institutions and individuals for whom they work. Offering accurate information on ways that yoga therapists are trained and can serve is of vital importance to the profession, as is contributing to the literature when possible.

Yoga therapists can now deliver care in a variety of settings, from solo private practice with varying focus to large clinic systems and grassroots non-profit organizations. As is clear from the work of the professionals featured in this chapter, these opportunities are still often uncovered through the yoga therapist's own creative initiative.

Common Threads

Those who contributed to this book universally expressed gratitude for being able to do their work. The variety of opportunities now available allows yoga therapists to forge creative individual paths. Tradeoffs include lack of stability and a clearly charted course to success.

Contributors spoke on common themes, including the importance of personal practice. As Judi Bar said, "[W]e must practice our yamas and niyamas to be open to what comes and goes with the flow." Although a full-time clinical practice can be rewarding, "clients are going through a lot medically, physically, spiritually, and mentally," noted Kelli Bethel. "It is important that the yoga therapist continue with their personal practice to prevent the fatigue and burnout we are seeing across the medical community."

A capacity for active listening and the ability to quickly cultivate meaningful therapeutic relationships are key skills, highlighted by Courtney D. Butler-Robinson, Tina Paul, and others.

Also important to practice success are communication skills that enable productive engagement with other kinds of professionals, and especially a deep understanding of the nuances of the care setting and its culture. It is essential to remain current on research and to be able to accurately and succinctly translate these findings—and yogic terms themselves—to biomedical language for an integrative care team.

Many of the yoga therapists featured here, like Shelly Prosko, described the benefits (and challenges) of a varied but self-determined schedule. They also highlighted the administrative considerations—financial pressures, time constraints—that inevitably accompany such independence. Boundary-setting skills are another basic asset required for a yoga therapist's toolkit.

Finally, the yoga therapists in this chapter offered encouragement, as exemplified by Pamela Stokes Eggleston:

> It can seem like you are the only one working hard to get clients or get a break. You have to keep pushing through the self-doubt, the imposter syndrome, and the denials. This is a voyage for the strong of heart and clear of purpose. Start every day with self-reflection and self-inquiry to realign with your purpose. This will keep you on the purposed path.

Broad Care in a Medical Clinic System

Judi Bar, C-IAYT, E-RYT 500 • Cleveland Clinic Center for Integrative and Lifestyle Medicine

When I heard that Cleveland Clinic was expanding its Integrative Medicine Department in 2006, I presented the idea of creating a yoga therapy class for chronic pain patients. With patience, perseverance, and observation on how best

I could serve, I was able to expand from one class in one area to many different departments and programs throughout the organization's system.

I was offered a full-time position several years later and am now the lead yoga therapist and yoga program manager. My workdays are quite varied, with some evenings and weekends. I teach shorter group yoga therapy classes in the course of shared medical appointments, where patients also work with medical staff, holistic psychologists, chiropractors, massage therapists, Chinese herbal medicine providers, and dietitians. In this context, we see patients with chronic pain, multiple sclerosis, breast cancer, and other conditions; those who need support for unhealthy eating patterns; and people seeking general information on new lifestyle practices. I also teach regular hour-long yoga therapy classes that are open to patients and the general public, and I offer one-to-one sessions with patients.

In addition to this client-facing work, with other departments I help to develop yoga programs for specific patient populations (e.g., epilepsy, irritable bowel disease, liver transplant) and for research. I plan classes for yoga teacher trainings and workshops and manage a team of ten part-time yoga therapists who support our yoga program for employees and patients.

Yoga therapists who want to work in healthcare settings need communication skills that enable them to interface with physicians in varied specialties, remembering that the medical team's information is as important as our observations. Part of my job is to develop new working relationships with physicians and other caregivers for potential future collaborations, and to get the word out about yoga in healthcare by speaking at integrative medicine conferences about the value and benefits of yoga. Strong skills as a yoga generalist are essential to allow yoga therapists in these clinical settings to step into any type of class or patient encounter and know what might support or hurt. Specifically, I think it's helpful to understand the difference between inpatient and outpatient teaching, how to interpret patients' needs quickly, and how to simplify accordingly. I sometimes find myself working in close quarters in short periods.

There's a lot to love about my job, including the variety that each day brings. It's rewarding to break yoga down into simple practices, making it accessible for anyone in any circumstance, and therefore reaching a population that might not ordinarily be introduced to yoga. I also love the ongoing challenges to grow personally and professionally as new situations present themselves with patients.

Hospital and Private Medical Practice Settings

Tina Paul, MS, C-IAYT, E-RYT 500 • Memorial Sloan Kettering Cancer Center and Manhattan Physical Medicine and Rehabilitation

I applied for a mind-body therapist position at Memorial Sloan Kettering (MSK) Cancer Center and originally joined the organization to support a randomized controlled trial on yoga for chemotherapy-induced peripheral neuropathy.

I now work at MSK a few days a week. I may have a few hour-long client appointments during the morning. I review notes and health records prior to the session, then update notes afterward. These clients are at various stages of their cancer journeys, from newly diagnosed to recovering or dealing with a recurrence; some are in active treatment or participating in research trials.

I also offer therapeutic workshop series throughout the year to support sleep, strength, anxiety-coping, and more. I teach a weekly chair yoga class at the hospital, too, open to both patients undergoing treatment or in recovery and their caregivers. We use whatever chairs are in the space—sometimes an open recreational environment, sometimes a quiet room—and sit in a circle. I invite participants to move at their own pace, skip movements, or simply sit and be with the group. From chair yoga, I head to the pediatrics department for a few hours, where I work with caregivers in 30-minute sessions, sometimes in patients' rooms but often in a mixed-use space that I convert into a yoga space by rearranging furniture.

I also work at Manhattan Physical Medicine and Rehabilitation, where Dr. Loren Fishman integrates yoga therapy into his private practice as a physiatrist—a medical doctor who specializes in physical medicine and rehabilitation.

I typically attend patient appointments, which can last from 30 to 60 minutes or more, and I'm often observing, listening, and asking questions alongside Dr. Fishman. I sometimes work with patients one-to-one after their appointments for an additional 30 or 60 minutes. One recent afternoon, for example, I saw people seeking help because of grief from the loss of a loved one, tennis-related rotator cuff tear, and lumbar disc herniation.

Although working in medical settings is deeply rewarding, it's not for everyone. Are you at ease in a clinical environment? Okay with regular flu shots? Things can move slowly, especially with the number of processes set up in larger systems, so how patient are you?

And, of course, witnessing a patient experience the death of a loved one, or losing a client myself, is a difficult part of the reality of working in a cancer center in particular. I learn so much from clients and caregivers, though, and I value the consistent reminders of our common mortality in this setting.

Neurological and Cancer Care in an Academic Medical Center

Kelli Bethel, DPT, PT, C-IAYT • University of Maryland School of Medicine

I work for the University of Maryland School of Medicine's Center for Integrative Medicine (CIM) as their director of yoga and yoga therapy. I started at CIM as a yoga trainer in the organization's 200- and 300-hour teacher training programs. Over time, these programs expanded to include yoga therapy as a clinical practice.

As director, my week varies, but includes administrative time, academic teaching, clinical practice, and research. The clinical practice portion of my work includes a weekly group yoga therapy program for stroke and brain injury, private yoga therapy clients, and supervision of yoga therapy programs for other clinical populations. As part of the integrative medicine team, I provide weekly yoga therapy to outpatients in the cancer center. In academics, I oversee CIM's Yoga Alliance-registered yoga teacher training programs and IAYT Approved Professional Development courses. I lecture on yoga therapy topics for patients and students in the University of Maryland, Baltimore graduate programs in the schools of medicine and nursing. I also implement a 30-credit continuing education course with the goal of helping nurses develop a self-care strategy to prevent professional burnout.

When beginning to work in a hospital setting or with special populations, I recommend that yoga therapists pick an area they know well. Those who have experience or additional training in cancer, for instance, might start with that area and expand. It is often overwhelming to try to do everything at once. When working with specific populations such as stroke or cancer survivors, advanced training is typically needed; even then, support and mentoring for clients with challenging conditions are necessary.

Additionally, we have to be clear in articulating what yoga therapy is and how it can benefit a client. For many in conventional medicine, yoga therapy is a new profession in the healthcare setting. It is important to be able to succinctly articulate how the practices can benefit specific patients. In holistic patient care, it's important for yoga therapists to remember that they are part of a team. Coordinating with other members of the team and communicating using medical terminology are helpful.

A portion of my salary is paid through grants and foundations, so funding isn't guaranteed forever. Another caveat: New administrations or changes in rules and requirements can also be the end of a program, regardless of how successful or meaningful it is to clients.

As a physical therapist, I have helped countless people return to function. As a yoga therapist, I am a guide who provides support for clients who wish to return to life.

Child and Adolescent Psychiatry

Shelley K. Goldman, MS, RN, LICDC-CS, CCM, MAC, C-IAYT • Cincinnati Children's Hospital and Medical Center

I was practicing as a psychiatric nurse when I discovered yoga and yoga therapy. I knew right away that I wanted to share this powerful gift with the patients and families I serve.

Because I am employed as a care manager, my day mostly looks like that of any psychiatric nurse filling such a role. However, I have been able to bring yoga therapy into my practice in a number of ways:

- I offer yoga therapy sessions one-to-one for inpatients (referred by behavioral specialists) and outpatients (referred by providers).
- I have conducted continuing education for care managers, stress-reduction classes for psychiatric social workers, and a self-care session for a Registered Nurse (RN) residency program.
- In addition to generally analyzing and presenting research on yoga therapy in mental health, I have spoken at our hospital's psychiatric symposium, offered breakout sessions on relaxation for a nurses' retreat, and given families a presentation on integrative modalities for mental health.
- I teach yogic breathing to patients and families during family meetings, and I've guided a mom and child through a meditation over the phone.

Through volunteering opportunities and planting seeds, I have become my department's mind-body expert, and people reach out when yoga, mindfulness, meditation, stress management, or self-care are discussed. I've even been asked by community healthcare providers to start meetings with a guided meditation.

Working in a hospital comes with innate challenges. There are a lot of policies and education requirements. Things like licenses, degrees, and experience matter. Those who want to work in the hospital setting need to know (and follow!) the dress code, expect to be fingerprinted, undergo drug screening, and get immunizations.

I need to be able to talk confidently about what I do using Western medical language. Research is respected. Trauma training is imperative. It can be difficult to break in to a medical model and be taken seriously, yet there are so many opportunities. I have been mostly celebrated and supported, although I was also mocked by a physician.

What I love the most is the look of peace and bliss on a child's face after a yoga therapy session. I love that I can find a way to bring yoga into so many conversations and ventures. Things can move slowly in a Midwestern medical center. Some day, though, I hope to have yoga therapy as my primary job description.

Cardiac Rehab and Cancer Recovery

Courtney D. Butler-Robinson, C-IAYT, E-RYT 500, RCYT, RPYT • Ornish Reversal Program at Saline Heart Group

As a "stress management specialist," I work with Dr. Allan Hatch at Saline Heart Group. We implement the Ornish Reversal Program, which focuses on intensive cardiac rehab and cancer recovery.

Before working as a yoga therapist, I volunteer-assisted with physical therapy in a medical setting and implemented therapies at a school for children with disabilities. When I became a yoga teacher, I wanted to help those who needed more than a general population class, often students who were living with a disability whom I met through both private instruction and a partner program at the college where I taught.

As my career grew and I opened a yoga school, I took a therapeutic approach to training teachers. As I expanded into workshops and retreats, I focused on practices that met the needs of those with health issues ranging from back pain to addiction and on working with disease processes like cancer and cardiovascular health.

These days, I spend quite a bit of time writing and speaking publicly about the field of yoga therapy, lately for the local college of medicine. Once or twice a year, I offer weekend workshops on yoga therapy classroom applications or present at conferences. Most weekdays, I'm a contractor at Saline, where I spend 2 to 4 hours teaching stress-management classes or presenting on yoga therapy's effects on the nervous system.

The key wisdom I'd share with new yoga therapists: Really get to know each client. No two are the same. There are so many types of cancer, for instance. In settings like the one where I work, you will have to understand how ports work and how they affect movement, or how the side-effects of chemo and other drugs make people feel, but it's just as important to know the client's lifestyle and what their home life is like. For example, I have one client who had a double mastectomy who is scared to move her arms or upper torso much, whereas another who had the same surgery tends to do too much, pushing herself to regain range of motion.

Often after about 3 weeks in our wellness clinic, I begin to see great changes. People become physically and emotionally stronger. They have more hope. One man recently told me, "I was in a deep dark place before I came here, but this program has changed my whole life." I see people reduce medication and the need for walkers all the time.

The cardiac program involves a regimented prescription, although I have a little latitude to address clients' individual needs in cancer recovery rehab. Sometimes this feels repetitive, but in the end it's amazing work.

Substance-Use Recovery

Durga Leela, C-IAYT, AP (NAMA), AYT (NAMA) • Yoga of Recovery

As the founder of Yoga of Recovery (YoR), I offer yoga therapy at retreats and in training courses, including as ayurvedic faculty for several IAYT-accredited programs. Like many others, I came to this work through my own need to heal in a deeper, more continuous, and integrative manner than conventional medicine could offer.

You must practice what you teach, so I show up for a disciplined daily schedule along with YoR retreat guests. Mornings start with optional meditation, then Hatha Yoga, pranayama, and savasana. Brunch is followed by a short period of karma yoga service. Afternoons include sharing, discussion, and practice over 2 to 3 hours. We practice yoga nidra before supper. An optional 12-step recovery meeting, open to all, is held in the evening. The days end similarly to how they begin, with meditation, the call-and-response chanting of *kirtan*, and a talk on yoga/ayurveda.

Having a regular sadhana (practice) is the only way I know to remain steady while teaching and to be able to listen with empathy and compassion to those who are suffering. Remaining current and curious about all pathways to recovery and understanding how yoga parallels them are also keys to effectively serving this population.

This work reframes self-destructive behaviors as natural, inherent energy and offers paths to express that energy more consciously. Attendees recognize the many ways we act out our spiritual seeking—through substance use as well as encouraged social behaviors that lead to insatiable craving. This perspective helps remove the shame and social stigma that can create fundamental blocks to recovery.

In this work one must be authentic, heart-based, and welcoming. I cultivate the skill of asking good questions—"What does recovery look like for you today?"—and allow space for moment-to-moment reactions and resistance as well as insights. I help clients understand that they are not just going to *do* yoga as a physical practice on the mat. Instead, I facilitate sessions that move toward deeper creative self-inquiry and transformational change. Using simple, practical, everyday experiences to help people reconnect the body and mind, and in turn the body-mind with the heart-soul, is very satisfying.

The most difficult part of YoR work is being heard over the pharmaceutical solutions that are amplified by channels the public trusts as scientific. This process emphasizes a reductionist diagnosis of addiction as a brain disease that can be cured by applying chemicals to balance neurochemical function. Such an approach is part of the solution for some, but addiction stems from biopsychosocial-spiritual as well as political, economic, and cultural conditions. This societal plague therefore requires a multimodal approach that yoga therapy can provide.

Solo Practice as a Physical Therapist, Yoga Therapist, and Educator

Shelly Prosko, PT, C-IAYT • Private practice in physical therapy

Through my business Prosko PhysioYoga Therapy, I work with clients in Sylvan Lake, Canada. I'm also a continuing education provider for yoga therapy and healthcare professionals.

I spent the first 14 years of my career working in five different salaried physical therapy (PT) settings. I appreciated the ability to focus on developing my skills as a therapist without having to attend so much to the business. I also appreciated having colleagues onsite; receiving support and mentorship is important. Opportunities to work alongside other healthcare professionals as a team are more readily available in a clinic or healthcare setting, too.

I had been integrating yoga therapy into my PT practice since 1998 in orthopedic rehab and long-term care settings. In 2012, I started building my own practice. Because I enjoyed teaching in-services about my integrative work, I also began to create workshops for health and yoga professionals. As time progressed, the demand for my work increased and I started offering more continuing education content, and this has become a significant part of my work.

As a continuing education provider, I choose the content I feel most passionate about teaching. I create online and in-person courses and resources, travel to guest lecture at yoga therapy and physical therapy training programs, speak at conferences, and provide online mentorship.

As a clinician, I get to help people gain insight into their own suffering and support them on their path to feeling empowered and living well. I value the amount of time I'm able to spend with clients: 1.5- to 2-hour sessions allow us to connect and give clients the chance to be seen, heard, and validated. They get to experience the practices without rushing, and I can make my setting conducive to co-creating a therapeutic, peaceful space.

I might see one to three people per day, plus spend time on recordkeeping, reflection, and planning. I rent a small space near my home, so travel time is negligible. As a small-business owner, I am grateful to set my own schedule and choose who I want to collaborate with, although I spend considerable time on networking, correspondence, and meetings. There is no "typical workday," but a non-travel day might include self-study and practice in the morning, administrative and marketing duties, an individual client session or two, an online mentoring session, and content creation (book chapters, articles/blogs, presentations, proposals, etc.).

Yoga therapists in business for themselves need to cultivate skills of boundary setting and time management. They'll also need patience, self-compassion, discipline, persistence, courage, humility, and an ability to communicate effectively and compassionately. Many healthcare providers in private practice are surprised by the amount of time they must spend on activities other than direct client care. But they may also be surprised by how much personal growth results from being a business owner!

Military Healthcare

Lynne Valdes, MS, C-IAYT • US Department of Defense contractor

I practice yoga therapy at Walter Reed National Military Medical Center in support of the Patient-Centered Medical Home model for delivery of primary care. As a "mind-body therapist," I work out of the General Internal Medicine Service. For me, this position is an opportunity to bring together my family military background and my professional yoga experience.

The patient population I work with is made up of active-duty service members, retirees, veterans, and dependent family members. Patients are referred by their primary or specialty care providers, or they can self-refer to see me. Most appointments are for symptom management of chronic pain and disease, sleep issues, anxiety and depression, posttraumatic stress disorder (PTSD), and general stress management.

My workday is from 7:30 a.m. to 4:00 p.m. Monday through Friday, structured into eight individual sessions per day. Regardless of whether it is an initial visit or a follow-up, I have 45 minutes for these back-to-back appointments, with a 90-minute break between morning and afternoon sessions. I have a 30-minute block at the beginning and end of my days for administrative purposes. There are also occasional opportunities to teach group classes as part of staff development and for training in clinical pathways for patient-care improvement.

The allotted 45-minute appointment time includes greeting the patient in the main clinic waiting area and walking back to the treatment room, so I end up with more like 30 to 35 minutes with each person. In this short span, I must build rapport, establish trust, assess, educate, and develop a plan of care. Time is of the essence, so preparation is essential. As in many settings, you may have only one opportunity to introduce and offer the practices of yoga.

Familiarity with military culture helps me to identify potential obstacles to yoga therapy and find common ground more quickly. From a clinical standpoint, I consider what I can identify and work on within this time frame that can have a meaningful effect. I prepare educational materials ahead of time, keeping things general so that I can tailor the delivery to suit the individual needs of each patient. I also keep in consideration that the practices I offer in this setting must be evidence-based.

For me, the best part of my position is the opportunity to work with this distinguished population. They have such amazing backgrounds and experiences, and their dedication to duty is inspiring. Being of service to this group far outweighs the inevitable organizational obstacles and daily challenges.

Yoga in Military Health Systems

Dorcia J. Tucker, PsyD, MS, C-IAYT • Department of Defense; formerly US Military

I previously incorporated therapeutic yoga practices into my psychology practice as an active-duty clinical psychologist and Alcohol and Drug Abuse Prevention and Treatment Program Manager for the US Air Force at various bases in the United States and Asia. Currently, I am a civilian clinical psychologist for the Department of Defense. I'm working to build a resilience center where active-duty and civilian employees can benefit from stress-management tools including meditation and biofeedback.

I entered the Air Force as a psychology intern and was able to use the pranamaya and meditation tools I'd learned in my own yoga practice to help patients manage stress and anxiety. These non-asana practices proved to be an excellent complement to the biofeedback and cognitive behavioral therapy of my psychology training.

Back then, my days included a mix of individual and group therapy sessions for anxiety, depression, substance abuse, work stress, symptoms related to medical conditions, and so on. Depending on the needs of the patient, I used a combination of psychotherapy, psychoeducation, behavioral coaching, biofeedback, meditation, and pranayama. I also supervised other clinical providers, attended case-consultation meetings, and taught weekly small-group yoga classes for the clinic's staff members.

Any issue that would be observed outside of the military can be found inside the military. Just as in civilian life, people are generally curious about new evidence-informed practices. Appropriate curiosity for military culture and each individual within it is a prerequisite to working in this setting. As in other positions that integrate yoga therapy with Western healthcare, necessary skills include familiarity with common biomedical conditions, efficient recordkeeping, ability to translate yogic concepts into common language, and being comfortable working with people from diverse backgrounds. A calm, unflappable demeanor is a plus.

One downside of working within a massive bureaucracy is that change and innovation can come slowly. Persistence and adaptability in the face of resistance are necessary for longevity in this environment.

In the military, I loved working in a medical system whose mission focuses on maintaining and restoring health rather than turning a profit. Many of the clinicians are open to collaboration and the use of complementary interventions they think will benefit their patients. One of the most exciting aspects of working in the military system is that processes are always evolving, which translates to more opportunities for complementary and integrative health practitioners to reach new audiences and to continue to refine their skills.

Entrepreneurship Through Service

Pamela Stokes Eggleston, MBA, MS, C-IAYT, E-RYT 500 • Yoga2Sleep; formerly Yoga Service Council

As the founder and director of Yoga2Sleep and co-founder of Retreat to Spirit, I practice yoga therapy in the Washington, DC, area and online.

I began my yoga journey in 2002 while working in corporate America and slowly burning out. My sister-in-law introduced me to a community yoga class, and the rest is history! During my training, I met a lot of veterans who felt that yoga had saved their lives. They connected me to organizations like Mindful Yoga Therapy for Veterans and the Give Back Yoga Foundation, and after receiving trauma-conscious yoga and yoga therapy training, I started working with veterans, the military, and their caregivers and family members in 2012. I continued cultivating and building on these initial relationships through work with the Omega Institute, Yoga Alliance, Yoga Service Council, the Omega Women's Leadership Center, Black Yoga Teachers Alliance, and Accessible Yoga.

As an entrepreneur, I now start the day with asana and meditation practice, no matter how short, to set the tone. Then, I make tea and review my day planner. Writing in it helps me to remember the meetings, paperwork, and projects inside. Previously, as co-executive director for a national yoga non-profit, I reviewed that daily schedule to prioritize what I was responsible for: grant writing and reporting, lots of meetings, relationship cultivation, and online education. I usually handle these business tasks in the morning, then see a few yoga therapy clients or continue working on Yoga2Sleep business.

It takes time and patience to build a yoga therapy practice with consistent clients and organizations that desire group yoga therapy. Relationship-building and networking in an authentic way help; a fake or forced demeanor will not help. The contracting and grant-writing skills I was fortunate to learn in my corporate career have carried over well, too.

Yoga therapists may not want as many clients as they think, and many of us will have to be flexible, maybe driving to the client, offering more group therapy, etc. I've also found that it's important to consider how my yoga therapy offerings can be diverse, not just in terms of populations, but also in the manner in which I serve the community as a whole. Retreat to Spirit, for example, presents innovative yoga-informed programming for those in service work and/or leadership roles.

I love working with clients who really need help, in my case all of them directly or indirectly with sleep deprivation or insomnia. It is a nice feeling to be able to empower someone to take back agency over their own health, happiness, and well-being.

A Virtual Nomad

Matthew J. Taylor, PT, PhD, C-IAYT • Integrated Systems

I live in Iowa City, Iowa, but through my organization, Integrated Systems, I work from around the world. In the words of Mary Catherine Bateson, PhD, yoga therapy is my "Adulthood Part II." The kids are grown, and the bills are paid. What next? Legacy work with meaning and purpose. The opportunities initially arrived from my close support of IAYT, and now through an expanding international network each project births new possibilities.

I work in a range of settings, including as a yoga therapy representative in interprofessional collaborations between IAYT and a number of groups, dissertation committee member, board member for yoga-related organizations, textbook and chapter author, adjunct university faculty and research writer, and even consultant to a UK parliamentary committee on yoga. My workdays include writing, research, videoconferencing, conference planning and participation, introducing colleagues, launching both non-profit and for-profit ventures involving yoga therapy, and mentoring. I select my work based on the ability to scale it up to help more people reduce future suffering. If it holds this promise and involves integrative healing or creativity, I'm in.

Beginning yoga therapists need to cultivate a broad network to work like this. When you promise to show up, show up and deliver beyond expectations. Praise publicly; complain/confront privately. Listen four times as much as you talk.

People with these qualities are rare, even in the yoga world (*especially* in the yoga world?). New yoga therapists might be surprised by how difficult the work can be, but also by what shows up after hard work, including new possibilities they never considered. They may also be amazed by the importance of self-care and practice and, unfortunately, by how many yogis are ego-filled.

With so many opportunities to choose from, I need to be especially clear about how things will be managed and decisions made in a project. It gets tiring some days, like any work, as well as frustrating. Things seem to change slowly unless I zoom out in perspective.

My work embodies a steep, ongoing learning arc that I love. It brings me into contact with wonderful, wise, and kind people from around the globe. I'm never bored. I can't wait to see what the next month and year will bring.

Index